FOURTH

ESSENTIALS OF
Epidemiology
IN PUBLIC HEALTH

Ann Aschengrau, ScD
Professor, Department of Epidemiology
Boston University School of Public Health
Boston, Massachusetts

George R. Seage III, DSc
Professor of Epidemiology
Harvard T.H. Chan School of Public Health
Boston, Massachusetts

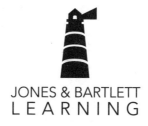

JONES & BARTLETT
LEARNING

World Headquarters
Jones & Bartlett Learning
5 Wall Street
Burlington, MA 01803
978-443-5000
info@jblearning.com
www.jblearning.com

Jones & Bartlett Learning books and products are available through most bookstores and online booksellers. To contact Jones & Bartlett Learning directly, call 800-832-0034, fax 978-443-8000, or visit our website, www.jblearning.com.

12843-7

Production Credits

VP, Product Management: David D. Cella
Director of Product Management: Michael Brown
Product Specialist: Carter McAlister
Production Manager: Carolyn Rogers Pershouse
Associate Production Editor, Navigate: Jamie Reynolds
Senior Marketing Manager: Sophie Fleck Teague
Manufacturing and Inventory Control Supervisor: Amy Bacus

Composition: codeMantra U.S. LLC
Cover Design: Kristin E. Parker
Rights & Media Specialist: John Rusk
Media Development Editor: Shannon Sheehan
Cover Image (Title Page, Chapter Opener):
    © Smartboy10/DigitalVision Vectors/Getty Images
Printing and Binding: LSC Communications
Cover Printing: LSC Communications

Library of Congress Cataloging-in-Publication Data
Names: Aschengrau, Ann, author. | Seage, George R., author.
Title: Essentials of epidemiology in public health / Ann Aschengrau, ScD,
    Professor of Epidemiology, Boston University School of Public Health,
    George R. Seage III, ScD, Professor of Epidemiology, Harvard T.H. Chan
    School of Public Health.
Description: Fourth edition. | Burlington, MA : Jones & Bartlett Learning,
    [2020] | Includes bibliographical references and index.
Identifiers: LCCN 2018023772 | ISBN 9781284128352 (paperback)
Subjects: LCSH: Epidemiology. | Public health. | Social medicine. | BISAC:
    EDUCATION / General.
Classification: LCC RA651 .A83 2020 | DDC 614.4–dc23
LC record available at https://lccn.loc.gov/2018023772

6048

Printed in the United States of America
22 21 20   10 9 8 7 6 5 4 3

Contents

Preface

What is epidemiology, and how does it contribute to the health of our society? Most people don't know the answer to this question. This is somewhat paradoxical because epidemiology, one of the basic sciences of public health, affects nearly everyone. It affects both the personal decisions we make about our lives and the ways in which governments, public health agencies, and medical organizations make policy decisions that affect how we live.

In recent years, the field of epidemiology has expanded tremendously in size, scope, and influence. The number of epidemiologists has grown rapidly along with the number of epidemiology training programs in schools of public health and medicine. Many subspecialties have arisen to study public health questions, from the molecular to the societal level.

Recent years have also witnessed an important evolution in the theory and methods of epidemiological research and analysis, causal inference, and the role of statistics (especially P values) in research.

Unfortunately, few of these changes have been taught in introductory epidemiology courses, particularly those for master's-level students. We believe this has occurred mainly because instructors have mistakenly assumed the new concepts were too difficult or arcane for beginning students. As a consequence, many generations of public health students have received a dated education.

Our desire to change this practice was the main impetus for writing this book. For nearly three decades we have successfully taught both traditional and new concepts to our graduate students at Boston University and Harvard University. Not only have our students successfully mastered the material, but they have also found that the new ideas enhanced their understanding of epidemiology and its application.

In addition to providing an up-to-date education, we have taught our students the necessary skills to become knowledgeable consumers of epidemiological literature. Gaining competence in the critical evaluation of this literature is particularly important for public health practitioners because they often need to reconcile confusing and contradictory results.

This textbook reflects our educational philosophy of combining theory and practice in our teaching. It is intended for public health students who will be consumers of epidemiological literature and those who will be practicing epidemiologists. The first five chapters cover basic epidemiological concepts and data sources. Chapter 1 describes the approach and evolution of epidemiology, including the definition, goals, and historical development of epidemiology and public health. Chapters 2 and 3 describe how epidemiologists measure and compare disease occurrence in populations. Chapter 4 characterizes the major sources of health data on the U.S. population and describes how to interpret these data appropriately. Chapter 5 describes how epidemiologists analyze disease patterns to understand the health status of a population, formulate and test hypotheses of disease causation, and carry out and evaluate health programs.

The next four chapters of the textbook focus on epidemiological study design.

Chapter 6 provides an overview of study designs—including experimental, cohort, case–control, cross-sectional, and ecological studies—and describes the factors that determine when a particular design is indicated. Each of the three following chapters provides a detailed description of the three main analytic designs: experimental, cohort, and case–control studies.

The next five chapters cover the tools students need to interpret the results of epidemiological studies. Chapter 10 describes bias, including how it influences study results and the ways in which it can be avoided. Chapter 11 explains the concept of confounding, methods for assessing its presence, and methods for controlling its effects. Chapter 12 covers random error, including hypothesis testing, P-value and confidence interval estimation and interpretation, and sample size and power calculations. We believe this chapter provides a balanced view of the appropriate role of statistics in epidemiology. Chapter 13 covers the concept of effect measure modification, an often neglected topic in introductory texts. It explains the difference between confounding and effect measure modification and describes the methods for evaluating effect measure modification. Chapter 14 pulls together the information from Chapters 10 through 13 by providing a framework for evaluating the literature as well as three examples of epidemiological study critiques.

Chapter 15 covers the epidemiological approach to causation, including the historical development of causation theories, Hill's guidelines for assessing causation, and the sufficient-component cause model of causation. Chapter 16 explains screening in public health practice, including the natural history of disease, characteristics of diseases appropriate for screening, important features of a screening test, and methods for evaluating a screening program. Finally, Chapter 17 describes the development

and application of guidelines to ensure the ethical conduct of studies involving humans. Up-to-date examples and data from the epidemiological literature on diseases of public health importance are used throughout the book. In addition, nearly 50 new study questions were added to the fourth edition.

Our educational background and research interests are also reflected in the textbook's outlook and examples. Ann Aschengrau received her doctorate in epidemiology from the Harvard School of Public Health in 1987 and joined the Department of Epidemiology at the Boston University School of Public Health shortly thereafter. She is currently Professor, Associate Chair for Education, and Co-Director of the Master of Science Degree Program in Epidemiology. For the past 30 years, she has taught introductory epidemiology to master's-level students. Her research has focused on the environmental determinants of disease, including cancer, disorders of reproduction and child development, and substance use.

George R. Seage III received his doctorate in epidemiology from the Boston University School of Public Health in 1992. For more than a decade, he served as the AIDS epidemiologist for the city of Boston and as a faculty member at the Boston University School of Public Health. He is currently Professor of Epidemiology at the Harvard T.H. Chan School of Public Health and Director of the Harvard Chan Program in the Epidemiology of Infectious Diseases. For over 30 years, he has taught courses in HIV epidemiology to master's and doctoral students. His research focuses on the biological and behavioral determinants of adult and pediatric HIV transmission, natural history, and treatment.

Drs. Aschengrau and Seage are happy to connect with instructors and students via email (aaschen@bu.edu and gseage@hsph.harvard.edu). Also check out Dr. Aschengrau's Twitter feed @AnnfromBoston.

▶ New to This Edition

- Completely updated with new examples and the latest references and public health statistics
- New section on process of investigating infectious disease outbreaks
- New section on the Ebola outbreaks and their investigation in Africa
- Introduction of the latest epidemiological terms and methods
- New figures depicting epidemiological concepts
- Expanded ancillary materials, including improved PowerPoint slides, an enlarged glossary, and new in-class exercises and test questions
- Over 50 new review questions

Acknowledgments

Our ideas about the principles and practice of epidemiology have been greatly influenced by teachers, colleagues, and students. We feel privileged to have been inspired and nurtured by many outstanding teachers and mentors, including Richard Monson, George (Sandy) Lamb, Steve Schoenbaum, Arnold Epstein, Ken Rothman, the late Brian MacMahon, Julie Buring, Fran Cook, Ted Colton, Bob Glynn, Adrienne Cupples, George Hutchison, and the late Alan Morrison. We are pleased to help spread the knowledge they have given us to the next generation of epidemiologists.

We are also indebted to the many colleagues who contributed to the numerous editions of this book in various ways, including clarifying our thinking about epidemiology and biostatistics, providing ideas about how to teach epidemiology, reviewing and commenting on drafts and revisions of the text, pilot testing drafts in their classes, and dispensing many doses of encouragement during the time it took to write all four editions of this book. Among these individuals are Bob Horsburgh, Herb Kayne, Dan Brooks, Wayne LaMorte, Michael Shwartz, Dave Ozonoff, Tricia Coogan, Meir Stampfer, Lorelei Mucci, Murray Mittleman, Fran Cook, Charlie Poole, Tom Fleming, Megan Murray, Marc Lipsitch, Sam Bozeman, Anne Coletti, Michael Gross, Sarah Putney, Sarah Rogers, Kimberly Shea, Kunjal Patel, and Kelly Diringer Getz. We are particularly grateful to Krystal Cantos for her many contributions to this edition, particularly the new sections on disease outbreaks, and Molly Pretorius Holme for contributing the chapter on ethics in human research. Ted Colton also deserves a special acknowledgment for originally recommending us to the publisher.

We thank our students for graciously reading drafts and earlier editions of this text in their epidemiology courses and for contributing many valuable suggestions for improvement. We hope that this book will serve as a useful reference as they embark on productive careers in public health. We also recognize Abt Associates, Inc., for providing George Seage with a development and dissemination grant to write the chapter on screening in public health practice. We are very grateful to the staff of Jones & Bartlett Learning for guiding the publication process so competently and quickly. Finally, we thank our son Gregory, an actor, for his patience and for providing many interesting and fun diversions along the way. Break a leg!

CHAPTER 1

The Approach and Evolution of Epidemiology

▶ Introduction

Most people do not know what epidemiology is or how it contributes to the health of our society. This fact is somewhat paradoxical given that epidemiology pervades our lives. Consider, for example, the following statements involving epidemiological research that have made headline news:

- Ten years of hormone drugs benefits some women with breast cancer.
- Cellular telephone users who talk or text on the phone while driving cause one in four car accidents.
- Omega-3 pills, a popular alternative medicine, may not help with depression.
- Fire retardants in consumer products may pose health risks.
- Brazil reacts to an epidemic of Zika virus infections.

The breadth and importance of these topics indicate that epidemiology directly affects the daily lives of most people. It affects the way that individuals make personal decisions about their lives and the way that the government, public health agencies, and medical organizations make policy decisions that affect how we live. For example, the results of epidemiological studies described by the headlines might prompt a person to use a traditional medication for her depression or to replace old furniture likely to contain harmful fire retardants. It might prompt an oncologist to determine which of his breast cancer patients would reap the benefits of hormone therapy, a manufacturer to adopt safer alternatives to fire retardants, public health agencies to monitor and prevent the spread of Zika virus infection, or a state legislature to ban cell phone use by drivers.

This chapter helps the reader understand what epidemiology is and how it contributes to important issues affecting the public's health. In particular, it describes the definition, approach, and goals of epidemiology as well as key aspects of its historical development, current state, and future challenges.

▶ Definition and Goals of Public Health

Public health is a multidisciplinary field whose goal is to promote the health of the population through organized community efforts.[1(pp3-14)] In contrast to medicine, which focuses mainly on treating illness in separate individuals, public health focuses on preventing illness in the community. Key public health activities include assessing the health status of the population, diagnosing its problems, searching for the causes of those problems, and designing solutions for them. The solutions usually involve community-level interventions that control or prevent the cause of the problem. For example, public health interventions include establishing educational programs to discourage teenagers from smoking, implementing screening programs for the early detection of cancer, and passing laws that require automobile drivers and passengers to wear seat belts.

Unfortunately, public health achievements are difficult to recognize because it is hard to identify people who have been spared illness.[1(pp6-7)] For this reason, the field of public health has received less attention and fewer resources than the field of medicine has received. Nevertheless, public health has had a greater effect on the health of populations than medicine has had. For example, since the turn of the 20th century, the average life expectancy of Americans has increased by about 30 years, from 47.3 to 78.8 years.[2] Of this increase, 25 years can be attributed to improvements in public health, and only 5 years can be attributed to improvements in the medical care system.[3] Public health achievements that account for improvements in health and life expectancy include the routine use of vaccinations for infectious diseases, improvements in motor vehicle and workplace safety, control of infectious diseases through improved sanitation and clean water, modification of risk factors for coronary heart disease and stroke (such as smoking cessation and blood pressure control), safer foods from decreased microbial contamination, improved access to family planning and contraceptive services, and the acknowledgment of tobacco as a health hazard and the ensuing antismoking campaigns.[4]

The public health system's activities in research, education, and program implementation have made these accomplishments possible. In the United States, this system includes federal agencies, such as the Centers for Disease Control and Prevention; state and local government agencies; nongovernmental organizations, such as Mothers Against Drunk Driving; and academic institutions, such as schools of public health. This complex array of institutions has achieved success through political action and gains in scientific knowledge.[1(pp5-7)] Politics enters the public health process when agencies advocate for resources, develop policies and plans to improve a community's health, and work to ensure that services needed for the protection of public health are available to all. Political action is necessary because the government usually has the responsibility for developing the activities required to protect public health.

▶ Sources of Scientific Knowledge in Public Health

The scientific basis of public health activities mainly comes from (1) the basic sciences, such as pathology and toxicology; (2) the clinical or medical sciences, such as internal medicine and pediatrics; and (3) the public health sciences, such as epidemiology, environmental health science, health education, and behavioral science. Research in these three areas provides complementary pieces of a puzzle that, when properly assembled, provide the scientific foundation for public health action. Other fields such as engineering and economics also contribute to public health. The three main areas approach research questions from different yet complementary viewpoints, and each field has its own particular strengths and weaknesses.

Basic scientists, such as toxicologists, study disease in a laboratory setting by conducting experiments on cells, tissues, and animals. The focus of this research is often on the disease mechanism or process. Because basic scientists conduct their studies in a controlled laboratory environment, they can regulate all important aspects of the experimental conditions. For example, a laboratory experiment testing the toxicity of a chemical is conducted on genetically similar animals that live in the same physical environment, eat the same diet, and follow the same daily schedule.[5(pp157-237)] Animals are assigned (usually by chance) to either the test group or the control group. Using identical routes of administration, researchers give the chemical under investigation to the test group and an inert chemical to the control group. Thus, the only difference between the two groups is the dissimilar chemical deliberately introduced by the investigator. This type of research provides valuable information on the disease process that cannot be obtained in any other way. However, the results are often difficult to extrapolate to real-life situations involving humans because of differences in susceptibility between species and differences in the exposure level between laboratory experiments and real-life settings. In general, humans are exposed to much lower doses than those used in laboratory experiments.

Clinical scientists focus their research questions mainly on disease diagnosis, treatment, and prognosis in individual patients. For example, they try to determine whether a diagnostic method is accurate or a treatment is effective. Although clinicians are also involved in disease prevention, this activity has historically taken a backseat to disease diagnosis and treatment. As a consequence, clinical research studies are usually based on people who come to a medical care facility, such as a hospital or clinic. Unfortunately, these people are often unrepresentative of the full spectrum of disease in the population at large because many sick people never come to the attention of healthcare providers.

Clinical scientists contribute to scientific knowledge in several important ways. First, they are usually the first to identify new diseases, the adverse effects of new exposures, and new links between an exposure and a disease. This information is typically published in case reports. For example, the epidemic of acquired immune deficiency syndrome (AIDS) (now called HIV for human immunodeficiency virus infection) officially began in the United States in 1981 when clinicians reported several cases of *Pneumocystis carinii* pneumonia and Kaposi's sarcoma (a rare cancer of the blood vessels) among previously healthy, young gay men living in New York and California.[6,7] These cases were notable because *Pneumocystis carinii* pneumonia had previously occurred only among individuals with compromised immune systems, and Kaposi's sarcoma had occurred mainly among elderly men. We now know that these case reports described symptoms of a new disease that would eventually be called HIV/AIDS. Despite their simplicity, case reports provide important clues regarding the causes, prevention, and cures for a disease. In addition, they are often used to justify conducting more sophisticated and expensive studies.

Clinical scientists also contribute to scientific knowledge by recording treatment and response information in their patients' medical records. This information often becomes an indispensable source of research data for clinical and epidemiological studies. For example, it would have been impossible to determine the risk of breast cancer following fluoroscopic X-ray exposure without patient treatment records from the 1930s through the 1950s.[8] Investigators used these records to identify the subjects for the study and gather detailed information about subjects' radiation doses.

Public health scientists study ways to prevent disease and promote health in the population at large. Public health research differs from clinical research in two important ways. First, it focuses mainly on disease prevention rather than disease treatment. Second, the units of concern

TABLE 1-1 Main Differences Among Basic, Clinical, and Public Health Science Research			
Characteristic	**Basic**	**Clinical**	**Public health**
What/who is studied	Cells, tissues, animals in laboratory settings	Sick patients who come to healthcare facilities	Populations or communities at large
Research goals	Understanding disease mechanisms and the effects of toxic substances	Improving diagnosis and treatment of disease	Prevention of disease, promotion of health
Examples	Toxicology, immunology	Internal medicine, pediatrics	Epidemiology, environmental health science

are groups of people living in the community rather than separate individuals visiting a healthcare facility. For example, a public health research project called the Home Observation and Measures of the Environment (HOME) injury study determined the effect of installing safety devices, such as stair gates and cabinet locks, on the rate of injuries among young children.[9] About 350 community-dwelling mothers and their children were enrolled in this home-based project.

The main differences between the three branches of scientific inquiry are summarized in **TABLE 1-1**. Although this is a useful way to classify the branches of scientific research, the distinctions between these areas have become blurred. For example, epidemiological methods are currently being applied to clinical medicine in a field called "clinical epidemiology." In addition, newly developed areas of epidemiological research, such as molecular and genetic epidemiology, include the basic sciences.

▶ Definition and Objectives of Epidemiology

The term *epidemiology* is derived from the Greek words *epi*, which means "on or upon"; *demos*, which means "the common people"; and *logy*, which means "study."[10(pp484,599,1029)] Putting these pieces together yields the following definition of epidemiology: "the study of that which falls upon the common people." Epidemiology can also be defined as the "branch of medical science which treats epidemics."[11] The latter definition was developed by the London Epidemiological Society, which was formed in 1850 to determine the causes of cholera and other epidemic diseases and methods of preventing them.[12] Over the past century, many definitions of epidemiology have been set forth. Some early definitions reflect the field's initial focus on infectious diseases, and later ones reflect a broader scope encompassing all diseases.[12]

We define **epidemiology** as follows: The study of the distribution and determinants of disease frequency in human populations and the application of this study to control health problems.[13(p1),14(p95)] Our definition is a combination of a popular one coined by MacMahon and Pugh in 1970 and another described by Porta in the sixth edition of *A Dictionary of Epidemiology*.[14(p95),15(p1)] Note that the term *disease* refers to a broad array of health-related states and events, including diseases, injuries, disabilities, and death.

We prefer this hybrid definition because it describes both the scope and ultimate goal of epidemiology. In particular, the objectives of epidemiology are to (1) study the natural course of disease from onset to resolution, (2) determine the extent of disease in a population, (3) identify patterns and trends in disease occurrence, (4) identify the causes of disease, and (5) evaluate the effectiveness of measures that prevent and treat disease. All of these activities contribute scientific knowledge for making sound policy decisions that protect public health.

Our definition of epidemiology has five key words or phrases: (1) population, (2) disease frequency, (3) disease distribution, (4) disease determinants, and (5) disease control. Each term is described in more detail in the following sections.

Population

Populations are at the heart of all epidemiological activities because epidemiologists are concerned with disease occurrence in groups of people rather than in individuals. The term *population* refers to a group of people with a common characteristic, such as place of residence, gender, age, or use of certain medical services. For example, people who reside in the city of Boston are members of a geographically defined population. Determining the size of the population in which disease occurs is as important as counting the cases of the disease because it is only when the number of cases is related to the size of the population that we know the true frequency of disease. The size of the population is often determined by a census—that is, a complete count—of the population. Sources of these data range from the decennial census, in which the federal government attempts to count every person in the United States every 10 years, to computerized records from medical facilities that provide counts of patients who use the facilities.

Disease Frequency

Disease frequency refers to quantifying how often a disease arises in a population. Counting, which is a key activity of epidemiologists, includes three steps: (1) developing a definition of disease, (2) instituting a mechanism for counting cases of disease within a specified population, and (3) determining the size of that population.

Diseases must be clearly defined to determine accurately who should be counted. Usually, disease definitions are based on a combination of physical and pathological examinations, diagnostic test results, and signs and symptoms. For example, a case definition of breast cancer might include findings of a palpable lump during a physical exam and mammographic and pathological evidence of malignant disease.

Currently available sources for identifying and counting cases of disease include hospital patient rosters; death certificates; special reporting systems, such as registries of cancer and birth defects; and special surveys. For example, the National Health Interview Survey is a federally funded study that has collected data on the health status of the U.S. population since the 1950s. Its purpose is to "monitor the health of the United States population" by collecting information on a broad range of topics, including health indicators, healthcare utilization and access, and health-related behaviors.[16]

disease frequency

Disease Distribution

Disease distribution refers to the analysis of disease patterns according to the characteristics of person, place, and time, in other words, who is getting the disease, where it is occurring, and how it is changing over time. Variations in disease frequency by these three characteristics provide useful information that helps epidemiologists understand the health status of a population; formulate hypotheses about the determinants of a disease; and plan, implement, and evaluate public health programs to control and prevent adverse health events.

Disease Determinants

Disease determinants are factors that bring about a change in a person's health or make a difference in a person's health.[14(p73)] Thus, determinants consist of both causal and preventive factors. Determinants also include individual, environmental, and societal characteristics. Individual determinants consist of a person's genetic makeup, gender, age, immunity level, diet, behaviors, and existing diseases. For example, the risk of breast cancer is increased among women who carry genetic alterations, such as BRCA1 and BRCA2; are elderly; give birth at a late age; have a history of certain benign breast conditions; or have a history of radiation exposure to the chest.[17]

Environmental and societal determinants are external to the individual and thereby encompass a wide range of natural, social, and economic events and conditions. For example, the presence of infectious agents, reservoirs in which the organism multiplies, vectors that transport the agent, poor and crowded housing conditions, and political instability are environmental and social factors that cause many communicable diseases around the world.

natural
progression
in
epidemiological
reasoning

Epidemiological research involves generating and testing specific hypotheses about disease determinants. A hypothesis is defined as "a tentative explanation for an observation, phenomenon, or scientific problem that can be tested by further investigation."[10(p866)] Generating hypotheses is a process that involves creativity and imagination and usually includes observations on the frequency and distribution of disease in a population. Epidemiologists test hypotheses by making comparisons, usually within the context of a formal epidemiological study. The goal of a study is to harvest valid and precise information about the determinants of disease in a particular population. Epidemiological research encompasses several types of study designs; each type of study merely represents a different way of harvesting the information.

Disease Control

Epidemiologists accomplish **disease control** through epidemiological research, as described previously, and through surveillance. The purpose of surveillance is to monitor aspects of disease occurrence that are pertinent to effective control.[18(p704)] For example, the Centers for Disease Control and Prevention collects information on the occurrence of HIV infection across the United States.[19] For every case of HIV infection, the surveillance system gathers data on the individual's demographic characteristics, transmission category (such as injection drug use or male-to-male sexual contact), and diagnosis date. These surveillance data are essential for formulating and evaluating programs to reduce the spread of HIV.

▶ Historical Development of Epidemiology

The historical development of epidemiology spans almost 400 years and is best described as slow and unsteady. Only since World War II has the field experienced a rapid expansion. The following sections, which are not meant to be a comprehensive history, highlight several historic figures and studies that made significant contributions to the evolution of epidemiological thinking. These people include John Graunt, who summarized the pattern of mortality in 17th-century London; James Lind, who used an experimental study to discover the cause and prevention of scurvy; William Farr, who pioneered a wide range of activities during the mid-19th century that are still used by modern epidemiologists; John Snow, who showed that cholera was transmitted by fecal contamination of drinking water; members of the Streptomycin in Tuberculosis Trials Committee, who conducted one of the first modern controlled clinical trials; Richard Doll and A. Bradford Hill, who conducted early research on smoking and lung cancer; and Thomas Dawber and William Kannel, who began the Framingham Study, one of the most influential and longest-running studies of heart disease in the world. It is clear that epidemiology has played an important role in the achievements of public health throughout its history.

John Graunt

The logical underpinnings for modern epidemiological thinking evolved from the scientific revolution of the 17th century.[20(p23)] During this period, scientists believed that the behavior of the physical universe was orderly and could therefore be expressed in terms of mathematical relationships called "laws." These laws are generalized statements based on observations of the physical universe, such as the time of day that the sun rises and sets. Some scientists believed that this line of thinking could be extended to the biological universe and reasoned that there must be "laws of mortality" that describe the patterns of disease and death. These scientists believed that the "laws of mortality" could be inferred by observing the patterns of disease and death among humans.

John Graunt, a London tradesman and founding member of the Royal Society of London, was a pioneer in this regard. He became the first epidemiologist, statistician, and demographer when he summarized the Bills of Mortality for his 1662 publication *Natural and Political Observations Mentioned in a Following Index, and Made Upon the Bills of Mortality.*[21] The Bills of Mortality were a weekly count of people who died that had been conducted by the parish clerks of London since 1592 because of concern about the plague. According to Graunt, the Bills were collected in the following manner:

> When any one dies, then, either by tolling, or ringing a Bell, or by bespeaking of a Grave of the Sexton, the same is known to the Searchers, corresponding with the said Sexton. The Searchers hereupon (who are ancient matrons, sworn to their office) repair to the place, where the dead Corps lies, and by view of the same, and by other enquiries, they examine by what Disease, or Casualty the Corps died. Hereupon they make their Report to the Parish-Clerk, and he, every Tuesday night, carries in an Accompt of all the Burials, and Christnings, happening that Week, to the Clerk of the Hall. On Wednesday the general Accompt is made up, and Printed, and on Thursdays published and dispersed to the several Families, who will pay four shillings per Annum for them.[21(pp25-26)]

This method of reporting deaths is not very different from the system used today in the United States. Like the "searchers" of John Graunt's time, modern physicians and medical examiners inspect the body and other evidence, such as medical records, to determine the official cause of death, which is recorded on the death certificate. The physician typically submits the certificate to the funeral director, who files it with the local office of vital records. From there, the certificate is transferred to the city, county, state, and federal agencies that compile death statistics. Although 17th-century London families had to pay four shillings for the Bills of Mortality, these U.S. statistics are available free of charge.

Graunt drew many inferences about the patterns of fertility, morbidity, and mortality by tabulating the Bills of Mortality.[21] For example, he noted new diseases, such as rickets, and he made the following observations:

- Some diseases affected a similar number of people from year to year, whereas others varied considerably over time.
- Common causes of death included old age, consumption, smallpox, plague, and diseases of teeth and worms.
- Many greatly feared causes of death were actually uncommon, including leprosy, suicide, and starvation.
- Four separate periods of increased mortality caused by the plague occurred from 1592 to 1660.
- The mortality rate for men was higher than for women.
- Fall was the "most unhealthful season."

Graunt was the first to estimate the number of inhabitants, age structure of the population, and rate of population growth in London and the first to construct a life table that summarized patterns of mortality and survival from birth until death (see **TABLE 1-2**). He found that the mortality rate for children was quite high; only 25 individuals out of 100 survived to age 26 years. Furthermore, even though mortality rates for adults were much lower, very few people reached old age (only 3 of 100 London residents survived to age 66 years).

Graunt did not accept the statistics at face value but carefully considered their errors and ambiguities. For example, he noted that it was often difficult for the "antient matron" searchers to determine the exact cause of death. In fact, by cleverly comparing the number of plague deaths and nonplague deaths, Graunt estimated that London officials had overlooked about 20% of deaths resulting from plague.[22]

Although Graunt modestly stated that he merely "reduced several great confused Volumes into a few perspicuous Tables and abridged such Observations as naturally flowed from them," historians consider his work much more significant. Statistician Walter Willcox summarized Graunt's importance:

> Graunt is memorable mainly because he discovered the numerical regularity of deaths and births, of ratios of the sexes at death and birth, and of the proportion of deaths from certain causes to all causes in successive years and in different areas; or in general terms, the uniformity and predictability of many important biological phenomena taken in the mass. In doing so, he opened the way both for the later discovery of uniformities in many social and volitional phenomena like marriage, suicide and crime, and for a study of these uniformities, their nature and their limits.[21(pxiii)]

TABLE 1-2 Life Table of the London Population Constructed by John Graunt in 1662

Age (years)	Number dying	Number surviving
Birth	0	100
6	36	64
16	24	40
26	15	25
36	9	16
46	6	10
56	4	6
66	3	3
76	2	1
86	1	0

Data from Graunt J. *Natural and Political Observations Made upon the Bills of Mortality*. Baltimore, MD: The Johns Hopkins Press; 1932:69.

James Lind

Only a few important developments occurred in the field of epidemiology during the 200-year period following the publication of John Graunt's Bills of Mortality. One notable development was the realization that experimental studies could be used to test hypotheses about the laws of mortality. These studies involve designed experiments that investigate the role of some factor or agent in the causation, improvement, postponement, or prevention of disease.[23] Their hallmarks are (1) the comparison of at least two groups of individuals (an experimental group and a control group) and (2) the active manipulation of the factor or agent under study by the investigator (i.e., the investigator assigns individuals either to receive or not to receive a preventive or therapeutic measure).

In the mid-1700s, James Lind conducted one of the earliest experimental studies on the treatment of scurvy, a common disease and cause of death at the time.[24(pp145-148)] Although scurvy affected people living on land, sailors often became sick and died from this disease while at sea. As a ship's surgeon, Lind had many opportunities to observe the epidemiology of this disease. His astute observations led him to dismiss the popular ideas that scurvy was a hereditary or infectious disease and to propose that "the principal and main predisposing cause" was moist air and that its "occasional cause" was diet.[24(pp64-67,85,91)] He evaluated his hypothesis about diet with the following experimental study:

> On the 20th of May, 1747 I took twelve patients in the scurvy, on board the Salisbury at sea. Their cases were as similar as I could have them. They all in general had putrid gums, the spots and lassitude, with weakness of their knees. They lay together in one place, being a proper apartment for the sick in the fore-hold; and had one diet common to all, viz, water-gruel sweetened with sugar in the morning; fresh mutton-broth often times for dinner; at other times puddings, boiled biscuit with sugar, etc.; and for supper barley and raisins, rice and currents, sago and wine, or the like. Two of these were ordered each a quart of cyder a day. Two others took twenty-five gutts of elixir vitriol three times a-day. . . . Two other[s] took two spoonfuls of vinegar three times a-day. . . . Two of the worst patients, with the tendons in the ham rigid (a symptom none of the rest had), were put under a course of sea-water. . . . Two others had each two oranges and one lemon given them every day. . . . They continued but six days under this course having consumed the quantity that could be spared. . . . The two remaining patients took bigness of a nutmeg three times a day, of an electuary recommended by an hospital-surgeon made of garlic, mustard seed.[24(pp145-148)]

After 4 weeks, Lind reported the following: "The consequence was, that the most sudden and visible good effects were perceived from the use of the oranges and lemons; one of those who had taken them being at the end of six days fit for duty. . . . He became quite healthy before we came into Plymouth which was on the 16th of June. . . . The other was the best recovered of any in his condition; and being now deem pretty well, was appointed nurse to the rest of the sick."[24(p146)] Lind concluded, "I shall here only observe, that the result of all my experiments was, that oranges and lemons were the most effectual remedies for this distemper at sea. I am apt to think oranges preferable to lemons though perhaps both given together will be found most serviceable."[24(p148)]

Although the sample size of Lind's experiment was quite small by today's standards (12 men divided into 6 groups of 2), Lind followed one of the most important principles of experimental research—ensuring that important aspects of the experimental conditions remained similar for all study subjects. Lind selected sailors whose disease was similarly severe, who lived in common quarters, and who had a similar diet. Thus, the main difference between the six groups of men was the dietary addition purposefully introduced by Lind. He also exhibited good scientific practice by confirming "the efficacy of these fruits by the experience of others."[24(p148)] In other words, Lind did not base his final conclusions about the curative powers of citrus fruits on a single experiment, but rather he gathered additional data from other ships and voyages.

Lind used the results of this experiment to suggest a method for preventing scurvy at sea. Because fresh fruits were likely to spoil and were difficult to obtain in certain ports and seasons, he proposed that lemon and orange juice extract be carried on board.[24(pp155-156)] The British Navy took 40 years to adopt Lind's recommendation; within several years of doing so, it had eradicated scurvy from its ranks.[24(pp377-380)]

William Farr

William Farr made many important advances in the field of epidemiology in the mid-1800s. Now considered one of the founders of modern epidemiology, Farr was the compiler of Statistical Abstracts for the General Registry Office in Great Britain from 1839 through 1880. In this capacity, Farr was in charge of the annual count of births, marriages, and deaths. A trained physician and self-taught mathematician,

> Farr pioneered a whole range of activities encompassed by modern epidemiology. He described the state of health of the population, he sought to establish the determinants of public health, and he applied the knowledge gained to the prevention and control of disease.[25(ppxi-xii)]

One of Farr's most important contributions involved calculations that combined registration data on births, marriages, and deaths (as the numerator) with census data on the population size (as the denominator). As he stated, "The simple process of comparing the deaths in a given time out of a given number" was "a modern discovery."[25(p170)] His first annual report in 1839 demonstrated the "superior precision of numerical expressions" over literary expressions.[25(p214)] For example, he quantified and arranged mortality data in a manner strikingly similar to modern practice (see **TABLE 1-3**). Note that the annual percentage of deaths increased with age for men and women, but for most age groups, the percentage was higher for men than for women.

Farr drew numerous inferences about the English population by tabulating vital statistics. For example, he reported the following findings:

- The average age of the English population remained relatively constant over time at 26.4 years.
- Widowers had a higher marriage rate than bachelors.
- The rate of illegitimate births declined over time.
- People who lived at lower elevations had higher death rates resulting from cholera than did those who lived at higher elevations.
- People who lived in densely populated areas had higher mortality rates than did people who lived in less populated areas.
- Decreases in mortality rates followed improvements in sanitation.

TABLE 1-3 Annual Mortality per Hundred Males and Females in England and Wales, 1838–1871		
Age (years)	Males	Female
0–4	7.26	6.27
5–9	0.87	0.85
10–14	0.49	0.50
15–24	0.78	0.80
25–34	0.99	1.01
35–44	1.30	1.23
45–54	1.85	1.56
55–64	3.20	2.80
65–74	6.71	5.89
75–84	14.71	13.43
85–94	30.55	27.95
95+	44.11	43.04

Data from Farr W. *Vital Statistics: A Memorial Volume of Selections from the Reports and Writings of William Farr.* New York, NY: New York Academy of Medicine; 1975:183.

Farr used these data to form hypotheses about the causes and preventions of disease. For example, he used data on smallpox deaths to derive a general law of epidemics that accurately predicted the decline of the rinderpest epidemic in the 1860s.[25(px)] He used the data on the association between cholera deaths and altitude to support the hypothesis that an unhealthful climate was the disease's cause, which was a theory that was subsequently disproved.

Farr made several practical and methodological contributions to the field of epidemiology. First, he constantly strove to ensure that the collected data were accurate and complete. Second, he devised a categorization system for the causes of death so that these data could be reduced to a usable form. The system that he devised is the antecedent of the modern International Classification of Diseases, which categorizes diseases and causes of death. Third, Farr made a number of important contributions to the analysis of data, including the invention of the "standardized mortality rate," an adjustment method for making fair comparisons between groups with different age structures.

John Snow

Another important figure in the development of epidemiological methods during the mid-1800s was John Snow (see **FIGURE 1-1**). A respected physician who was a successful anesthetist and researcher on anesthetic gases, Snow was also interested in the cause and spread of cholera.[26(pxxxiv)] Although Farr mistakenly thought that an unhealthful climate accounted for the variation in cholera mortality by altitude, Snow used these data to support an innovative hypothesis that cholera was an infectious disease spread by fecal contamination of drinking water.

Snow argued,

> Cholera must be a poison acting on the alimentary canal by being brought into direct contact with the alimentary mucous surface . . . the symptoms are primarily seated in the alimentary canal and all the after-symptoms of a general kind are the results of the flux from the canal.[26(ppxxxiv-xxxv)]

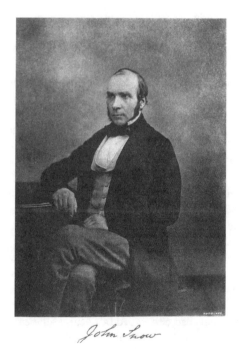

John Snow

FIGURE 1-1 John Snow investigated the cause and spread of cholera in 19th-century London.

His inference from this was that the poison of cholera is taken directly into the canal by mouth. This view led him to consider the media through which the poison is conveyed and the nature of the poison itself. Several circumstances lent their aid in referring him to water as the chief, though not the only, medium and to the excreted matters from the patient already stricken with cholera as the poison.

In 1849, Snow published his views on the causes and transmission of cholera in a short pamphlet titled *On the Mode of Communication of Cholera*. During the next few years, he continued groundbreaking research testing the hypothesis that cholera was a waterborne infectious disease. The second edition of his pamphlet, published in 1855, describes in greater detail "the whole of his inquiries in regard to cholera."[26(pxxxvi)] The cholera investigations for which Snow is best known are described in the following paragraphs.

One such investigation focused on the Broad Street epidemic. During August and September of 1854, one of the worst outbreaks of cholera occurred in the London neighborhood surrounding Broad Street. Almost 500 fatalities from cholera occurred within a 10-day period within 250 yards of the junction between Broad and Cambridge Streets (see **FIGURE 1-2**). According to Snow, "The mortality in this limited area probably equals any that was ever caused in this country, even by the plague; and it was much more sudden, as the greater number of cases terminated in a few hours."[26(p38)] Snow continued,

> As soon as I became acquainted with the situation and extent of this irruption of cholera, I suspected some contamination of the water of the much-frequented street-pump in Broad Street, near the end of Cambridge Street; but on examining the water, on the evening of the 3rd of September, I found so little impurity in it of an organic nature that I hesitated to come to a conclusion. Further inquiry, however, showed me that there was no other circumstance or agent common to the cholera occurred, and not extending beyond it, except the water of the above mentioned pump.[26(p39)]

His subsequent investigations included a detailed study of the drinking habits of 83 individuals who died between August 31 and September 2, 1854.[26(pp39-40)] He found that 73 of the 83 deaths occurred among individuals living within a short distance of the Broad Street pump and that 10 deaths occurred among individuals who lived in houses that were near other pumps. According to the surviving relatives, 61 of the 73 individuals who lived near the pump drank the pump water and only 6 individuals did not. (No data could be collected for the remaining 6 people because everyone connected with these individuals had either died or departed the city.) The drinking habits of the 10 individuals who lived "decidedly nearer to another street pump" also implicated the Broad Street pump. Surviving relatives reported that 5 of the 10 drank water from the Broad Street pump because they preferred it, and 2 drank its water because they attended a nearby school.

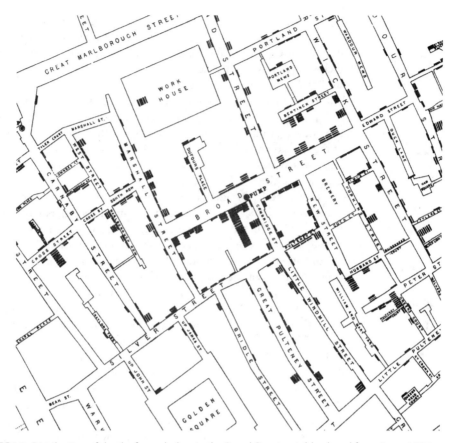

FIGURE 1-2 Distribution of deaths from cholera in the Broad Street neighborhood from August 19 to September 30, 1854. "A black mark or bar for each death is placed in the situation of the house in which the fatal attack took place. The situation of the Broad Street Pump is also indicated, as well as that of all the surrounding Pumps to which the public had access."

Courtesy of The Commonwealth Fund. In: Snow J. *Snow on Cholera*. New York, NY; 1936.

Snow also investigated pockets of the Broad Street population that had fewer cholera deaths. For example, he found that only 5 cholera deaths occurred among 535 inmates of a workhouse located in the Broad Street neighborhood.[26(p42)] The workhouse had a pump well on its premises, and "the inmates never sent to Broad Street for water." Furthermore, no cholera deaths occurred among 70 workers at the Broad Street brewery who never obtained pump water but instead drank a daily ration of malt liquor.

Although Snow never found direct evidence of sewage contamination of the Broad Street pump well, he did note that the well was near a major sewer and several cesspools. He concluded, "There had been no particular outbreak or increase of cholera, in this part of London, except among the persons who were in the habit of drinking the water of the above-mentioned pump-well."[26(p40)] He presented his findings to the Board of Guardians of St. James's Parish on September 7, and "the handle of the pump was removed on the following day."[26]

Snow's investigation of the Broad Street epidemic is noteworthy for several reasons. First, Snow was able to form a hypothesis implicating the Broad Street pump after he mapped the geographic distribution of the cholera deaths and studied that distribution in relation to the surrounding public water pumps (see Figure 1-2). Second, he collected data on the drinking water habits of unaffected as well as affected individuals, which allowed him to make a comparison that would support or refute his hypothesis. Third, the results of his investigation were so convincing that they led to immediate action to curb the disease, namely, the pump handle was removed. Public health action to prevent disease seldom occurs so quickly.

Another series of Snow's groundbreaking investigations on cholera focused on specific water supply companies. In particular, he found that districts supplied by the Southwark and Vauxhall Company and the Lambeth Company had higher cholera mortality rates than all of the other water companies.[26(pp63-64)] A few years later, a fortuitous change occurred in the water source of several of the south districts of London. As Snow stated, "The Lambeth Company removed their water works, in 1852, from opposite Hungerforth Market to Thames Ditton; thus obtaining a supply of water quite free from the sewage of London."[26(p68)]

Following this change, Snow obtained data from William Farr to show that "districts partially supplied with the improved water suffered much less than the others"[26(p69)] (see **TABLE 1-4**). Districts with a mixture of the clean and polluted drinking water (Southwark and Vauxhall Company and Lambeth Company combined) had 35% fewer cholera deaths (61 versus 94 deaths per 100,000) than districts with only polluted drinking water (Southwark and Vauxhall Company alone).

TABLE 1-4 Mortality from Cholera in Relation to the Water Supply Companies in the Districts of London, November 1853

Water supply company	Number of cholera deaths	Size of population	Death rate resulting from cholera
Southwark and Vauxhall	111	118,267	94/100,000
Southwark and Vauxhall, Lambeth	211	346,363	61/100,000

Data from Snow J. *Snow on Cholera*. New York, NY: Hafner Publishers; 1965:69. With permission from the Commonwealth Fund, New York, NY.

TABLE 1-5 Mortality from Cholera in Relation to the Water Supply Companies in the Subdistricts of London, 1853

Water supply company	Number of cholera deaths	Size of population	Death rate resulting from cholera
Southwark and Vauxhall alone	192	167,654	114/100,000
Southwark and Vauxhall and Lambeth combined	182	301,149	60/100,000
Lambeth alone	0	14,632	0/100,000

Data from Snow J. *Snow on Cholera*. New York, NY: Hafner Publishers; 1965: 73. With permission from the Commonwealth Fund, New York, NY.

Snow next analyzed the cholera mortality data in smaller geographic units—London subdistricts—to make an even clearer distinction between the polluted and clean water supplies. In particular, he examined the death rates in the London subdistricts supplied by (1) the Southwark and Vauxhall Company alone (heavily polluted water), (2) the Lambeth Company alone (nonpolluted water), and (3) both companies combined (a mixture of polluted and nonpolluted water). The cholera death rates were highest in subdistricts supplied by the heavily polluted water of the Southwark and Vauxhall Company and were intermediate in subdistricts supplied by the mixed water from the Southwark and Vauxhall Company and Lambeth Company combined. No cholera deaths were observed in subdistricts supplied with the nonpolluted water of the Lambeth Company (see **TABLE 1-5**).

Although Snow thought that these data provided "very strong evidence of the powerful influence which the drinking of water containing the sewage of a town exerts over the spread of cholera, when that disease is present," he thought that further study of the people living in the subdistricts supplied by both companies would "yield the most incontrovertible proof on one side or another."[26] Snow understood that the differences in cholera death rates between the two companies might not have been caused by the water supply itself but rather by differences between the groups, such as differences in gender, age, and socioeconomic status. Fortunately for Snow, further study revealed that the two groups were strikingly similar.

Snow made the following observation:

In the subdistricts enumerated in the above table [Table 1-5] as being supplied by both companies, the mixing of the supply is of the most intimate kind. The pipes of each Company go down all the street, and into nearly all the courts and alleys. A few houses are supplied by one Company and a few by the other, according to the decision of the owner or occupier at that time when the water companies were in active competition. In many cases a single house has a supply different from that on either side. Each company supplied both rich and poor, both large houses and small; there is no difference either in the condition or occupation of the persons receiving the water of different companies. . . . As there is no difference whatsoever, either in the houses or the people receiving the supply of the two Water Companies, or in any of the physical conditions with which they are surrounded, it is obvious that no experiment could have been devised which would more thoroughly test the effect of water supply on the progress of cholera than this, which circumstances placed ready made before the observer. The experiment, too, was on the grandest scale. No fewer than three hundred thousand people of both sexes, of every age and occupation, and of every rank and station, from gentlefolks down to the very poor, were divided into two groups without their choice, and, in most cases, without their knowledge; one group being supplied with water containing the sewage of London, and amongst it, whatever might have come from the cholera patients, the other group having water quite free from such impurity.[26(pp74-75)]

Snow's next step was to obtain a listing from the General Register Office of the addresses of persons dying of cholera in the subdistricts that used water from both suppliers. Then, he had the difficult task of going door to door to inquire about the drinking water supplier. According to Snow,

The inquiry was necessarily attended with a good deal of trouble. There were very few instances in which I could get the information I required. Even when the water-rates are paid by the residents, they can seldom remember the name of the Water Company till they have looked for the receipt.[26(p76)]

However, Snow found an ingenious solution to this problem:

It would, indeed, have been almost impossible for me to complete the inquiry, if I had not found that I could distinguish the water of the two companies with perfect certainty by a chemical test. The test I employed was founded on the great difference in the quantity of chloride of sodium contained in the two kinds of water. On adding solution of nitrate of silver to a gallon of water of the Lambeth Company . . . only 2.28 grains of chloride of silver were obtained. . . . On treating the water of Southwark and Vauxhall Company in the same manner, 91 grains of chloride of silver were obtained.[26(pp77-78)]

Thus, Snow identified the drinking water source of each household and was able to link the death rate from cholera to the water supply companies (see **TABLE 1-6**). He concluded, "The mortality in the houses supplied by the Southwark and Vauxhall Company was therefore between eight and nine times as great as in the houses supplied by the Lambeth Company."[26(p86)]

Based on his findings, Snow made a series of recommendations for the prevention of cholera. For example, he recommended,

> Care should be taken that the water employed for drinking and preparing food . . . is not contaminated with the contents of cesspools, house-drains, or sewers; or in the event that water free from suspicion cannot be obtained, is [sic] should be well boiled, and if possible, also filtered.[26(pp133-134)]

Even though his results and recommendations were reported at once to William Farr and others, it took several years for Snow's theories to be accepted.[27]

Fortunately, over time we have come to recognize the importance of John Snow's contributions to our understanding of infectious diseases, in general, and cholera, in particular. For several reasons, Snow's investigations are considered "a nearly perfect model" for epidemiological research.[26(pix)] First, Snow organized his observations logically so that meaningful inferences could be derived from them.[20(p29)] Second, he recognized that "a natural experiment" had occurred in the subdistricts of London that would enable him to gather unquestionable proof either for or against his hypothesis. Third, he conducted a quantitative analysis of the data contrasting the occurrence of cholera deaths in relation to the drinking water company.

TABLE 1-6 Mortality from Cholera in Relation to the Water Supply Companies in the Subdistricts of London, July–August 1854

Water supply company	Number of cholera deaths	Number of houses	Death rate resulting from cholera
Southwark and Vauxhall Company	1,263	40,046	315/10,000
Lambeth Company	98	26,107	37/10,000
Rest of London	1,422	256,423	55/10,000

Adapted from Snow J. *Snow on Cholera*. New York, NY: Hafner Publishers; 1965: 86. With permission from the Commonwealth Fund, New York, NY; and Carvalho FM, Lima F, Kriebel D. Re: on John Snow's unquestioned long division. *Am J Epidemiol*. 2004;159:422.

Modern Experimental Studies

The development and application of epidemiological methods advanced slowly during the late 1800s and early 1900s. Only during the 1930s and 1940s did physicians begin to realize that it was necessary to refine the methods used to evaluate the effectiveness of disease treatments.[28] Although some physicians still thought that they could assess the usefulness of a treatment merely by observing the patient's response and comparing it with what they expected on the basis of their education and experience, many realized that "modern" experimental studies with comparable treatment and control groups of patients and comparable methods for assessing the disease changes were needed to yield correct conclusions.[29]

Streptomycin Tuberculosis Trial

In the late 1940s, the Streptomycin in Tuberculosis Trials Committee of the British Medical Research Council conducted one of the first modern experimental studies on the use of streptomycin to treat pulmonary tuberculosis.[30] According to the investigators,

> The natural course of pulmonary tuberculosis is . . . so variable . . . that evidence of improvement or cure following the use of a new drug in a few cases cannot be accepted as proof of the effect of that drug. The history of chemotherapeutic trials in tuberculosis is filled with errors. . . . It had become obvious that . . . conclusions regarding the clinical effect of a new chemotherapeutic agent . . . could be considered valid only if based on . . . controlled clinical trials.[30(p4582)]
>
> Medical Research Council. Streptomycin in Tuberculosis Trials Committee. Streptomycin treatment of pulmonary tuberculosis. *Br Med J.* 1948;2:769-782.

This controlled clinical trial of streptomycin included 107 patients with acute progressive bilateral pulmonary tuberculosis.[30] The investigators decided to include only cases of tuberculosis that were unsuitable for other forms of treatment "to avoid having to make allowances for the effect of forms of therapy other than bed-rest."[30] In addition, they excluded cases in which spontaneous regression was likely and cases in which there was little hope of improvement.

One group of 55 patients was treated with bed rest and streptomycin, and a second group of 52 patients was treated with bed rest alone.[30] Patients were assigned to these groups by an innovative method known as randomization, which is defined as "an act of assigning or ordering that is the result of a random process."[23(p220)] Random assignment methods include flipping a coin or using a sequence of random numbers. The exact process used in the Streptomycin Tuberculosis Trial was as follows:

> Determination of whether a patient would be treated by streptomycin and bed rest (S case) or by bed rest alone (C case) was made by reference to a statistical series based on random

sampling numbers drawn up for each sex at each centre by Professor Bradford Hill; the details of the series were unknown to any of the investigators or to the co-ordinator and were contained in a set of sealed envelopes.[30(p770)]

Patients in the streptomycin group received the drug by injection four times a day.[30] Although investigators observed toxic effects in many patients, these effects were not so severe as to require the termination of treatment. During the 6-month follow-up period, 7% of the streptomycin patients died, and 27% of the control patients died. Investigators observed X-ray evidence of considerable pulmonary improvement in 51% of the streptomycin patients and only 8% of the control patients. Clinical improvement was also more common in the streptomycin group. The investigators reached the following conclusion:

> The course of bilateral acute progressive disease can be halted by streptomycin therapy. . . . That streptomycin was the agent responsible for this result is attested by the presence in this trial of the control group of patients, among whom considerable improvement was noted in only four (8%).[30(p780)]

According to Richard Doll, "Few innovations have made such an impact on medicine as the controlled clinical trial that was designed by Sir Austin Bradford Hill for the Medical Research Council's Streptomycin in Tuberculosis Trials Committee in 1946."[29(p343)] Four features of the trial were particularly innovative. First and foremost was its use of randomization to assign patients to the streptomycin and control groups. Although randomization had been used in agriculture and laboratory research, this trial was one of the first instances in which it was used in medical research. The main advantage of randomization is that the order of future assignments cannot be predicted from that of past ones. Lack of predictability is the key to minimizing bias, which is defined as a systematic error in the study that causes a false conclusion.

The second innovation was the placement of restrictions on the type of patient eligible for the trial.[29] Patients with the type of tuberculosis that was unsuitable for therapies other than bed rest were excluded so that the results would not be obscured by the effects of other treatments. Patients who were likely to get better without any treatment or who were so ill that the streptomycin was unlikely to help were also excluded.

Third, the data collection methods helped ensure that the results would be free of bias.[29] These methods included using a precise and objective endpoint, such as death, and masking the investigators who were assessing the radiological improvements. Masking means that the investigators who reviewed the X-rays were unaware of the person's treatment assignment and therefore the chances of their making a biased judgment were reduced.

Fourth, the investigators considered the ethical issues involved in conducting the trial, including whether it was ethical to withhold the streptomycin treatment from the control group.[29] Before the trial was conducted, researchers had already shown that streptomycin inhibited the tubercle bacillus *in vitro* and reduced experimental infections of guinea pigs. Preliminary results of clinical studies had also been encouraging. However, only a small amount of the drug was available in Britain, and it was impossible to treat all patients with tuberculosis. Thus, the committee reasoned, "It would . . . have been unethical not to have seized the opportunity to design a strictly controlled trial, which could speedily and effectively reveal the value of the treatment."[29(p339)]

Doll and Hill's Studies on Smoking and Lung Cancer

Most epidemiologists consider Richard Doll and A. Bradford Hill's 1950 study on smoking and lung cancer to be one of the major milestones of epidemiology.[31] Doll and Hill undertook the study because of the striking increase in lung cancer death rates in England and Wales during the 25-year period following World War I.[32] Some scientists argued that the increase was the result of improvements in lung cancer diagnosis. However, Doll and Hill believed that improved diagnosis could not be entirely responsible because the number of lung cancer deaths had increased in areas with and without modern diagnostic facilities. Thus, Doll and Hill thought it was "right and proper" to justify searching for an environmental cause. Their work is emblematic of an important shift in epidemiology following World War II that redirected the focus of epidemiological research from infectious to chronic diseases.[31] The shift was fueled by the idea that chronic diseases were not merely degenerative disorders of old age but rather were potentially preventable diseases with environmental origins.

Doll and Hill's first study was a "case–control study,"[32] which included 709 subjects who had lung cancer (the cases) and 709 subjects who had diseases other than cancer (the controls). Control patients were purposely selected to be of the same gender, within the same 5-year age group, and in the same hospital at approximately the same time as the lung cancer patients.

Patients from each group were interviewed while in the hospital for treatment about their smoking habits. In particular, they were asked,

(a) if they had smoked at any period of their lives; (b) the ages at which they had started and stopped; (c) the amount they were in the habit of smoking before the onset of the illness which had brought them to the hospital; (d) the main changes in their smoking history and the maximum they had ever been in the habit of smoking; (e) the varying proportions smoked in pipes and cigarettes; and (f) whether or not they inhaled.[32(p741)]

Doll and Hill found that proportionately more lung cancer patients than noncancer patients were smokers.[32] In particular, 99.7% of male lung cancer patients and 95.8% of male noncancer patients smoked; 68.3% of female lung cancer patients and only 46.7% of female noncancer patients were smokers. Furthermore, a higher proportion of patients with lung cancer described themselves as heavy smokers. For example, 26.0% of the male lung cancer patients and 13.5% of the male noncancer patients reported that they had smoked 25 or more cigarettes per day before their illness began. Although the authors acknowledged that they did not know what carcinogens in tobacco smoke might be responsible, they concluded that "smoking is an important factor in the cause of lung cancer."

Three other case–control studies published in 1950 also showed an association between smoking and lung cancer. However, modern epidemiologists consider the Doll and Hill study to be "a classic exemplar for the investigation of a given outcome and an array of exposures. . . . No previous research paper lays out the essentials of the case–control method with such understanding and meticulous care."[31(p163)] Far in advance of their peers, Doll and Hill considered a wide range of problems in the design and analysis of their study, including errors that may have occurred when they recruited and interviewed their subjects.

In the years following the 1950 Doll and Hill study, several more studies were conducted using the case–control approach of comparing the smoking histories of patients with and without lung cancer (such as Wynder and Cornfeld's 1953 study).[33] These studies all found that the proportion of smokers, particularly heavy smokers, was higher among lung cancer patients than among noncancer patients. However, Doll and Hill believed that additional "retrospective" studies were "unlikely to advance our knowledge materially or to throw any new light upon the nature of the association." (Retrospective studies investigate diseases that have already occurred.) They asserted that if there were "any undetected flaw in the evidence that such studies have produced, it would be exposed only by some entirely new approach."[32] The new approach that they proposed was a "prospective" study—a study that follows participants into the future to observe the occurrence of disease.

Doll and Hill initiated a prospective study in 1951 by inviting 59,600 male and female members of the British Medical Association to complete a short questionnaire about their smoking habits.[34] The investigators then divided the respondents into four groups on the basis of their answers: nonsmokers, light smokers, moderate smokers, and heavy smokers. The investigators obtained information on the causes of death among those who answered the questionnaire from the General Register Office in the United Kingdom.

During the 29-month period following the administration of the questionnaire, 789 deaths were reported among the 24,389 male doctors aged 35 years and older. Of these deaths, 36 were reported to have died of lung cancer as either the direct or contributory cause. After accounting for age differences between the smoking groups, the investigators found that death rates caused by lung cancer increased from 0.0 per 1,000 among nonsmokers to 0.48 per 1,000 among light smokers, 0.67 per 1,000 among moderate smokers, and 1.14 per 1,000 among heavy smokers.[34]

The investigators continued to follow the doctors for the next 50 years.[35] During this period, they updated the smoking and mortality data. Of the 34,439 men studied, 25,346 were known to have died from 1951 through 2001. Death rates were about two to three times as high among cigarette smokers as among lifelong nonsmokers. The causes of death related to smoking included not only lung cancer but also heart disease, chronic obstructive lung disease, and a variety of vascular diseases.

Because the proportion of doctors who smoked cigarettes declined over the 50-year period, the investigators were also able to examine the death rate among former smokers who had stopped smoking for various lengths of time. They found that, as compared with lifelong nonsmokers, the risk of lung cancer death among ex-smokers steadily declined in relation to the number of years since they had stopped smoking. However, those who had smoked until about age 40 before they stopped still had some excess of lung cancer at older ages.

Like their first case–control study, Doll and Hill's prospective study broke new ground. First, the study included tens of thousands of subjects, and therefore it had adequate "power" to examine numerous health effects of several levels of smoking. Second, the investigators followed the subjects for a long period of time. A long follow-up period is particularly important in the study of diseases such as cancer that take decades to develop. Third, Doll and Hill incorporated changes in smoking habits over time and therefore were able to examine the health benefits of smoking cessation.

The Framingham Study

Like the work of Doll and Hill, the Framingham Study is notable for bringing about a shift in focus from infectious to noninfectious diseases following World War II. Considered "the epitome of successful epidemiologic research," this study "has become the prototype and model of the cohort study."[31(p157)] The cohort study is one of the three main study designs used in epidemiological research.

According to Susser, the Framingham Study is "undisputedly the foundation stone for current ideas about risk factors in general and the prevention of ischemic heart disease in particular." In addition, it has provided the impetus for solving difficult design and analysis issues in epidemiological research, including the development of appropriate methods for measuring the major risk factors for coronary heart disease (such as high blood pressure, elevated serum cholesterol levels, physical activity, and life stress) and for solving problems associated with measurements that vary over time.[31(pp157-161)] The study has also served as a stimulus for developing other cohort studies of cardiovascular disease and other topics.

When the Framingham Study was started in 1947, its goal was to develop ways of identifying latent cardiovascular disease among healthy volunteers.[31] Within a few years, investigators expanded the study's purpose to include determining the causes of cardiovascular disease. The study now investigates a wide variety of diseases, including stroke, diabetes, Alzheimer's disease, and cancer, and includes the offspring and grandchildren of the original participants.

Initially, the investigators enrolled about 5,000 healthy adult residents in Framingham, Massachusetts, a town located about 18 miles west of Boston.[36(pp14-29)] In the late 1940s, Framingham was a self-contained community of about 28,000 residents who obtained their medical care from local physicians and two hospitals near the center of town. Framingham residents were considered an excellent population for a community-based prospective study because (1) the town's population was stable, (2) the investigators could identify a sufficient number of people with and without risk factors for heart disease, and (3) local medical doctors were eager to help recruit study subjects.

For more than half a century, Framingham Study participants have undergone interviews, physical exams, laboratory tests, and other tests every 2 years.[37] The interviews have gathered information on each subject's medical history and history of cigarette smoking, alcohol use, physical activity, dietary intake, and emotional stress. The physical exams and laboratory tests have measured characteristics such as height and weight, blood pressure, vital signs and symptoms, cholesterol levels, glucose levels, bone mineral density, and genetic characteristics. These data-gathering efforts have left an immeasurable legacy of research findings on numerous topics. The contributions of the Framingham Study will only multiply in coming years with the addition of offspring, third-generation, and multiethnic cohorts.[38]

▶ Modern Epidemiology

The field of epidemiology has expanded tremendously in size, scope, and influence since the early days of the modern era. The number of epidemiologists has grown rapidly along with the number of epidemiology training programs in schools of public health and medicine. Many subspecialties have been established that are defined either by (1) disease, (2) exposure, or (3) population being studied. Disease-specific subspecialties include reproductive, cancer, cardiovascular, infectious disease, and psychiatric epidemiology. Exposure-specific subspecialties include environmental, behavioral, and nutritional epidemiology and pharmaco-epidemiology. Population-specific subspecialties include pediatric and geriatric epidemiology.

In addition, the scope of epidemiological research has expanded in several directions. First, some epidemiologists examine health determinants at the genetic and molecular level and therefore combine the basic and public health sciences. For example, human genome epidemiology uses "epidemiological methods to assess the impact of human genetic variation on disease occurrence" and plays an essential role in the discovery of genes that cause disease and the use of genetic testing for "diagnosing, predicting, treating and preventing disease."[39] Molecular epidemiology involves the use of biolological markers to improve the measurement of exposures, disease susceptibility, and health outcomes.[40(pp564-579)] For example, biomarkers such as serum micronutrient levels can determine a person's fruit and vegetable intake more accurately than can personal interviews.

The second direction of epidemiological research has involved the study of determinants at the societal level.[41] Social epidemiology is the study of exposures and disease susceptibility and resistance at diverse levels, including the individual, household, neighborhood, and region. For example, social epidemiologists investigate how neighborhoods, racial discrimination, and poverty influence a person's health.

The third new direction of epidemiological research has involved the analysis of determinants across the life span. Life course epidemiology, which involves the study of lasting effects of exposures during gestation, childhood, adolescence, and young adulthood on disease risk in later adult life, is based on the notion that exposures throughout life influence health in adult life.[14(p74)] For example, life course epidemiolgists investigate how undernutrition during gestation increases the risk of chronic diseases among adults.

Theories and methods of epidemiological research have also evolved over time. For example, epidemiologists have developed new views on disease causation, and the theoretical framework underlying epidemiological study designs has matured. Finally, the availability of high-powered computer hardware and software has facilitated the analysis of large electronic datasets (now termed "big data") with substantial numbers of people and many risk factors, enabling epidemiologists to explore new public health questions and assess the effects of multiple risk factors simultaneously.

Not surprisingly, epidemiology is currently being used to investigate a wide range of important public health topics. Noteworthy topics that have been examined recently include the risk of adult-onset asthma among Black women experiencing racism,[42] social determinants of multidrug-resistant tuberculosis,[43] the role of exercise in reducing deaths from breast cancer,[44] the numerous genetic determinants of Alzheimer's disease,[45] the effectiveness of a popular diet for diabetes prevention,[46] the effect of prenatal exposure to air pollution on the risk of autism,[47] and the effectiveness of mindfulness therapy in the treatment of posttraumatic stress disorder.[48]

The 21st century poses even more challenging problems for epidemiologists, such as "air, water and soil pollution; global warming; population growth; poverty and social inequality; and civil unrest and violence."[49(p5)] Recently, some of these challenges came to the forefront in the United States when the drinking water in Flint, Michigan, became highly contaminated with lead, a potent neurotoxin, and when an alarming string of mass shootings highlighted the country's inadequate gun control laws. An editorial on epidemiology in the 21st century noted that, like public health achievements of the past, solutions to these problems will occur through "the complementary contributions of different facets of epidemiology: calculating disease trends and probabilities, communicating findings to the public and policy makers, and designing and implementing interventions based on data."[50(p1154)] The editorialists went on to observe,

> Epidemiology's full value is achieved only when its contributions are placed in the context of public health action, resulting in a healthier populace. . . . Like others in epidemiology's rich history, we should keep our eyes on the prizes of preventing disease and promoting health.[50(p1155)]

The prospect of preventing disease and death through "analytic prowess" has attracted many great minds to epidemiology throughout its history, and it will undoubtedly continue to attract them in the coming century.

Summary

Disease prevention and health promotion are the main goals of public health, a multidisciplinary field that focuses on populations and communities rather than on separate individuals. Epidemiology, one of the basic sciences of public health, is defined as "the study of the distribution and determinants of disease frequency in human populations and the application of this study to control health problems."[13(p1),14(p55)] Epidemiology has played an important role in the public health achievements of the past 400 years. Key historic figures and studies have included John Graunt, who summarized the patterns of mortality in 17th-century London; James Lind, who discovered the cause and prevention of scurvy using an experimental study design in the 18th century; William Farr, who originated many modern epidemiological methods in the 19th century, including the combination of numerator and denominator data; John Snow, who demonstrated that contaminated drinking water was the mode of cholera transmission in the 19th century; members of the Streptomycin in Tuberculosis Trials Committee, who conducted one of the first modern controlled clinical trials in the 1940s; Doll and Hill, who conducted case–control studies on smoking and lung cancer in the 1950s;

and investigators who have worked on the Framingham Study, which was started in 1947 and has become one of the most influential studies of heart disease in the world. In recent years, the field of epidemiology has greatly expanded in size, scope, and influence, and epidemiologists currently investigate a wide range of important public health problems. The 21st century will pose even more challenging problems for epidemiologists. Like past public health achievements, the solutions to these problems will be found by placing the contributions of epidemiology in the context of public health action.

References

1. Schneider MJ. *Introduction to Public Health*. 5th ed. Burlington, MA: Jones & Bartlett Learning; 2017.
2. National Center for Health Statistics. *Health, United States, 2015, With Special Feature on Racial and Ethnic Health Disparities*. Hyattsville, MD: Government Printing Office; 2016.
3. Bunker JP, Frazier HS, Mosteller F. Improving health: measuring effects of medical care. *Milbank Q*. 1994; 72:225-258.
4. Centers for Disease Control and Prevention. Ten great public health achievements—United States, 1900-1999. *MMWR*. 1999;48:241-243.
5. Loomis TA. *Essentials of Toxicology*. 3rd ed. Philadelphia, PA: Lea & Febiger; 1978.
6. Gottlieb MS, Schanker HM, Fan PT, Saxon A, Weisman JD, Pozalski I. *Pneumocystis* pneumonia— Los Angeles. *MMWR*. 1981;30:250-252.
7. Friedman-Kien A, Laubenstein L, Marmor M, et al. Kaposi's sarcoma and *Pneumocystis* pneumonia among homosexual men—New York City and California. *MMWR*. 1981;30:305-308.
8. Boice JD, Monson RR. Breast cancer in women after repeated fluoroscopic examination of the chest. *J Natl Cancer Inst*. 1977;59:823-832.
9. Phelan KJ, Khoury K, Xu Y, Liddy S, Hornung R, Lanphear BP. A randomized controlled trial of home injury hazard reduction: the HOME injury study. *Arch Pediatr Adolesc Med*. 2011;165:339-345.
10. Pickett JP (ed.). *The American Heritage Dictionary of the English Language*. 4th ed. Boston, MA: Houghton Mifflin; 2000.
11. *Oxford English Dictionary* (OED) Online. Oxford University Press; 2016. Accessed September 7, 2016.
12. Lilienfeld D. Definitions of epidemiology. *Am J Epidemiol*. 1978;107:87-90.
13. MacMahon B, Trichopoulos D. *Epidemiology: Principles and Methods*. 2nd ed. Boston, MA: Little, Brown and Co; 1996.
14. Porta M. *A Dictionary of Epidemiology*. 6th ed. New York, NY: Oxford University Press; 2014.
15. MacMahon B, Pugh TF. *Epidemiology: Principles and Methods*. Boston, MA: Little, Brown and Co; 1970.
16. About the National Health Interview Survey. cdc.gov. http://www.cdc.gov/nchs/nhis/about_nhis.htm. Accessed September 6, 2016.
17. *Breast Cancer Facts & Figures—2017-2018*. cancer.org. https://www.cancer.org/content/dam/cancer-org /research/cancer-facts-and-statistics/breast-cancer -facts-and-figures/breast-cancer-facts-and-figures -2017-2018.pdf. Accessed June 8, 2018.
18. Heymann DL (ed.). *Control of Communicable Diseases Manual*. 20th ed. Washington, DC: American Public Health Association; 2015.
19. HIV/AIDS: Surveillance Overview. cdc.gov. https:// www.cdc.gov/hiv/statistics/surveillance/index .html?s_cid=cs_2519. Accessed June 20, 2017.
20. Lilienfeld DE, Stolley PD. *Foundations of Epidemiology*. 3rd ed. New York, NY: Oxford University Press; 1994.
21. Graunt J. *Natural and Political Observations Mentioned in a Following Index, and Made Upon the Bills of Mortality*. Willcox, WF (ed.). Baltimore, MD: The Johns Hopkins Press; 1939.
22. Rothman KJ. Lessons from John Graunt. *Lancet*. 1996;347:37-39.
23. Meinert CL. *Clinical Trials Dictionary, Terminology and Usage Recommendations*. Baltimore, MD: The Johns Hopkins Center for Clinical Trials; 1996.
24. Stewart CP, Guthrie D (eds.). *Lind's Treatise on Scurvy. A Bicentenary Volume Containing a Reprint of the First Edition of a Treatise of the Scurvy by James Lind, MD, with Additional Notes*. Edinburgh, Scotland: Edinburgh University Press; 1953.
25. Farr W. *Vital Statistics: A Memorial Volume of Selections from the Reports and Writings of William Farr*. New York, NY: New York Academy of Medicine; 1975.
26. Snow J. *On the Mode of Communication of Cholera*. 2nd ed. London, England: Churchill, 1855. Reprinted as Snow J. *Snow on Cholera*. New York, NY: Hafner Publishing Co; 1965.

27. Winkelstein W. A new perspective on John Snow's communicable disease theory. *Am J Epidemiol.* 1995;142:S3-S9.

28. Vandenbroucke JP. Second thoughts: a short note on the history of the randomized controlled trial. *J Chron Dis.* 1987;40:985-987.

29. Doll R. Clinical trials: retrospect and prospect. *Stat Med.* 1982;1:337-44.

30. Medical Research Council. Streptomycin in Tuberculosis Trials Committee. Streptomycin treatment of pulmonary tuberculosis. *Br Med J.* 1948;2:769-782.

31. Susser M. Epidemiology in the United States after World War II: the evolution of technique. *Epidemiol Rev.* 1985;7:147-177.

32. Doll R, Hill AB. Smoking and carcinoma of the lung. *Br Med J.* 1950;2:739-748.

33. Wynder EL, Cornfeld J. Cancer of the lung in physicians. *New Engl J Med.* 1953;248:441-444.

34. Doll R, Hill AB. The mortality of doctors in relation to their smoking habits. *Br Med J.* 1954;1:1451-1455.

35. Doll R, Peto R, Boreham J, Sutherland I. Mortality in relation to smoking: 50 years' observations on male British doctors. *Br Med J.* 2004;328(7455):1519.

36. Dawber TR. *The Framingham Study: The Epidemiology of Atherosclerotic Disease.* Cambridge, MA: Harvard University Press; 1980.

37. Kannel WB. The Framingham Study: its 50-year legacy and future promise. *J Atheroscler Thromb.* 2000;6:60-66.

38. About the Framingham Heart Study. framinghamheartstudy.org. https://www.framinghamheartstudy.org/about-fhs/index.php. Accessed June 20, 2017.

39. Khoury MJ, Millikan R, Little J, Gwinn M. The emergence of epidemiology in the genomics age. *Intl J Epidemiol.* 2004;33:936-944.

40. Khoury MJ, Millikan R, Gwinn M. Genetic and molecular epidemiology. In: Rothman KJ, Greenland S, Lash TL, eds. *Modern Epidemiology.* 3rd ed. Philadelpia, PA: Wolters Kluwer/Lippincott Williams and Wilkins; 2008.

41. Kreiger N. Epidemiology and social sciences: towards a critical reengagement in the 21st century. *Epidemiol Rev.* 2000;22:155-163.

42. Coogan PF, Yu J, O'Connor GT, Brown TA, Cozier YC, Palmer JR, et al. Experiences of racism and the incidence of adult-onset asthma in the Black Women's Health Study. *Chest.* 2014;145:480-485.

43. Odone A, Calderon R, Becerra MC, Zhang Z, Contreras CC, Yataco R, et al. Acquired and transmitted multidrug resistant tuberculosis: the role of socal determinants. *PLoS One.* 2016;11(1):e0146642.

44. Ammitzboll G, Sogaard K, Karlsen RV, Tjonneland A, Johansen C, Frederiksen K, et al. Physical activity and survival in breast cancer. *Eur J Cancer.* 2016;66:67-74.

45. Chouraki V, Reitz C, Maury F, Bis JC, Bellenguez C, Yu L, et al. Evaluation of a genetic risk score to improve risk prediction for Alzheimer's disease. *J Alzheimers Dis.* 2016;53:921-932.

46. Marrero DG, Palmer KN, Phillips EO, Miller-Kovach K, Foster GD, Saha CK. Comparison of commercial and self-initiated weight loss programs in people with prediabetes: a randomized control trial. *Am J Public Health.* 2016;106:949-956.

47. Volk HE, Hertz-Picciotto I, Delwiche L, Lumann F, McConnell R. Residential proximity to freeways and autism in the CHARGE study. *Environ Health Perspect.* 2011;119:873-877.

48. Polusny MA, Erbes CR, Thuras P, Moran A, Lamberty GJ, Collins RC, et al. Mindfulness-based stress reduction for posttraumatic stress disorder among veterans: a randomized clinical trial. *JAMA.* 2015;314:456-465.

49. Winkelstein W. Interface of epidemiology and history: a commentary on past, present, and future. *Epidemiol Rev.* 2000;22:2-6.

50. Koplan JP, Thacker SB, Lezin NA. Epidemiology in the 21st century: calculation, communication, and intervention. *Am J Public Health.* 1999;89:1153-1155.

Chapter Questions

1. Define each of the following terms:
   a. Public health
   b. Epidemiology
   c. Population
   d. Disease frequency
   e. Disease distribution
   f. Disease determinants
   g. Disease control
   h. Hypothesis

2. What is the primary difference between public health and medicine?

3. What public health achievements have accounted for improved life expectancy in the United States over the past century?
4. What are the main objectives of epidemiology?
5. How do epidemiologists quantify the disease frequency in a population?
6. State the contribution that was made by each of the following historical figures:
    a. John Graunt
    b. John Snow
    c. Richard Doll and Austin Bradford Hill
    d. James Lind
    e. William Farr

7. How are the many subspecialities of modern epidemiology typically defined?
8. In which three directions has modern epidemiological research expanded?

CHAPTER 2

Measures of Disease Frequency

LEARNING OBJECTIVES

By the end of this chapter the reader will be able to:

- Define and provide examples of a population.
- Distinguish between a fixed and dynamic (or open) population.
- Explain how epidemiologists create a case definition, and discuss how the definition of acquired immunodeficiency syndrome (AIDS) has changed over time.
- Describe the key aspects of measuring disease occurrence.
- Define and distinguish between cumulative incidence, incidence rate, and prevalence.
- Describe the mathematical relationship between the measures of disease frequency.
- Provide examples of commonly used measures of disease frequency in public health.

▶ Introduction

Epidemiologists study the distribution and determinants of **disease** frequency in human populations to control health problems.[1(p1),2(p95)] Thus, the objectives of epidemiology are to determine the extent of disease in a population, identify patterns and trends in disease occurrence, identify the causes of disease, and evaluate the effectiveness of prevention and treatment activities. Measuring how often a disease arises in a population is usually the first step in achieving these goals.

This chapter describes how epidemiologists quantify the occurrence of disease in a population. Readers will learn that this quantification process involves developing a definition of a particular disease, counting the number of people who are affected by the disease, determining the size of the population from which the diseased cases arose, and accounting for the passage of time.

▶ Definition of a Population

Because epidemiology is concerned with the occurrence of disease in groups of people rather than in individuals, populations are at the heart of epidemiologists' measurements. A **population** can be defined as a group of people with a common characteristic, such as place of residence, religion, gender, age, use of hospital services, or life event (such as giving birth).

Location of residence, such as a country, state, city, or neighborhood, is one of the most common ways to define a population. For example, the people who reside in the Brooklyn borough of New York City, the city of Boston, the state of Oregon, and the country of Sweden are members of distinct populations defined by geopolitical entities ranging in size from a neighborhood to an entire country. Residence near natural geographic features, such as rivers, mountains, lakes, or islands, can also be used to define a population. For example, people who live along the 2,350-mile length of the Mississippi River, around Mount St. Helens in Washington State, and on Nantucket Island off the coast of Massachusetts are members of populations defined by geographic formations.

Because epidemiology focuses on disease occurrence, populations are commonly defined in relation to a medical facility, such as a medical professional's office, clinic, or hospital. The service population of a medical facility (also called **catchment population**) consists of the people who use the facility's services. This population is often difficult to define because an individual's decision to use a facility may depend on how far it is from home, the person's particular medical condition, his or her type of medical insurance, and so forth.

Consider a situation in which a county has only one general hospital that provides the complete range of medical services, including preventive care, birthing services, and diagnostic and therapeutic services for acute and chronic conditions. The catchment population for this general hospital is likely to consist of all people who live in the county where the hospital is located (see **FIGURE 2-1**).

Now, suppose that this hospital enhances its cardiology department, adding many well-trained clinicians and the latest diagnostic equipment. As the cardiology department's reputation for excellent care grows, patients travel from greater distances to receive care. As a result, the catchment population for the cardiology department expands to the surrounding counties, whereas the catchment population for the other hospital services, particularly those dealing with acute conditions requiring prompt treatment, remains the single county where the hospital is situated (see Figure 2-1).

Socioeconomic status is still another determinant of hospital catchment populations. Consider a city in which there are two hospitals—one public and one private—located within a few miles of each other. The private hospital generally treats patients with medical insurance, and the public hospital mainly treats patients without insurance. Even though each catchment population resides roughly within the same geographic

Single county hospital with local
catchment population

County hospital specialty clinic with
broad catchment population

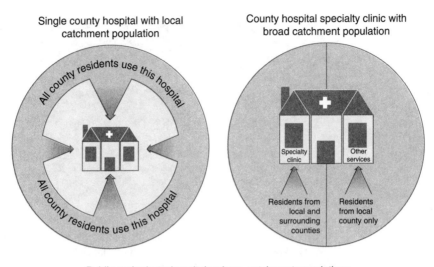

Public and private hospitals whose catchment populations
vary by socioeconomic status

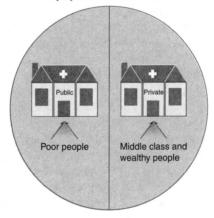

FIGURE 2-1 Types of hospital catchment areas.

area, the two service groups are distinct in terms of income and probably many other factors (see Figure 2-1).

Still another way that a population can be defined is by the occurrence of a life event, such as undergoing a medical procedure, giving birth to a child, entering or graduating from school, or serving in the military. For example, students who graduated from college in 2017 are members of the population known as the "Class of '17," and the men and women who served in the U.S. military during the War in Iraq are members of the population known as Iraq War veterans. Populations are often defined by other characteristics such as age, gender, religion, or type of job.

A unifying framework for thinking about a population is whether its membership is permanent or transient (see **TABLE 2-1**). A population whose membership is permanent is called a **fixed population**. Its membership is always defined by a life event. For example, the people who

Hiroshima ⊃
atomic bomb.
never Δ.

TABLE 2-1 Types of Populations

Type of population	Key element	Example
Fixed	Membership is based on an event and is permanent.	Japanese atomic bomb survivors
Dynamic or open	Membership is based on a condition and is transitory.	Residents of a city, hospital patients

were in Hiroshima, Japan, when the atomic bomb exploded at the end of World War II are members of a fixed population. This population will never gain any new members because only people who were at this historical event can be members.

The opposite of a fixed population is a **dynamic population**, also called an open population. Its membership is defined by a changeable state or condition and therefore is transient. A person is a member of a dynamic population only as long as he or she has the defining state or condition. For example, the population of the city of Boston is dynamic because people are members only while they reside within the city limits. Turnover is always occurring because people enter the city by moving in or by birth, and people leave the city by moving away or by death. The term *steady state* describes a situation in which the number of people entering the population is equal to the number leaving. Dynamic populations include groups defined by geographic and hospital catchment areas, religious groups, and occupations.

Boston residents

Regardless of the way in which it is defined, a population can be divided into subgroups on the basis of any characteristic. For example, men who undergo coronary bypass surgery are a gender subgroup of a fixed population defined by a life event, and all children up to 6 years of age who live along the Mississippi River are an age subgroup of a dynamic population defined by a geographic formation.

▶ Definitions of Health and Disease

In 1948, the World Health Organization defined **health** as "a state of complete physical, mental and social well-being and not merely the absence of disease or infirmity."[3] More recently, a national plan for improving the health of the American people stated that health is a key aspect of the quality of life and that it "reflects a personal sense of physical and mental health and the ability to react to factors in the physical and social environments." The plan also states that the "health-related quality of life is more subjective than life expectancy and therefore can be more difficult to measure."[4]

Because measurement is a cornerstone of epidemiology and "health" and "a sense of well-being" are nonspecific and difficult to quantify, epidemiologists have almost entirely focused their activities on the "absence of health," such as specific diseases, injuries, disabilities, and death. Consequently, epidemiologists must first compose a definition of the "absence of health" or "disease" before they can begin measuring its frequency.

The definition of a disease is usually based on a combination of physical and pathological examinations, diagnostic test results, and signs and symptoms. Which and how many criteria are used to define a "case" (a person who meets the disease definition) has important implications for accurately determining who has the disease.

Consider the various criteria that can be used to define a heart attack case. One could use the symptoms of chest pain; the results of diagnostic tests, such as electrocardiograms; or blood enzyme tests for cardiac damage. What are the implications of using only chest pain to define heart attack cases? Using only this nonspecific symptom will capture most but not all people who have heart attacks because it will miss people who have "silent" heart attacks, which occur without chest pain. In addition, it will erroneously include many people who have other conditions that produce chest pain, such as indigestion.

A definition that includes more specific criteria, such as the results of diagnostic tests, will be more accurate. For example, if positive blood enzyme tests are included, silent heart attacks are likely to be picked up and the other conditions that cause chest pain omitted. In practice, epidemiologists use all available information from physical and pathological examinations and laboratory and other tests to define a case of a disease as accurately as possible.

▶ Changes in Disease Definitions

Even when clear-cut criteria are used, disease definitions often change over time as more is learned about a disease and its various manifestations. For example, the official definition of HIV/AIDS (human immunodeficiency virus infection/acquired immune deficiency syndrome) has been changed several times as researchers have gained knowledge about the disease's cause and natural course (see **TABLE 2-2**).

The story began in the summer of 1981 when the Centers for Disease Control and Prevention (CDC) reported that Kaposi's sarcoma and *Pneumocystis carinii* pneumonia had been observed among previously healthy gay men.[5] Previously, Kaposi's sarcoma, a malignant neoplasm of the blood vessels, had been seen primarily among elderly males, and opportunistic infections, such as *Pneumocystis carinii* pneumonia, had occurred almost exclusively in people with compromised immune systems.

In 1982, the CDC composed the first definition of AIDS for national reporting as "a disease, at least moderately predictive of a defect in cell-mediated immunity, occurring in a person with no known

TABLE 2-2 Changes in the Definition of HIV/AIDS over Time

Year	State of knowledge and practices	Criteria for case definition
1982	Knowledge very limited	Only a few conditions, including Kaposi's sarcoma, *Pneumocystis carinii* pneumonia, and other severe opportunistic infections
1985	HIV virus discovered as cause of AIDS; antibody test developed	23 clinical conditions with laboratory evidence of infection
1993	Discovered importance of CD4 T lymphocytes in monitoring immunodeficiency and disease progression	26 clinical conditions and asymptomatic HIV infected cases with low CD4 T lymphocyte counts
2008	HIV testing widely available and diagnostic testing improved	Single case definition for HIV infection that includes AIDS and requires laboratory evidence of infection; 26 clinical conditions retained
2014	Further improvements in diagnotic testing, including recognition of early HIV infection	Single case definition ranging from early HIV infection to AIDS diagnosis; 27 AIDS-defining opportunistic illnesses included

Data from Centers for Disease Control and Prevention. Update on acquired immune deficiency syndrome (AIDS)—United States. *MMWR*. 1982;31:507-514; Centers for Disease Control and Prevention. Revision of the case definition of acquired immune deficiency syndrome for national reporting—United States. *MMWR*. 1985;34:373-375; Centers for Disease Control and Prevention. 1993 revised classification system for HIV infection and expanded surveillance case definition for AIDS among adolescents and adults. *MMWR*. 1992;44:1-19; Centers for Disease Control and Prevention. Revised surveillance case definitions for HIV infection among adults, adolescents, and children aged < 18 months and for HIV infection and AIDS among children aged 18 months to < 13 years—United States, 2008. *MMWR*. 2008;57:1-12; and Centers for Disease Control and Prevention. Revised surveillance case definition for HIV infection–United States, 2014. *MMWR*. 2014; 63:1-10.

cause for diminished resistance to that disease … including Kaposi's sarcoma, *Pneumocystis carinii* pneumonia, and serious other opportunistic infections."[6] Even then, the CDC acknowledged that the case definition was imperfect because it could possibly miss the full range of AIDS manifestations and falsely include individuals who were not truly immunodeficient. However, because the cause of AIDS was unknown at that time, the definition at least served as a consistent tool for monitoring the epidemic.

The CDC made the first major change in the official AIDS case definition in 1985 after HIV was determined to be the cause of AIDS and a highly accurate laboratory test was developed to detect the antibody to the HIV virus.[7] Because epidemiologists now knew what to look for and how to find its trail, it was possible to expand the AIDS case definition from a few severe clinical conditions to a wide range of conditions accompanied by laboratory evidence of HIV infection. Conversely, it also became possible to exclude patients who had AIDS-like symptoms but had negative HIV antibody test results.

At the end of 1992, the CDC changed the AIDS case definition again after natural history studies revealed the importance of lymphocytes in the HIV infection.[8] The new definition was expanded to include individuals who had no disease symptoms but had low levels of CD4 T lymphocytes, a type of white blood cell that is responsible for fighting off infections. (These cells are the primary target of HIV and an excellent marker of disease progression.) In 2008, the CDC further refined the disease definition by combining HIV infection and AIDS into a single case definition and requiring laboratory confirmation of infection.[9] In 2014, further refinements were made primarily to recognize early HIV infection.[10]

In summary, as epidemiologists discovered the cause of AIDS, learned more about its manifestations, and developed a test to detect HIV, the case definition was expanded from a few severe diseases to many varied conditions and the results of sophisticated laboratory tests (see Table 2-2).

What effect did these changes in case definition have on the number of reported HIV/AIDS cases? In general, any expansion in the case definition will increase the number of reportable cases, and any contraction will decrease that number. With HIV/AIDS, the definition changes increased the number of people who were officially counted as cases in national statistics from the 1980s until 1993.[8] However, incidence subsequently declined despite the 1993 expanded case definition because of HIV testing and prevention programs, which reduced the rate of transmission, and treatment programs that included highly effective antiretroviral therapy.[11]

▶ Measuring Disease Occurrence

Epidemiologists must always consider three factors when they measure how commonly a disease occurs in a group of people: (1) the number of people who are affected by the disease, (2) the size of the population from which the cases of disease arise, and (3) the length of time that the population is followed. Failure to consider all three components will give a false impression about the effect of the disease on a population.

Consider the following hypothetical data on the frequency of breast cancer in two counties. In County A, with a population of 50,000, a total of 100 new cases of breast cancer occurred over a 1-year period. In County B, with a population of 5,000, 75 new cases occurred over a 3-year period. Which county has a higher frequency of new breast cancer cases? If one considers only the number of new cases, it appears that County A has a higher frequency (100 versus 75). However, simply comparing the number of cases in each county does not provide a full picture because the cases occurred over different lengths of time (1 versus 3 years) and among populations of different sizes (50,000 versus 5,000) (see TABLE 2-3).

TABLE 2-3 Hypothetical Data on the Frequency of Breast Cancer in Two Counties

Type of data	County A	County B
Number of cases	100	75
Population size	50,000	5,000
Follow-up period	1 year	3 years
Comparable disease frequency	200/100,000/year	500/100,000/year

To make a meaningful comparison between the two counties, it is necessary to convert the data into the same population size and time period. Let us estimate the frequency of breast cancer in the two counties over a 1-year period and as if each population consisted of 100,000 people. The frequency of breast cancer in County A is 100 cases/50,000 population/1 year; if the county's population were 100,000, the frequency would double to become 200 cases/100,000 population/1 year.

Two steps are needed to make a similar conversion for County B: (1) divide the numerator by 3 to convert the frequency of breast cancer from a 3- to a 1-year period: 25 cases/5,000 population/1 year; (2) multiply both the numerator and denominator by 20 to estimate the frequency for a population of 100,000. Thus, the frequency of new cases in County B is 500 cases/100,000 population/1 year.

Now, it is clear that the "rate" at which new cases are occurring is much higher in County B than County A (500 cases/100,000 population/1 year versus 200 cases/100,000 population/1 year, respectively) and that examining only the number of new cases gives a false impression. Note that the decision to convert the frequencies to a population size of 100,000 and a 1-year time period, although commonly done, is arbitrary. Other population sizes (such as 1,000 or 10,000) and time periods (such as 1 month or 5 years) could be used. The guiding principle is that the same population size and time period should be used for the compared groups.

▶ Types of Calculations: Ratios, Proportions, and Rates

Three types of calculations are used to describe and compare measures of disease occurrence: ratios, proportions, and rates (see **TABLE 2-4**). A **ratio** is simply one number divided by another. The entities represented by the two numbers are not required to be related to one another. In other words, the individuals in the numerator can be different from those in

TABLE 2-4 Types of Calculations	
Type of calculation	**Characteristics**
Ratio	Division of two unrelated numbers
Proportion	Division of two related numbers; numerator is a subset of denominator
Rate	Division of two numbers; time is always in denominator

the denominator. For example, the "gender ratio" is a ratio of two unrelated numbers: the number of males divided by the number of females, usually expressed as the number of males per 100 females. According to 2016 U.S. Census estimates, the gender ratio among U.S. residents in Florida was 95.5 males per 100 females.[12]

A **proportion** is also one number divided by another, but the entities represented by these numbers are related to one another. In fact, the numerator of a proportion is always a subset of the denominator. Proportions, also known as fractions, are often expressed as percentages and range from 0 to 1 or 0% to 100%. For example, the proportion of U.S. residents who are Black is the number of Black residents divided by the total number of U.S. residents of all races. According to 2016 U.S. Census estimates, the proportion of Black U.S. residents was 0.141, or 14.1%.[12]

A **rate** is also one number divided by another, but time is an integral part of the denominator. We are familiar with rates in our daily travels because a rate is a measure of how fast we travel. For example, in many areas of the United States, the maximum speed or rate at which cars are permitted to travel is 55 miles per hour. This rate can also be written as 55 miles/1 hour. The measure of time in the denominator is what makes this number a rate. The measures of disease occurrence calculated previously for Counties A and B are also rates (200 cases/100,000 population/1 year and 500 cases/100,000 population/1 year, respectively). Unfortunately, the term *rate* is often incorrectly used to describe ratios and proportions.[13]

▶ Measures of Disease Frequency

The two basic measures of disease frequency in epidemiology are incidence and prevalence. **Incidence** measures the occurrence of new disease, and **prevalence** measures the existence of current disease. Each measure describes an important part of the natural course of a disease. Incidence deals with the transition from health to disease, and prevalence focuses on the period of time that a person lives with a disease.

Incidence

Incidence is defined as the occurrence of new cases of disease that develop in a candidate population over a specified time period. There are three key ideas in this definition.

First, incidence measures *new disease events*. For diseases that can occur more than once, it usually measures the first occurrence of the disease. Second, new cases of disease are measured in a **candidate population**, which is a population of people who are "at risk" of getting the disease. Someone is at risk because he or she has the appropriate body organ, is not immune, and so forth. For example, a woman who still has an intact uterus (i.e., she has not undergone a hysterectomy) is a candidate for getting uterine cancer, and a child who has not been fully immunized against the measles virus is a candidate for contracting a measles infection. Although it is possible to define and measure the incidence of disease in a population not at risk (e.g., the incidence of uterine cancer in women who have undergone hysterectomies is, by definition, zero), it is not a particularly interesting pursuit.

Third, incidence takes into account the *specific amount of time* that the members of the population are followed until they develop the disease. Because incidence measures a person's transition from a healthy to a diseased state, time must pass for this change to occur and be observed. As described in the following sections, there are two types of incidence measures: cumulative incidence and incidence rate. Although closely related, each measure has different strengths and weaknesses and is used in different settings.

Cumulative Incidence

Cumulative incidence is defined as the proportion of a candidate population that becomes diseased over a specified period of time. Mathematically, it is expressed as follows:

$$\frac{\text{Number of new cases of disease}}{\text{Number in candidate population}} \text{ Over a specified time period}$$

Note that the numerator (new cases of disease) is a subset of the denominator (candidate population) and therefore the possible value of cumulative incidence ranges from 0 to 1, or if expressed as a percentage, from 0% to 100%. Time is not an integral part of this proportion but rather is expressed by the words that accompany the numbers of the cumulative incidence measure. Thus, cumulative incidence is dimensionless (see **TABLE 2-5**).

Cumulative incidence can be thought of as the average risk of getting a disease over a certain period of time. (A risk is the probability of getting a disease.) A commonly cited measure of cumulative incidence is the "lifetime risk of breast cancer" among women. Currently estimated at "one in eight" among U.S. women, it means that about 12% of women will develop breast cancer sometime during the course of their lives.[14]

TABLE 2-5 Distinguishing Characteristics of Incidence and Prevalence						
Measure	**Type of number**	**Units**	**Range**	**Numerator**	**Denominator**	**Major uses**
Cumulative incidence	Proportion	None	0 to 1	New cases	Population at risk	Research on causes, prevention, and treatment of disease
Incidence rate	True rate	1/time, or t^{-1}	0 to infinity	New cases	Person-time at risk	Research on causes, prevention, and treatment of disease
Prevalence	Proportion	None	0 to 1	Existing cases	Total population	Resource planning

Cumulative incidence is influenced by the length of time to which it applies. Generally, the cumulative incidence over a long period of time (such as a lifetime) will be higher than that over a few years.

Cumulative incidence is mainly used in fixed populations when there are no or small losses to follow-up. Consider, for example, the estimated 255,000 residents of Hiroshima, Japan, who were present in the city when the atomic bomb was dropped on August 6, 1945 (see **FIGURE 2-2**). During the blast and in the weeks and months immediately thereafter, an estimated 65,000 people died from physical trauma, burns, and acute radiation sickness, resulting in a 25% cumulative incidence of mortality over a 4-month period.[15] Officials estimate that another 21% of the population died during the year following that initial 4-month period. During the subsequent years and decades, the cumulative incidence of death was much lower, and different causes of death, such as cancer and circulatory disease, predominated.[16] The cumulative incidence of death was 58% over the 53-year period from 1950 through 2003 among Hiroshima and Nagasaki survivors who were enrolled in the Life Span Cohort Study of the effects of high-dose radiation on the incidence of disease and death.[16]

Note that the cumulative incidence of death during the first 16 months after the bomb was dropped (25% + 21% = 46%) was close to that during the 53-year follow-up period of the Life Span Cohort Study (58%). In addition, the size of the candidate population dwindles as members die. For example, all 255,000 residents were at risk of dying when the bomb was dropped in August 1945, whereas approximately 190,000 survivors of the initial period were at risk of dying during the subsequent years (see Figure 2-2).

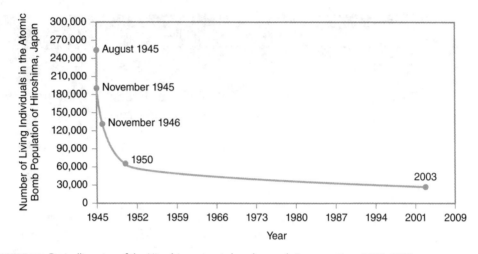

FIGURE 2-2 Dwindling size of the Hiroshima atomic bomb population over time: 1945–2003.

Data from Liebow, AA. *Encounter with Disaster: A Medical Diary of Hiroshima*. New York, NY: WW Norton and Co; 1970:175-176; Committee for the Compilation of Materials on Damage Caused by the Atomic Bombs in Hiroshima and Nagasaki. *Hiroshima and Nagasaki: The Physical, Medical, and Social Effects of the Atomic Bombings*. New York, NY: Basic Books; 1981:113; and Ozasa K, Shimizu Y, Suyama A, Kasagi F, Soda M, Grant EJ, et al. Studies of the mortality of atomic bomb survivors, Report 14, 1950-2003: an overview of cancer and noncancer diseases. *Radiat Res.* 2012;177:229-243.

The following hypothetical example further highlights the importance of selecting the appropriate time period for measuring cumulative incidence measure. Suppose that a pharmaceutical company has developed a new drug for the treatment of acute migraine headaches. Before the U.S. Food and Drug Administration (FDA) will approve its use, the company is required to conduct a small study (N = 20 patients) to determine whether the new drug is more effective than the most popular drug currently approved for migraine treatment. The FDA requests that the study answer two key questions: First, what proportion of patients experience symptom relief within 10 hours of taking the new drug as compared to the current drug? Second, does the new drug relieve symptoms faster than the current drug? As the study results indicate in **FIGURE 2-3**, the proportion of patients who experience symptom relief within 10 hours is identical for the two drugs. Stated in epidemiologic terms, the 10-hour cumulative incidence of relief is 60% for both drugs. However, all patients who took the new drug had symptom relief within 3 hours, whereas those who took the current drug had symptom relief several hours later. Note that the 10-hour measure of cumulative incidence misses this important finding and makes the drugs appear equally effective. Only when you examine the timing of relief can you see this important difference. Furthermore, if a 5-hour cumulative incidence had been selected as the measure of symptom relief instead of the 10-hour measure, this notable difference would have been captured.

A final critical assumption that underlies the cumulative incidence measure is that everyone in the candidate population has been followed for the specified time period. Thus, in the examples above, the cumulative incidence measures assume that everyone in the migraine study population was followed for 10 hours and that everyone in the Hiroshima Life Span

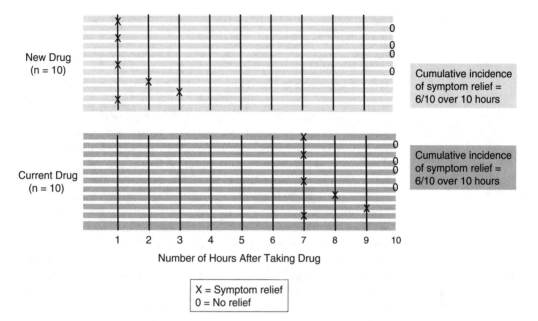

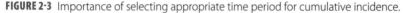

FIGURE 2-3 Importance of selecting appropriate time period for cumulative incidence.

Cohort Study was followed for 53 years. Clearly, the former is much easier to accomplish than the latter. In fact, complete follow-up is difficult to attain when there is a long follow-up period, particularly in a dynamic population in which members are continually entering and exiting. Thus, cumulative incidence is usually reserved for fixed populations, particularly when the follow-up period is short and there are no or few losses to follow-up.

Incidence Rate

Incidence rate is defined as the occurrence of new cases of disease that arise during **person-time** of observation. Mathematically, the incidence rate is expressed as follows:

defined pop / defined time

$$\frac{\text{Number of new cases of disease}}{\text{Person-time of observation in candidate population}}$$

Note that the numerator for incidence rate is identical to that of cumulative incidence. The difference between the two measures lies in the denominator. The incidence rate's denominator integrates time (t) and therefore is a true rate.[13] Thus, its dimension is 1/t, or t^{-1}, and its possible values range from zero to infinity (Table 2-5). An incidence rate of infinity is possible if all members of a population die instantaneously.

The concept of person-time can be difficult to understand. Person-time is accrued only among candidates for the disease. Thus, a person contributes time to the denominator of an incidence rate only up until he or she is diagnosed with the disease of interest. However, unlike cumulative incidence, the incidence rate is not based upon the assumption that everyone in the candidate population has been followed for a specified time period. Person-time is accrued only while the candidate is being followed. Accrual of person-time stops when the person dies or is lost to follow-up (such as when a person moves to an unknown community). The incidence rate can be calculated for either a fixed or dynamic population. However, because it directly takes into account population changes (such as migration, birth, and death), it is especially useful as a measure of the transition between health and disease in dynamic populations.

Consider the following population of a hypothetical town (**FIGURE 2-4**). This dynamic population of five individuals is followed for the 10-year period from 2006 to 2016. Person A moved into town in 2007, was diagnosed with disease in 2011, and therefore accrued 4 years of person-time. Person B was a resident of the town at the start of the observation period in 2006, died in 2012, and therefore accrued 6 person-years. Person C moved to town in 2008 and remained healthy until he moved away in 2011. The investigator could not determine where he moved and therefore could not learn whether he became diseased later. Person C was considered lost to follow-up as of the time he moved and therefore accrued 3 person-years. Person D was a resident of the town at the start of the observation period, remained healthy for the entire period, and therefore accrued 10 years of person-time. Person E was born to Person A in 2009, remained healthy for the entire observation period, and therefore accrued 7 person-years.

The incidence rate in this hypothetical population is 1/30 person-years. Only one person became diseased, and 30 person-years of observation were accrued by the population. The denominator of the incidence rate is the sum of person-time accrued by each member of the population at risk.

Now, consider an actual population of 59,000 U.S. Black women who were studied to quantify the effect of racism and segregation on

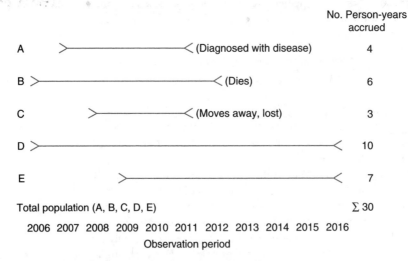

	No. Person-years accrued
A ──────< (Diagnosed with disease)	4
B ───────< (Dies)	6
C ────< (Moves away, lost)	3
D ──────────<	10
E ───────<	7
Total population (A, B, C, D, E)	Σ 30

2006 2007 2008 2009 2010 2011 2012 2013 2014 2015 2016
Observation period

FIGURE 2-4 Measurement of person-time in a hypothetical population.

the incidence of obesity.[17] The women were enrolled in 1995 and followed through 2009 to determine their weight over time. Each woman's follow-up time began with the date of return of her questionnaire in 1997 when questions of racism were first asked and continued until one of the following events occurred: the occurrence of obesity (defined as a body mass index ≥ 30 kg/m^2), loss to follow-up, death, or the end of follow-up for the study, whichever came first. Investigators identified 1,105 incident cases of obesity among 33,235 person-years of follow-up (33.2/1,000 person-years) among women who experienced the lowest levels of daily racism in contrast to 1,043 incident cases of obesity among 23,403 person-years of follow-up (44.6/1,000 person-years) among women who experienced the highest levels of daily racism. Although it is the most accurate to determine person-time on an individual basis, as was done in this study, this method is very time consuming and labor intensive. Thus, researchers sometimes use shortcuts, such as multiplying the number of people under observation by an estimate of the average follow-up time.

In the hypothetical example portrayed in Figure 2-4, five individuals who were followed for varying amounts of time accrued 30 person-years of follow-up. However, depending on the size of the population and length of follow-up, the 30 person-years could have been accrued in many ways, such as 5 people each contributing 6 years, 3 people each contributing 10 years, and so forth. Regardless of how the person-time is accrued (e.g., from 5 or 50 people), the person-time units are assumed to be equivalent. This assumption is usually reasonable, except in extreme situations in which a small number of people are followed for a long period of time.

The particular time unit used to measure person-time can vary, but decisions are guided by how long it takes for the disease to develop. For example, person-years are commonly used for diseases that take many years to develop (such as cancer), and person-months or person-days are used for diseases that develop rapidly (such as infection).

The number of person-time units in the denominator is arbitrary. For example, the same incidence rate can be expressed in terms of 1 person-year, 10 person-years, or 100 person-years. Epidemiologists generally use 100,000 person-years for rare diseases and those that take a long time to develop.

Relationship Between Cumulative Incidence and Incidence Rate

It is possible to obtain cumulative incidence from an incidence rate. The simplest situation to demonstrate this relationship is in a fixed population with a constant incidence rate and small cumulative incidence (less than 10%). Here, the mathematical relationship is as follows:

$$CI = IR_i \times t_i$$

where CI is cumulative incidence, IR_i is incidence rate, and t_i is the specified period of time.

When the incidence rate is not constant, it is necessary to take into account the different rates that prevail during each time period:

$$CI = \sum (IR_i \times t_i)$$

For example, the **mortality rate** (a type of incidence rate) among Hiroshima residents was much higher shortly after the atomic bomb explosion than during subsequent years (see Figure 2-2).

Incidence Summary

In summary, two measures of disease frequency—cumulative incidence and incidence rate—focus on measuring the transition from health to disease. These measures have complementary strengths and weaknesses. The cumulative incidence is easy to calculate and understand, although it is less accurate when its assumptions are not met. Although the incidence rate has greater accuracy, its person-time denominator is more difficult to calculate and understand. Finally, the incidence rate is more useful for dynamic populations, and cumulative incidence is usually reserved for fixed populations.

Prevalence

Whereas incidence measures the frequency with which new disease develops, prevalence measures the *frequency of existing disease*. It is simply defined as the proportion of the total population that is diseased. There are two types of prevalence measures—point prevalence and period prevalence—that relate prevalence to different amounts of time (see **FIGURE 2-5**). **Point prevalence** refers to the proportion of the population that is diseased at a single point in time and can be thought of as a single snapshot of the population. The point can be either a particular calendar date such as July 1, 2017, or a point in someone's life, such as college graduation. **Period prevalence** refers to the proportion of the population that is diseased during a specified duration of time, such as

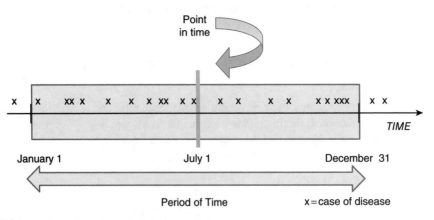

FIGURE 2-5 Time frame for point and period prevalence.

during the year 2017. The period prevalence includes the number of cases that were present at any time over the course of the year.

Mathematically, point prevalence is expressed as follows:

$$\frac{\text{Number of existing cases of disease}}{\text{Number in total population}} \text{ At a point in time}$$

Period prevalence can be expressed as follows:

$$\frac{\text{Number of existing cases of disease}}{\text{Number in total population}} \text{ During a period of time}$$

Let's use these formulas to calculate the point and period prevalence of pneumonia in a nursing home population. The point and period of interest are July 1, 2017, and January 1 through December 31, 2017, respectively. On July 1, 2017, there were 5 cases of pneumonia among the 500 nursing home residents. Thus, the point prevalence of pneumonia was 5/500, or 1%, on that date. During the period January 1 through December 31, 2017, there were 45 cases of pneumonia among the 500 nursing home residents; therefore, the period prevalence was 45/500, or 9%, during the year. Note that, in this example, the size of the nursing home population remained stable over the year, but if it had gained or lost members, the average size of the nursing home population during 2017 would have been the appropriate denominator for the period prevalence measure.

Note that the numerator (existing cases) is a subset of the denominator (total population). Unlike the numerator for the two incidence measures, the prevalence numerator includes all currently living cases regardless of when they first developed. The denominator includes everyone in the population—sick, healthy, at risk, and not at risk. Because prevalence is a proportion, it is dimensionless, and its possible values range from 0 to 1, or 0% to 100% (see Table 2-5).

Relationship Between Prevalence and Incidence

Prevalence depends on the rate at which new cases of disease develop (the incidence rate) as well as the duration or length of time that individuals have the disease. The duration of a disease starts at the time of diagnosis and ends when the person either is cured or dies. Mathematically, the relationship between prevalence and incidence is as follows:

$$\frac{P}{(1-P)} = IR \times D$$

where P is prevalence (the proportion of the total population with the disease), $(1 - P)$ is the proportion of the total population without the disease, IR is incidence rate, and D is the average duration (or length of time) that an individual has the disease.

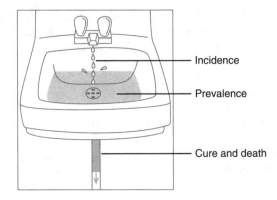

FIGURE 2-6 Relationship among incidence, prevalence, mortality, and cure.

This equation assumes that the population is in steady state (i.e., inflow equals outflow) and that the incidence rate and duration do not change over time. If the frequency of disease is rare (i.e., less than 10%), the equation simplifies to

$$P = IR \times D$$

To better understand this relationship, think of the variables that influence the level of water in a sink (see **FIGURE 2-6**). The water level is influenced by both the inflow from the faucet and the outflow down the drain. The water level will be high if the inflow is large, if the outflow is low, or if both occur. The water level will be low if inflow is low, outflow is high, or both. Now, consider the water level in the sink as prevalence, the incoming water as incidence, and the outflowing water as diseased people who either are cured or die. The number of cases of people currently living with a disease (prevalence) will be influenced by the rate at which new cases develop as well as by the rate at which they are eliminated through cure or death.

Uses of Incidence and Prevalence

Epidemiologists and other public health professionals use each measure of disease frequency for specific purposes (see Table 2-5). Incidence is most useful for evaluating the effectiveness of programs that try to prevent disease from occurring in the first place. In addition, researchers who study the causes of disease prefer to study new cases (incidence) over existing ones (prevalence) because they are usually interested in exposures that lead to developing the disease. Prevalence obscures causal relationships because it combines incidence and survival. In addition, many researchers prefer to use incidence because the timing of exposures in relation to disease occurrence can be determined more accurately.

On the other hand, prevalence is useful for estimating the needs of medical facilities and allocating resources for treating people who already have a disease. In addition, researchers who study diseases such as birth defects (wherein it is difficult to gather information on defects present in miscarried and aborted fetuses) and chronic conditions such as arthritis (whose beginnings are difficult to pinpoint) have no choice but to use prevalence. Unfortunately, results of such studies are difficult to interpret because it is unclear how much the association is influenced by using a group of survivors.

▶ Commonly Used Measures of Disease Frequency in Public Health

There are many measures of disease frequency that are commonly used in the public health disciplines. Some are incidence measures, some are prevalence measures, some are ratios. Descriptions and examples of the major measures follow. Note that the word *rate* is often used incorrectly to describe a proportion or ratio.

Crude mortality (or death) rate: Total number of deaths from all causes per 100,000 population per year. The term *crude* means that the rate is based on raw data. In 2015 the crude mortality rate in the United States was 844.0/100,000 population/year.[18]

Cause-specific mortality rate: Number of deaths from a specific cause per 100,000 population per year. In 2015, the cause-specific mortality rate from heart disease in the United States was 197.2/100,000/year.[18]

Age-specific mortality rate: Total number of deaths from all causes among individuals in a specific age category per 100,000 population per year in the age category. In 2015, the age-specific death rate was 589.6/100,000/year among U.S. children under the age of 1 year.[18]

Years of potential life lost: The number of years that an individual was expected to live beyond his or her death. In 2015, a total of 957 years were lost from heart disease, 1,283 years were lost from cancer, and 1,172 were lost from unintentional injuries before age 75 per 100,000 population younger than 75 years of age in the United States.[18] The number of years of potential life lost reflects both the number of individuals who died of a particular cause and the age at which the death occurred. For example, a cause of death that is more common among children and young adults (such as unintentional injuries) will result in more years of life lost per individual than a cause of death that is common among the elderly (such as heart disease).

Livebirth rate: Total number of livebirths per 1,000 population per year. A livebirth is a pregnancy that results in a child who, after separation, breathes or shows any other evidence of life. Sometimes, the denominator includes only women of childbearing age. In 2015, the crude livebirth rate among women who were residents of the United States was 12.4/1,000/year.[18]

Infant mortality rate: Number of deaths of infants less than 1 year of age per 1,000 livebirths per year. This statistic is often divided into neonatal deaths (those occurring during the first 27 days following birth) and postneonatal deaths (those occurring from 28 days through 12 months). In 2014, the infant mortality rate in the United States was 5.8/1,000 livebirths/year, the neonatal mortality rate was 3.9/1,000 livebirths/year, and the postneonatal death rate was 1.9/1,000 livebirths/year.[17]

Birth defect rate *(also called congenital anomaly or malformation rate):* Number of children born with defects, usually per 10,000 births. The numerator and denominator often include both livebirths and stillbirths. In 2016–2017, the prevalence of brain malformations, including microcephaly, was 5% among women with evidence of recent possible Zika virus infection.[19]

Morbidity rate: Number of existing or new cases of a particular disease or condition per 100 population. The time period that is covered and the population size in the denominator vary. *Morbidity* is a general word that can apply to a disease, condition, or event. For example, from 2011 to 2014, the prevalence of physician-diagnosed diabetes among U.S. adults aged 65 years and over was 20.6%.[18]

Attack rate: Number of new cases of disease that develop (usually during a defined and short time period) per the number in a healthy population at risk at the start of the period. This cumulative incidence measure is usually reserved for infectious disease outbreaks. For example, the 24-hour attack rate for food poisoning was 50% among people who ate chicken salad at the banquet.

Case fatality rate: Number of deaths per number of cases of disease. Note that this measure is a type of cumulative incidence and therefore it is necessary to specify the length of time to which it applies. For example, in 2014 in the Democratic Republic of Congo, the 5-month case fatality rate among individuals with Ebola virus disease was 74.2%.[20]

Survival rate: Number of living cases per number of cases of disease. This rate is the complement of the case fatality rate and is also a cumulative incidence measure. Five-year relative survival rates for cancer compare people with a particular cancer to similar people in the general population. For example, from 2007 to 2013, 5-year relative survival rates for prostate cancer were 100% among men diagnosed while the tumor was still confined to the prostate or had spread only to the regional lymph nodes and 29.8% among men whose tumor had metastasized to distant sites.[14]

Summary

A population is defined as a group of people with a common characteristic, such as place of residence, age, or the occurrence of an event. There are two main types of populations, fixed and dynamic (or open). The membership of a fixed population is defined by a life event and is permanent, whereas the membership of a dynamic population is defined by a changeable characteristic and is transient.

Three factors should always be considered when measuring how commonly a disease occurs in a population: (1) the number of affected individuals or cases, (2) the size of the population from which the cases arise, and (3) the amount of time that this population is followed. Before epidemiologists can count the number of affected cases, they must compose a disease definition that is usually based on physical and pathological examinations, diagnostic tests, and signs and symptoms. Disease definitions often change over time as more is learned about a disease and its manifestations. For example, the official case definition of HIV/AIDS expanded when its cause was discovered and improvements in detection were made.

Incidence and prevalence are the two basic measures of disease frequency. Incidence measures the occurrence of new disease and therefore captures the transition from health to disease. Cumulative incidence and incidence rate are the two main types of incidence measures. Cumulative incidence is defined as the proportion of a candidate population that becomes diseased over a specified time period. It is a dimensionless proportion that measures the average risk of contracting a disease over a certain time period. Incidence rate is the occurrence of new cases of disease that arise during person-time of observation; therefore, it is a true rate. It is important to remember that person-time accumulates only among candidates for disease. Cumulative incidence and incidence rate are related mathematically. Both measures are most useful for evaluating the effectiveness of disease-prevention activities and for etiologic studies of disease.

Prevalence measures existing disease and therefore focuses on the period when a person is ill. Prevalence measures the proportion of the total population that is diseased at a point in time or during a period of time. Its numerator consists of the number of existing cases, and its denominator includes the total population, including sick, healthy, at-risk, and immune individuals. Point prevalence refers to a single point in time and is like a snapshot. Period prevalence refers to a specific duration of time that may be derived from a series of snapshots. Prevalence is typically used for estimating the needs of medical facilities and allocating resources for treating diseased individuals. The incidence rate and prevalence are mathematically related.

Many measures of disease frequency are commonly used in public health, including the crude, cause-specific, and age-specific mortality rates; morbidity rate; livebirth rate; infant mortality rate; attack rate; case fatality rate; and survival rate. Note that the term *rate* is often incorrectly used to refer to proportions and ratios.

References

1. MacMahon B, Trichopoulos D. *Epidemiology: Principles and Methods.* 2nd ed. Boston, MA: Little, Brown and Co; 1996.
2. Porta M. *A Dictionary of Epidemiology.* 6th ed. New York, NY: Oxford University Press; 2014.
3. *Constitution of the World Health Organization.* who.int. http://www.who.int/governance/eb/who _constitution_en.pdf. Accessed June 8, 2018.
4. U.S. Department of Health and Human Services. *Healthy People 2010: Understanding and Improving Health.* 2nd ed. Washington, DC: U.S. Government Printing Office; 2000.
5. Centers for Disease Control and Prevention. Kaposi's sarcoma and *Pneumocystis* pneumonia among homosexual men—New York City and California. *MMWR.* 1981;30:305-308.
6. Centers for Disease Control and Prevention. Update on acquired immune deficiency syndrome (AIDS)—United States. *MMWR.* 1982;31:507-514.
7. Centers for Disease Control and Prevention. Revision of the case definition of acquired immune deficiency syndrome for national reporting—United States. *MMWR.* 1985;34:373-375.
8. Centers for Disease Control and Prevention. *HIV/ AIDS Surveillance Report.* 1997;9(2): 1-43. https:// www.cdc.gov/hiv/pdf/library/reports/surveillance /cdc-hiv-surveillance-report-1997-vol-9-2.pdf. Accessed June 8, 2018.
9. Centers for Disease Control and Prevention. Revised surveillance case definitions for HIV infection among adults, adolescents, and children aged < 18 months and for HIV infection and AIDS among

children aged 18 months to < 13 years—United States, 2008. *MMWR.* 2008;57:1-12.

10. Centers for Disease Control and Prevention. Revised surveillance case definition for HIV infection—United States, 2014. *MMWR.* 2014;63:1-10.

11. New HIV Infections in the United States. December 2012. cdc.gov. https://www.cdc.gov/nchhstp/newsroom/docs/2012/hiv-infections-2007-2010.pdf. Accessed September 12, 2016.

12. Annual Estimates of the Resident Population by Sex, Race Alone or in Combination, and Hispanic Origin for the United States, States and Counties: April 1, 2010 to July 1, 2016. census.gov. https://factfinder.census.gov/faces/tableservices/jsf/pages/productview.xhtml?src=bkmk. Accessed December 2017.

13. Elandt-Johnson RC. Definition of rates: some remarks on their use and misuse. *Am J Epidemiol.* 1975;102:267-271.

14. Howlander N, Noone AM, Krapcho M, et al. (eds.). *SEER Cancer Statistics Review, 1975-2014.* cancer.gov. https://seer.cancer.gov/csr/1975_2014/. Published April 2017. Accessed December 2017.

15. Liebow AA. *Encounter with Disaster: A Medical Diary of Hiroshima.* New York, NY: W. W. Norton & Co; 1970.

16. Ozasa K, Shimizu Y, Suyama A, et al. Studies of the mortality of atomic bomb survivors, report 14, 1950-2003: an overview of cancer and noncancer diseases. *Radiat Res.* 2012;229-243.

17. Cozier YC, Yu J, Coogan PF, Bethea TN, Rosenberg L, Palmer JR. Racism, segregation, and risk of obesity in the Black Women's Health Study. *Am J Epidemiol.* 2014;179:875-883.

18. Centers for Disease Control and Prevention. *Health, United States, 2016, With Chartbook on Long-term Trends in Health.* https://www.cdc.gov/nchs/data/hus/hus16.pdf. Accessed June 8, 2018.

19. Shapiro-Mendoza CK, Rice ME, Galang RR, et al. Pregnancy outcomes after maternal Zika virus infection during pregnancy—U.S. territories, January 1, 2016–April 25, 2017. *MMWR.* 2017;66:615-621.

20. Nanclares NC, Kapetshi J, Lionetto F, de la Rosa O, Tamfun JJ, Alia M, et al. Ebola virus disease, Democratic Republic of the Congo, 2014. *Emerg Infect Dis.* 2016;22:1579-1586.

Chapter Questions

1. What measure of disease frequency is each of the following?
   a. The percentage of freshman girls who become pregnant over the course of their high school years
   b. The percentage of senior boys who are fathers at the time of graduation
   c. The number of live-born babies who die of sudden infant death syndrome during the first year of life per 100,000 baby-years of follow-up
   d. The percentage of infants weighing less than 2500 grams at birth
   e. The lifetime risk of breast cancer

2. Briefly describe the main similarities and differences between each of the following:
   a. Prevalence and incidence
   b. Incidence rate and cumulative incidence
   c. Fixed and dynamic populations

3. What are the lowest and highest possible values of each of the following measures of disease frequency?
   a. Prevalence
   b. Cumulative incidence
   c. Incidence rate

4. Suppose that there were 2900 new cases of breast cancer diagnosed among women in Boston, Massachusetts, and 200 new cases diagnosed among women in Anchorage, Alaska, in 2017. Based on these data, is it accurate to say that the incidence rate of breast cancer is higher in Boston than Anchorage? Why or why not?

5. A study of 100 injection drug users who tested negative for HIV infection at enrollment had their HIV status retested at 3-month intervals over a 2-year follow-up period. All of the injection drug users were followed for the entire 2-year period. None died and none were lost to follow-up. Which of the following frequency measures of HIV infection can be calculated at the end of the study?

    a.   Prevalence

    b.   Cumulative incidence

    c.   Incidence rate

    d.   All of the above

6. Consider a class with 100 enrolled students. None of the students were ill at the beginning of the school year. On September 30, a total of 5 students reported having gastroenteritis. All 5 continued to be ill on October 1, but all 5 recovered within 3 days. On October 14, another 3 students developed gastroenteritis. All of these students continued to be ill on October 15, but all 3 recovered 5 days later. In this example, assume that a person cannot get gastroenteritis more than once.
   a. Calculate the prevalence of gastroenteritis in the class on October 1.
   b. Calculate the prevalence of gastroenteritis in the class on October 30.
   c. Calculate the cumulative incidence of gastroenteritis in the class during the month of October.

7. The incidence rate of a nonfatal disease is 500/100,000 person-years. People usually have the disease for an average of 3 years, at which time the disease resolves spontaneously. Estimate the prevalence of this disease using this information. Assume that the population is in steady state.

8. A population of 100 healthy men was followed for the development of prostate cancer. After being followed for 5 years, 20 men developed prostate cancer. Another 10 men were followed for 1 year and then were lost. The remaining men who never developed the disease were followed for 10 years. Calculate the number of person-years of observation accrued by this population.

9. Consider the following hypothetical data on the occurrence of hepatitis in two cities:

City	New cases	Observation period	Starting population at risk
City A	25	January–December 2017	25,000
City B	30	January–December 2017	50,000

   a. Calculate the cumulative incidence of hepatitis in each city.
   b. Which city has the higher cumulative incidence?

10. A total of 60 cases of myocardial infarction were reported over a period of 2 years in a city with a population of 100,000 people. Using these data, estimate the incidence rate of myocardial infarction per 100,000 person-years. State any assumptions that are needed.

11. The incidence rate of postpartum depression among 250,000 women who recently experienced a pregnancy was 12 cases per 100,000 woman-years of follow-up. Exactly how many incident cases of postpartum depression developed in this population?

12. State the type of population (fixed or dynamic) that best describes each of the following:
   a. People who live in New York City
   b. Male residents of Paris who had coronary bypass surgery between 2010 and 2017
   c. Children residing in California who were vaccinated against polio in 1955
   d. Women who are practicing physicians in the United States

13. How does each of the following conditions influence the prevalence of a disease in a population? For each scenario, assume that no other changes occur. Your choices are increases prevalence, decreases prevalence, or has no effect on prevalence.

a.   A cheap new clinical test becomes widely available that allows doctors to diagnose previously latent (i.e., hidden) disease.

b.   A new treatment is developed that cures people of the disease very soon after they are diagnosed.

c.   There is migration of a large number of healthy people into the population.

14.   Indicate whether the following statements are true or false:

a.   Only the population at risk contributes to the denominator of the cumulative incidence.

b.   When calculating the incidence rate of a disease, it is necessary to follow all subjects for the same length of time.

c.   If the incidence rate of a very serious disease is 75/100,000 person-years and the prevalence of this disease in the population is 25/100,000, then the average duration of this disease must be 3 years.

d.   All other things being equal, when a new prevention measure for a disease is developed, the prevalence of the disease will decrease over time.

e.   All other things being equal, when a treatment is developed that prolongs the life of people suffering from a disease, the prevalence of the disease will increase over time.

15.   An epidemiological investigation that was started on January 1, 2017, identified a population of 1,000 individuals among whom 4 were found to have the disease under study. During the year of the study, 6 new cases were found. Among the total of 10 cases, there were 6 deaths during the year. For the 10 cases, the diagram indicates the time of case recognition, periods of observation during the study, and vital status at the time of the termination of observation. An arrow at the start of the diagram (subjects 1, 2, 3, 4) indicates that the start of disease occurred before the study began. Assume that the 990 remaining individuals in the study did not become ill or die during the year of observation. From the information and diagram given, calculate the following:

a.   Prevalence of the disease on January 1, 2017; July 1, 2017; and December 31, 2017

b.   Cumulative incidence of disease during 2017

c.   Cumulative incidence of death during 2017

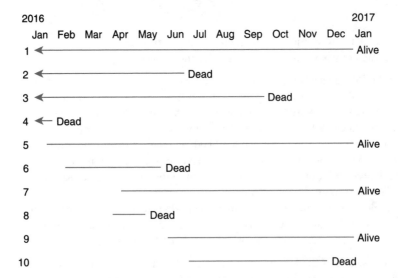

CHAPTER 3

Comparing Disease Frequencies

LEARNING OBJECTIVES

By the end of this chapter the reader will be able to:
- Organize disease frequency data into a two-by-two table.
- Describe and calculate absolute and relative measures of comparison, including rate/risk difference, population rate/risk difference, attributable proportion among the exposed and the total population and rate/risk ratio.
- Verbally interpret each absolute and relative measure of comparison.
- Describe the purpose of standardization and calculate directly standardized rates.

▶ Introduction

Measures of disease frequency are the building blocks epidemiologists use to assess the effects of a disease on a population. Comparing measures of disease frequency organizes these building blocks in a meaningful way that allows one to describe the relationship between a characteristic and a disease and to assess the public health effect of the exposure.

Disease frequencies can be compared between different populations or between subgroups within a population. For example, one might be interested in comparing disease frequencies between residents of France and the United States or between subgroups within the U.S. population according to demographic characteristics, such as race, gender, or socio-economic status; personal habits, such as alcoholic beverage consumption or cigarette smoking; and environmental factors, such as the level of air pollution.

For example, one might compare incidence rates of coronary heart disease between residents of France and those of the United States or among U.S. men and women, Blacks and Whites, alcohol drinkers and nondrinkers, and areas with high and low pollution levels.

Usually, people who have a particular characteristic (e.g., they drink alcoholic beverages) are compared with people who do not share the characteristic. Very often, the characteristic is called the *exposure*. Those who have it form the **exposed group**, and those who do not have it form the **unexposed group**. The exposed group can also be called the index group, and the unexposed group can also be called the reference, or comparison, group. The terms *index* and *referent group* are more generic terms and tend to be used when a characteristic with no clearly exposed and unexposed categories is being examined, as for example, when different racial groups are being compared. Furthermore, in instances in which no group is clearly unexposed, the group with the lowest exposure is typically used as the reference group. In addition, whenever possible, the exposure is divided into levels such as light, moderate, and heavy. Here, individuals at each exposure level would be compared with the reference group.

For example, to test the hypothesis that secondhand tobacco smoke increases the risk of childhood asthma, one could compare the frequency (e.g., 10-year cumulative incidence) of asthma among children whose parents smoke cigarettes (the exposed group) to that of children whose parents are nonsmokers (the unexposed group). Using detailed data on parental smoking, one could compare the cumulative incidence of asthma among children with two smoking parents (high level of exposure), children with only one smoking parent (low level of exposure), and children of nonsmokers. Depending on the type of comparison made, this analysis could provide information on the degree to which secondhand smoke increases a child's risk of developing asthma and the number of cases of childhood asthma that might have been prevented if parents did not smoke.

This chapter describes the various ways that epidemiologists compare measures of disease frequency and the methods they use to ensure that these comparisons are "fair." The chapter focuses not only on mathematical calculations but also on interpretation of these numbers with words.

▶ Data Organization

To compare disease frequencies, epidemiologists first organize the data in a "two-by-two" or "fourfold" table, so called because data are cross tabulated by two categories of exposure (yes or no) and two categories of disease (yes or no). **TABLE 3-1** depicts a **two-by-two table** that might be used in a study comparing proportions, such as prevalence or cumulative incidence.

The outermost row and column numbers are called the margins of the table (e.g., a + b), and the numbers in the inner area are called the cells (a, b, c, d). Note that some epidemiologists prefer to arrange the

TABLE 3-1 General Organization of Cumulative Incidence or Prevalence Data in a Two-by-Two Table

Exposure	Disease		
	Yes	**No**	**Total**
Yes	a	b	a + b
No	c	d	c + d
Total	a + c	b + d	a + b + c + d

Where:

Total number in the study = a + b + c + d
Total number exposed = a + b
Total number unexposed = c + d
Total number diseased = a + c
Total number not diseased = b + d
Number exposed and diseased = a
Number exposed but not diseased = b
Number not exposed but diseased = c
Number neither exposed nor diseased = d

table with the exposure status across the top and the disease status along the side. If you also prefer this arrangement, be sure to make the appropriate changes to the formulas for the disease frequencies.

TABLE 3-2 is a two-by-two table that describes data from a groundbreaking cohort study of air pollution and mortality among U.S. residents.[1] The "Six Cities" Study was based on 8,111 randomly selected adults who lived in one of six U.S. cities with various levels of air pollution. Investigators followed study participants for about 15 years and then determined the number and causes of death. This two-by-two table describes the cumulative incidence of mortality for the cities with the highest and lowest pollution levels—Steubenville, Ohio, and Portage, Wisconsin, respectively. A total of 2,982 participants resided in these two cities (a, b, c, d). Of these, 1,351 lived in Steubenville (a, b) and 1,631 lived in Portage (c, d). By the end of the study, 523 deaths had been observed among the participants (a, c). Of the total number of deaths, 291 occurred among residents of Steubenville (a) and 232 occurred among residents of Portage (c). Based on these data, the cumulative incidence of mortality was 291/1,351 (or 215.4/1,000) in Steubenville and 232/1,631 (or 142.2/1,000) in Portage. The combined cumulative incidence for the two cities was 523/2,982 (or 175.4/1,000).

The two-by-two table is slightly modified when incidence rates are compared (see **TABLE 3-3**). The modifications include omission of the number of people without disease (these data are unnecessary for

TABLE 3-2 Six Cities Study Cumulative Incidence of Mortality Data Arranged in a Two-by-Two Table

	Dead		
Exposure	**Yes**	**No**	**Total**
Lived in most polluted city (Steubenville, Ohio)	291	1,060	1,351
Lived in least polluted city (Portage, Wisconsin)	232	1,399	1,631
Total	523	2,459	2,982

Data from Dockery DW, Pope A, Xu X, et al. An association between air pollution and mortality in six U.S. cities. *New Engl J Med.* 1993;329:1755.

TABLE 3-3 Organization of Incidence Rate Data in a Two-by-Two Table

	Disease		
Exposure	**Yes**	**No**	**Person-time (PT)**
Yes	a	–	PT exposed
No	c	–	PT unexposed
Total	a + c	–	Total PT

incidence rate calculations) and substitution of counts with person-time in the margin. Note again that some epidemiologists prefer to arrange the table with the exposure status across the top and the disease status along the side. If you also prefer this arrangement, be sure to make the appropriate changes to the incidence rate formulas.

Because the Six Cities investigators also calculated person-time of follow-up for every study subject, it is possible to describe the incidence rate of mortality in a modified two-by-two table (see **TABLE 3-4**). In this study, person-time of follow-up began when subjects were enrolled in the study and ended at either the date of their death (for subjects who died), the date of their last follow-up contact (for subjects who were lost), or the ending date of the study (for subjects who survived and were not lost).

TABLE 3-4 Six Cities Study Incidence Rate of Mortality Data Arranged in a Two-by-Two Table

	Dead		
Exposure	**Yes**	**No**	**Person-time**
Lived in most polluted city (Steubenville, Ohio)	291	–	17,914
Lived in least polluted city (Portage, Wisconsin)	232	–	21,618
Total	523	–	39,532

Data from Dockery DW, Pope A, Xu X, Spengler JD, Ware JH, Fay ME, et al. An association between air pollution and mortality in six U.S. cities. *New Engl J Med*. 1993;329:1755.

Using this information, the incidence rates of mortality were 291/17,914 person-years (or 16.24/1,000 person-years) in Steubenville and 232/21,618 person-years (or 10.73/1,000 person-years) in Portage. The combined incidence rate of mortality for the two cities was 523/39,532 person-years (or 13.23/1,000 person-years).

▶ Measures of Comparison

Measures of disease frequency can be compared in two ways. They can be subtracted from one another or divided by one another. The subtracted measures of disease frequency are termed *absolute comparisons*, and the divided ones are known as *relative comparisons*. Absolute comparisons generally give information about the public health impact of an exposure, and relative comparisons generally give information about the strength of the relationship between an exposure and a disease. Each measure of comparison is described in more detail in the sections that follow.

Absolute Measures of Comparison

An absolute comparison is based on the difference between two measures of disease frequency. A general term for this comparison is the risk difference or rate difference. More precise terms based on the measure of disease frequency used for the calculation include incidence rate difference, cumulative incidence difference, and prevalence difference. Although the term *attributable risk* or *rate* is commonly used, some epidemiologists think that this term should be discarded because it implies a definite causal relationship.[2(p16)]

Absolute comparisons can be calculated for either exposed individuals or the total population. When exposed individuals are the focus, the absolute difference measure is calculated as follows:

$$RD = R_e - R_u$$

where RD is the **rate or risk difference** (such as incidence rate difference, cumulative incidence difference, or prevalence difference), R_e is the rate or risk (incidence rate, cumulative incidence, or prevalence) in the exposed group, and R_u is the rate or risk (incidence rate, cumulative incidence, or prevalence) in the unexposed group.

The RD describes the disease burden associated with exposure among the people who are exposed. Interpreted narrowly, the RD is simply the excess risk or rate of disease associated with the exposure. However, there is a broader interpretation that makes the assumption of causality. If the exposure is considered a cause of the disease, the RD can be used to calculate the number of disease cases that would be eliminated if the exposure were eliminated (or reduced to the level of the reference group).

Let us use the Six Cities data to calculate the mortality incidence rate difference for the least and most polluted cities (see Table 3-4).

$$\text{Incidence rate difference} = IR_{\text{most polluted city}} - IR_{\text{least polluted city}}$$

$$IRD = \frac{16.24}{1,000}\text{person-years} - \frac{10.73}{1,000}\text{person-years}$$

$$IRD = \frac{5.51}{1,000}\text{person-years}$$

Interpreted narrowly, there are 5.51 excess deaths per 1,000 person-years among Steubenville residents. Or, more broadly, if pollution caused the deaths, then 5.51 deaths among Steubenville residents for every 1,000 person-years of observation would be eliminated if the pollution level were reduced to that of Portage. See **FIGURE 3-1** for a graphical depiction of this association. The excess risk or rate can be multiplied by the number of exposed people to obtain the actual number of excess cases.

A population usually consists of exposed and unexposed people. Thus, it is useful to know the impact of the exposure not only on the exposed but also on the total population. A general term used to describe this comparison is the population risk difference (or population rate difference).

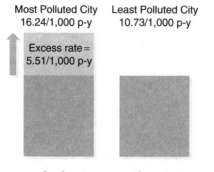

FIGURE 3-1 Interpreting an **absolute measure of comparison**: mortality rate difference in the Six Cities Study.

Data from Dockery DW, Pope A, Xu X, Spengler JD, Ware JH, Fay ME, et al. An association between air pollution and mortality in six U.S. cities. *New Engl J Med.* 1993;329:1755.

When the total population is of interest, the absolute difference measure is calculated as follows:

$$PRD = R_t - R_u$$

where PRD is the population rate difference (or population risk difference), R_t is the rate or risk (incidence rate, cumulative incidence, or prevalence) in the total population, and R_u is the rate or risk (incidence rate, cumulative incidence, or prevalence) in the unexposed group.

It is also possible to obtain the population rate difference by multiplying the risk or rate difference (RD) by the proportion of the population that is exposed (P_e):

$$PRD = RD \times P_e$$

where RD is the incidence rate difference, cumulative incidence difference, or prevalence difference, and P_e is the proportion of the population that is exposed.

The disease rate in the total population (R_t) or the proportion exposed (P_e) may be obtained from either the study population or the general population. However, before the study population is used as the source of this information, the study design must be examined carefully. Studies in which the exposed proportion has been arbitrarily set by the investigator will give inaccurate data because the percentage exposed in the study population does not reflect real life. For example, in the Six Cities Study, the investigators arbitrarily included three more and three less polluted cities.

Just as the rate or risk difference describes the public health impact of the exposure among the exposed, the population rate difference (or population risk difference) describes the impact among the total population. The PRD describes the excess number of cases in the total population that is associated with the exposure. Or, more broadly, if one believes that there is a causal relationship between the exposure and disease, the PRD identifies the number of cases of disease that would be eliminated in the total population if the exposure were eliminated (or reduced to the level in the reference group). The PRD helps public health officials determine which exposures are most important to a given population and to prioritize prevention activities. Later investigations in the Six Cities population found that mortality was more strongly associated with fine particles from automobiles and coal-burning combustion sources and therefore provide a focus for public health intervention.[3]

Note in the second PRD formula that the impact of an exposure on a population is a function of both the rate difference (RD) and the proportion of exposed individuals in the population (P_e). Thus, even if the rate difference is relatively high, the PRD will not be high if the exposure is rare. On the other hand, even if the rate difference is relatively low, the PRD will be high if the exposure is common.

For example, assume that 10% of the U.S. population is exposed to air pollution levels as high as those in Steubenville, Ohio, which is the most polluted city in the Six Cities Study. Using this information, one would calculate the population rate difference for the United States as follows:

$$PRD = RD \times P_e$$

$$PRD = \left(\frac{5.5}{1,000} \text{ person-years} \right) \times 0.10 = \frac{0.55}{1,000} \text{ person-years}$$

Thus, 0.55 additional deaths for every 1,000 person-years of observation in the entire U.S. population can be attributed to pollution. Or, if pollution were the cause of death, then 0.55 deaths for every 1,000 person-years of observation in the U.S. population would be eliminated if pollution were reduced.

What would the PRD be if high pollution levels were more common? Let us apply the Six Cities results to Krakow, which is considered to be one of the most polluted cities in Poland.[4] If we assume that 40% of the population in Krakow is exposed to air pollution levels as high as those in Steubenville, Ohio, population rate difference would be calculated as follows:

$$\left(\frac{5.5}{1,000} \text{ person-years} \right) \times 0.40 = \frac{2.2}{1,000} \text{ person-years}$$

This means that cleaning up air pollution in this area of Eastern Europe would save even more lives than it would in the United States.

One can see from the formulas that, unless everyone in the population is exposed, the impact of the exposure is always smaller in the total population than in the exposed group and therefore the PRD is always smaller than the RD. Also, note that the units and range of the absolute measures of comparison (RD and PRD) depend on the measure of disease frequency that is used for the calculation. For example, if incidence rates are used, then the measure will have person-time units and can range from negative infinity to positive infinity. On the other hand, if one uses cumulative incidence or prevalence, the measure is dimensionless and can range from −1 to +1.

Two parallel measures of comparison that express the public health impact of an exposure as proportions are the attributable proportion among the exposed[5] (also called the etiologic fraction[6]) and the attributable proportion among the total population. The **attributable proportion among the exposed (APe)** describes the proportion of disease among the exposed that would be eliminated if the exposure were eliminated. It assumes a causal relationship between the exposure and disease. Mathematically, it is expressed as follows:

$$AP_e = \left(\frac{(R_e - R_u)}{R_e} \right) \times 100$$

where AP_e is the attributable proportion among the exposed; R_e is the incidence rate, cumulative incidence, or prevalence in the exposed group; and R_u is the incidence rate, cumulative incidence, or prevalence in the unexposed population.

For example, using the Six Cities data,

$$AP_e = \left(\frac{(16.24 \,/\, 1{,}000 \text{ person-years} - 10.73 \,/\, 1{,}000 \text{ person-years})}{16.24 \,/\, 1{,}000 \text{ person-years}} \right) \times 100$$

$$AP_e = 33.9\%$$

This means that 33.9% of the deaths among participants from Steubenville may be attributed to the high pollution level and thus could be eliminated if the pollution level were reduced.

The **attributable proportion among the total population (APt)** describes the proportion of disease among the total population that would be eliminated if the exposure were eliminated. It is expressed as follows:

$$AP_t = \left(\frac{(R_t - R_u)}{R_t} \right) \times 100$$

where R_t is the incidence rate, cumulative incidence, or prevalence in the total population and R_u is the incidence rate, cumulative incidence, or prevalence in the unexposed population.

For example, using the Six Cities data,

$$AP_t = \left(\frac{(12.87 \,/\, 1{,}000 \text{ person-years} - 10.73 \,/\, 1{,}000 \text{ person-years})}{12.87 \,/\, 1{,}000 \text{ person-years}} \right) \times 100$$

$AP_t = 16.6\%$

Note that the incidence rate for the total population was derived from the incidence rate among participants in all six cities, not just Portage and Steubenville. The AP_t means that 16.6% of the deaths in the total study population may be attributed to high pollution levels and thus could be eliminated if the pollution levels were reduced.

The attributable proportion among the total population is very useful for determining priorities for public health action.[7] In the example just given, the elimination of the pollution would lead to a substantial reduction in deaths, and therefore public health policymakers would probably rate it as a priority. On the other hand, if an exposure had a much lower attributable proportion, policymakers would probably not use limited health dollars to eliminate it.

If there is no relationship between the exposure and disease (in other words, the rate or risk of disease among the exposed is exactly the same as that among the unexposed), the numeric value for all of the absolute comparisons (rate difference, population rate difference, attributable proportion among the exposed, and attributable proportion among the total population) is zero.

The attributable proportion is used when an exposure is considered a cause of the disease. When an exposure is thought to protect against the disease, the prevented fraction (PF)[6] can be calculated according to the following formula:

$$PF = \left(\frac{(R_u - R_e)}{R_u} \right) \times 100$$

where R_u is the incidence rate, cumulative incidence, or prevalence in the unexposed group and R_e is the incidence rate, cumulative incidence, or prevalence in the exposed group.

For example, a pioneering study published in 1950 found that the addition of fluoride to drinking water supplies reduced the incidence of dental caries. The incidence of dental caries in Newburgh, New York, a fluoridated area, was 14.8%, whereas the incidence in Kingston, New York, a nonfluoridated area, was 21.3%.[8] Thus, the preventive fraction was 30.5%. This means that almost 31% of caries in Newburgh were prevented because of fluoridation.

Relative Measures of Comparison

A **relative measure of comparison** is based on the ratio of two measures of disease frequency. This measure is generally called the risk ratio, rate ratio, relative rate, or relative risk. More precise terms that are based on the measure of disease frequency used for the calculation include incidence rate ratio, cumulative incidence ratio, and prevalence ratio.

Mathematically, the relative measure is expressed as follows:

$$RR = \frac{R_e}{R_u}$$

where RR is the **rate or risk ratio**; R_e is the incidence rate, cumulative incidence, or prevalence in the exposed group; and R_u is the incidence rate, cumulative incidence, or prevalence in the unexposed group.

A relative comparison gives information about the strength of the relationship between the exposure and disease and is most useful for etiologic research. For example, the relative rate of death in the Six Cities Study is (16.24/1,000 person-years)/(10.73/1,000 person-years), or 1.51. This means that, compared with the residents of Portage, there is a 1.51-fold increased rate of death among residents of Steubenville. Another interpretation is that the death rate in Steubenville is 1.51 times that of Portage. See **FIGURE 3-2** for a graphical depiction of this association.

If there is no relationship between the exposure and disease, the numeric value for the relative measure is 1.0. If there is a positive relationship between the exposure and disease (i.e., the exposure increases the rate of disease), the numeric value is greater than 1.0. Another way to express this information is in terms of the excess relative rate, which is mathematically equal to $(RR - 1) \times 100$.[5] For example, using the Six Cities relative rate of 1.51, the excess relative rate is $(1.51 - 1) \times 100$, or 51%. Thus, compared with the residents of Portage, the residents of Steubenville have a 51% increased rate of death.

If the exposure prevents disease, the numeric value of the relative comparison measure is less than 1.0. For example, a relative risk of 0.5

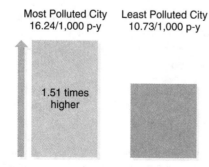

Most Polluted City
16.24/1,000 p-y

Least Polluted City
10.73/1,000 p-y

1.51 times
higher

FIGURE 3-2 Interpreting a relative measure of comparison: mortality rate ratio in the Six Cities Study.

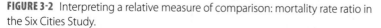

Data from Dockery DW, Pope A, Xu X, Spengler JD, Ware JH, Fay ME, et al. An association between air pollution and mortality in six U.S. cities. *New Engl J Med.* 1993;329:1755.

means that the exposed group has one-half the risk of the unexposed group, or a 50% decreased risk of disease. A relative risk of 0.33 means that the exposed group has one-third the risk, or a 67% reduction in risk, and so on. For example, the relative risk of dental caries in Newburgh versus Kingston is 0.69.[8] This means that residents of Newburgh had a 31% reduced risk of dental caries $(1.0 - 0.69 = 0.31)$. Note that the relative measure of comparison is always dimensionless and can range from zero to infinity.

Most epidemiologists prefer to use the relative method of comparison for etiologic research because of the way it is anchored by a baseline value. In other words, it indicates how many times higher or lower the disease risk is among the exposed as compared with the baseline risk among the unexposed. However, because of this anchoring, interpretation of the relative risk requires caution in several situations. First, when the baseline risk or rate of disease is high, maximum value of the relative risk is limited. For example, if the baseline risk is 50% among the unexposed, then the highest possible value of the relative risk is 2.0 (because disease risk among the exposed cannot exceed 100%). Second, when cumulative incidence or prevalence is used for the comparison, the relative risk will approach 1.0 as the disease frequency increases. As the prevalence or cumulative incidence approaches 100% in the exposed and unexposed groups, the ratio (the relative risk) approaches 1.0. This often occurs with cumulative incidence when the population is followed for a long period of time. The ratio of incidence rates is not affected in this manner because incidence rates can range up to infinity.

Note that the relative measure of comparison can also be used to calculate both the attributable proportion among the exposed and the attributable proportion among the total population. The formula for the attributable proportion among the exposed is expressed as follows:

$$AP_e = \left[\frac{(RR - 1)}{RR} \right] \times 100$$

where AP_e is the attributable proportion among the exposed and RR is the relative measure of comparison.

The formula for the attributable proportion among the total population is expressed as follows:

$$AP_t = \left[\frac{P_e(RR - 1)}{P_e(RR - 1) + 1} \right] \times 100$$

where AP_t is the attributable proportion among the total population, RR is the relative measure of comparison, and P_e is the exposed proportion in either the study or general population.

As discussed previously, before the study population is used as the source of the exposed proportion (P_e), the study design must be examined

TABLE 3-5 Absolute and Relative Measures of Comparison

Type of measure	Formula	Interpretation
Rate or risk difference	$R_e - R_u$	Excess rate or risk of disease (RD) among exposed population
Population rate difference (PRD)	$R_t - R_u$ or $RD \times P_e$	Excess rate or risk of disease in total population
Attributable proportion among exposed (AP_e)	$[(R_e - R_u)/R_e] \times 100$ or $[(RR - 1)/RR] \times 100$	Excess proportion of disease among exposed population; if causal, proportion of disease among exposed that would be eliminated if the exposure were eliminated
Attributable proportion among total population (AP_t)	$[(R_t - R_u)/R_t] \times 100$ or $[P_e(RR - 1)/P_e(RR - 1) +1] \times 100$	Excess proportion of disease in total population; if causal, proportion of disease in total population that would be eliminated if the exposure were eliminated
Rate or risk ratio (RR)	R_e/R_u	Strength of relationship between exposure and disease; the number of times higher or lower the rate or risk is among exposed as compared with rate or risk among unexposed population

carefully. Studies in which the exposed proportion has been arbitrarily set (e.g., 50% exposed) will give inaccurate data because the percentage exposed in the study population does not reflect the underlying population.

The formulas given in this chapter and summarized in **TABLE 3-5** can be used for most types of epidemiological studies, including cohort studies, experimental studies, and cross-sectional studies. Other formulas are used for case–control studies because of the way the subjects are selected.

▶ Direct Standardization

Crude rates are summary measures of disease frequency that are based on the raw data. For example, a crude prevalence is calculated by dividing the total number of cases in the population by the total number of individuals in that population at a point in time (point prevalence) or during a period of time (period prevalence). It is difficult to interpret absolute and relative measures of comparison that are based on crude rates when the compared groups differ on a characteristic that affects the rate of disease (such as age, gender, or race). This difference between the groups may result in an unfair comparison and distort the results.

For example, let us compare the crude mortality rates among people living in Alaska with the rates of Florida residents (see **TABLE 3-6**). The crude mortality rate among Florida residents (945.9 per 100,000) is much higher than that among Alaska residents (584.5 per 100,000), and the excess crude rate is 361.4 per 100,000 (945.9 − 584.5 per 100,000).

TABLE 3-6 Number of Deaths, Estimated Population Size, and Crude Mortality Rates in Alaska and Florida in 2015

	Alaska	Florida
Number of deaths	4,316	191,737
Number in population	738,432	20,271,272
Crude mortality rate (per 100,000 persons)*	584.5	945.9

*The crude mortality rate is calculated by dividing the number of deaths by the number in the population.

Data from Centers for Disease Control and Prevention. Compressed Mortality, 1999-2016. http://wonder.cdc.gov/cmf-icd10.html. Published December 2016. Accessed November 2017.

TABLE 3-7 Census Population Estimates and Age-Specific Mortality Rates for Alaska and Florida in 2015

Age group (years)	Alaska			Florida		
	Number in category	% of total	Death rate per 100,000	Number in category	% of total	Death rate per 100,000
Younger than 5	55,449	7.5	182.1	1,101,071	5.4	151.1
5–24	211,440	28.6	68.1	4,762,781	23.5	47.1
25–44	210,642	28.5	178.5	5,062,786	25.0	153.5
45–64	188,064	25.5	658.8	5,402,166	26.7	653.7
65 and older	72,837	9.9	3,371.9	3,942,468	19.4	3,671.2
Total	738,432	100.00	584.5	20,271,272	100.00	945.9

Data from Centers for Disease Control and Prevention. Compressed Mortality, 1999-2016. http://wonder.cdc.gov/cmf-icd10.html. Published December 2016. Accessed November 2017.

What explains the difference between the crude mortality rates of the two states? One possible answer is the different age structures of the populations. Note in **TABLE 3-7** that Florida has relatively fewer residents in the younger age categories and more residents in the oldest age category. There is a strong association between mortality and age; therefore, it is possible that these age differences account for the mortality differences between the states.

However, let us examine the age-specific mortality rates also shown in Table 3-7. Note that Florida has higher mortality rates than Alaska in those 65 years and older, whereas Alaska has higher mortality rates than Florida in the remaining age groups. Thus, a side-by-side comparison of the five age-specific mortality rates suggests that the age difference may account for the difference in the crude mortality rate between the two populations.

Side-by-side comparisons of age-specific rates give a more accurate picture of the mortality rates than do crude rates. However, because there are many age groups to examine, this method results in a cumbersome number of comparisons. Furthermore, comparing age-specific rates can give a confusing picture if some of the rates are higher in one state and some are higher in the other. For this reason, epidemiologists commonly use an alternative method in which the rates in each state are summarized in a single number that adjusts for the age differences between the populations. These summary rates, which are known as age-standardized or age-adjusted rates, answer the question, "What would the death rate be in each state if the populations had identical age distributions?"

The two methods for calculating age-standardized rates are known as direct and indirect methods of standardization. This chapter describes only the direct method, which requires the following information: (1) age-specific rates in each group (in this case, each state) and (2) age structure of a "standard" population (see **TABLE 3-8**). The choice of the standard population is arbitrary. The total population of the United States is typically used as the standard population for standardization of U.S. rates, and the world standard population is used for standardization of international rates.

Age-standardized rates are weighted averages of the age-specific rates, with the weights equal to the proportion of the standard population in each age category. Thus, the age-standardized rate for Alaska is calculated as follows:

$$\left(0.062 \times \frac{182.1}{100,000}\right) + \left(0.264 \times \frac{68.1}{100,000}\right) + \left(0.264 \times \frac{178.5}{100,000}\right)$$

$$+ \left(0.261 \times \frac{658.8}{100,000}\right) + \left(0.149 \times \frac{3,371}{100,000}\right) = \frac{750.8}{100,000}$$

Likewise, the age-standardized rate for Florida is calculated as follows:

$$\left(0.062 \times \frac{151.1}{100,000}\right) + \left(0.264 \times \frac{47.1}{100,000}\right) + \left(0.264 \times \frac{153.5}{100,000}\right)$$

$$+ \left(0.261 \times \frac{653.7}{100,000}\right) + \left(0.149 \times \frac{3,671.2}{100,000}\right) = \frac{780.0}{100,000}$$

Note that the weights used for both of the calculations are the same: the proportion of the entire U.S. population in each age category. Thus, the age-standardized rates are hypothetical rates that would have occurred if each state had the age structure of the entire U.S. population in 2015.

TABLE 3-8 Age-Specific Mortality Rates for Alaska and Florida and U.S. Census Population Estimates for 2015

| Age group (years) | Age-specific death rate per 100,000 | | 2015 U.S. Census | |
	Alaska	Florida	Population estimates	% of Total
Younger than 5	182.1	151.1	19,907,281	6.2
5–24	68.1	47.1	84,957,722	26.4
25–44	178.5	153.5	84,726,985	26.4
45–64	658.8	653.7	84,065,980	26.1
65 and older	3,371.9	3,671.2	47,760,852	14.9
Total	584.5	945.9	321,418,820	100.00

Data from Centers for Disease Control and Prevention. Compressed Mortality, 1999-2016. http://wonder.cdc.gov/cmf-icd10.html. Published December 2016. Accessed November 2017.

The excess age-adjusted mortality rate in Florida is 29.2 per 100,000 (780.0 − 750.8 per 100,000). This is considerably smaller than the excess crude mortality rate of 361.4 per 100,000. This finding suggests that age accounts for most but not all of the difference in the crude mortality rates between the two populations. The remaining difference may be from other factors, such as race, socioeconomic status, and access to health care. Note that these are hypothetical rates whose actual values depend on the standard that is used. Thus, they should be used only for comparisons.

Summary

Measures of disease frequency are contrasted in either absolute or relative terms, depending on the goals of the epidemiologist. Absolute measures of comparison, which are based on the difference between two measures of disease frequency, describe the public health impact of an exposure. Absolute measures include the rate or risk difference, the **population rate or risk difference**, and attributable proportion among the exposed and the total population. Relative measures of comparison, which are based on the ratio of two measures of disease frequency, describe the strength of the relationship between the exposure and disease. Relative measures include the rate or risk ratio. Comparing measures of disease frequency in either absolute or relative terms is facilitated by organizing the data into a two-by-two table.

It is often difficult to make fair comparisons of crude measures of disease frequency because of key differences between the groups that affect the disease rates. To overcome this problem, a technique known as **direct standardization** is used to adjust for these differences. For example, direct standardization for age involves taking a weighted average of age-specific rates with the weights being equal to the proportion of the standard population in each age category. The choice of the standard population is arbitrary, but U.S. population census data are typically used.

References

1. Dockery DW, Pope CA, Xu X, et al. An association between air pollution and mortality in six U.S. cities. *New Engl J Med*. 1993;329:1753-1759.
2. Walker AM. *Observation and Inference: An Introduction to the Methods of Epidemiology*. Chestnut Hill, MA: Epidemiology Resources Inc; 1991.
3. Laden F, Neas LM, Dockery DW, Schwartz J. Association of fine particulate matter from different sources with daily mortality in six U.S. cities. *Environ Health Perspect*. 2000;108:941-947.
4. Samek L. Overall human mortality and morbidity due to exposure to air pollution. *Int J Occup Med Environ Health*. 2016;29:417-426.
5. Cole P, MacMahon B. Attributable risk percent in case-control studies. *Br J Prev Soc Med*. 1971;25:242-244.
6. Miettinen OS. Proportion of disease caused or prevented by a given exposure, trait or intervention. *Am J Epidemiol*. 1974;99:325-332.
7. Northridge ME. Annotation: public health methods—attributable risk as a link between causality and public health action. *Am J Public Health*. 1995;85:1202-1204.
8. Ast DB, Finn SB, McCaffrey I. The Newburgh-Kingston caries fluorine study. *Am J Public Health*. 1950;40:716-724.

Chapter Questions

1. Describe the main similarity and difference between each of the following:
   a. Incidence rate ratio and incidence rate difference
   b. Risk difference and population risk difference

2. Suppose that an investigation of the association between regular physical activity and ovarian cancer revealed that the incidence rate of ovarian cancer among women who engaged in regular physical activity was 30 per 100,000 woman-years of follow-up, whereas the rate among women who did not engage in regular activity was 45 per 100,000 woman-years of follow-up.
   a. Use these data to compute the incidence rate ratio of ovarian cancer for women who are physically active versus women who are not.
   b. State in words your interpretation of this measure.
   c. Compute the incidence rate difference of ovarian cancer for women who are physically active versus women who are not.
   d. State in words your interpretation of this measure.
   e. If there were no association between regular physical activity and ovarian cancer, what would be the numeric values of the incidence rate ratio and incidence rate difference?

3. State the main difference between a crude rate and an age-adjusted rate.
4. State the main difference between an age-specific rate and an age-adjusted rate.
5. Consider the following heart disease mortality data from two hypothetical countries, including a low-income and a high-income country.

Age group (years)	Percentage of population in age group	Death rate from heart disease
Hypothetical low-income country		
0–20	30%	2/100,000 person-years
21–50	40%	20/100,000 person-years
51–85	30%	40/100,000 person-years
Hypothetical high-income country		
0–20	20%	2/100,000 person-years
21–50	30%	20/100,000 person-years
51–85	50%	40/100,000 person-years

   a. Use these data to calculate the overall crude death rates from heart disease in the hypothetical high- and low-income countries.
   b. Based on these data, do you think that it is better to compare the heart disease death rates in the two countries using the overall crude rate or the age-standardized rate for each country? Briefly justify your answer.

6. The 58th annual convention of the American Legion was held in Philadelphia from July 21 until July 24, 1976. People at the convention included American Legion delegates, their families, and other Legionnaires who were not official delegates. Between July 20 and August 30, some of those who had been present became ill with a type of pneumonia that was subsequently named Legionnaires' disease. No one attending the convention developed the disease after August 30. The numbers of delegates and nondelegates who developed Legionnaires' disease during the period July 20 to August 30 (a 41-day period) are as follows:

Convention status	Developed Legionnaires' disease		
	Yes	No	Total
Delegate	125	1724	1849
Nondelegate	3	759	762

Data from Fraser DW, Tsai TR, Orenstein W, et al. Legionnaires' disease: description of an epidemic of pneumonia. *New Engl J Med.* 1977;297:1189-1197.

    a. Compute the cumulative incidence of Legionnaires' disease among delegates and nondelegates.

    b. Calculate the cumulative incidence ratio of Legionnaires' disease among delegates compared with nondelegates.

    c. State in words the meaning of this measure.

    d. Calculate the cumulative incidence difference of Legionnaires' disease among delegates compared with nondelegates.

    e. State in words the meaning of this measure.

    f. Calculate the attributable proportion of Legionnaires' disease among the delegates.

    g. State in words the meaning of this measure.

7. Indicate whether the following statements are true or false.

    a. When there is no association between an exposure and a disease, the numerical value of the risk ratio will be zero.

    b. When there is no asssociation between an exposure and a disease, the numerical value of the risk difference will be 1.0.

    c. A study examined the relationship between air pollution and the risk of having a baby with low birth weight. The investigators found that the risk ratio comparing pregnant women exposed to high versus low levels of air pollution was 1.35. This means that women exposed to high air pollution levels were 35% more likely to have a baby with low birth weight.

    d. A study examined the autopsied brains of 100 professional football players with a history of repeated concussions. The investigators found that abnormal protein deposits were present in nearly 100% of the brains. This means that there was an association between repeated concussions and abnormal protein deposits in the brains of these athletes.

    e. A study examined the relationship between swimming in an unchlorinated pool and the risk of developing diarrhea. The investigators found a 15% excess risk among people who swam in the pool compared with those who did not. This means that 15% of the diarrhea cases among pool users could have been prevented if they had refrained from swimming in the unchlorinated pool.

    f. A study examined the relationship between vitamin supplementation and the occurrence of asthma among children. The investigators found that compared with children who did not take vitamins, children who took vitamins on a daily basis were 0.8 times as likely to develop asthma. This means that children who took vitamins were 80% less likely to develop asthma.

8. The incidence rate of migraine headaches was 1.5/100 person-years among overweight women and 1.0/100 person-years among normal weight women. Using only this information, state whether you can calculate each of the following measures:

    a. Rate difference

    b. Rate ratio

    c. Attributable proportion among the exposed

    d. Attributable proportion among the total population

9. Consider the following data from a British study of cigarette smoking and mortality among male physicians (Doll R, Peto R, Boreham J, Sutherland I. Mortality in relation to smoking:

50 years' observations on male British doctors. *Br Med J.* 2004;328:1519. doi:10.1136 /bmj.38142.554479.AE). The age-standardized mortality rates (per 100,000 person-years) from lung cancer and ischemic heart disease are 249 and 1001, respectively, among current smokers and 17 and 619 among lifelong nonsmokers.

a. Use these data to calculate the mortality rate ratio and mortality rate difference for each disease comparing current smokers to lifelong nonsmokers.

b. Based on your answer to part A, is smoking a stronger risk factor for deaths from lung cancer or ischemic heart disease?

c. Based on your answer to part A, does smoking have a greater public health impact via deaths from lung cancer or ischemic heart disease? In other words, if smoking were the cause of mortality, how many deaths from each cause would have been averted if these individuals had never smoked?

d. Describe the reason(s) for your answers to parts B and C.

CHAPTER 4

Sources of Public Health Data

LEARNING OBJECTIVES

By the end of this chapter the reader will be able to:
- Describe the major sources of health data on U.S. and international populations.
- Describe the issues involved in appropriately interpreting these data sources.

▶ Introduction

There is a wealth of easily accessible information on the health status of the U.S. population. Most of these public health data are collected by governmental and nongovernmental agencies on a routine basis or by special surveys. Information is obtainable on deaths and a wide variety of diseases and conditions, including acute illnesses and injuries, chronic illnesses and impairments, birth defects, and other adverse pregnancy outcomes. Data are also available on characteristics that influence a person's risk of illness (such as ambient air pollution levels; nutritional habits; immunizations; and the use of cigarettes, alcohol, and drugs) and on the effect of these illnesses on the utilization of health services, including hospitalizations and visits to office-based medical professionals and hospital emergency and outpatient departments. Several sources of international data are compiled by the World Health Organization and the United Nations. Although the international data are not as extensive as those about the United States, they include information about births, deaths, and major health indicators.

This chapter provides short descriptions of the major sources of descriptive public health data, including the data collection methods. It is important for epidemiologists to understand data collection methods to interpret the information appropriately. In particular, it is important to know the specific population that is covered by a data collection system. For example, although U.S. birth and death data pertain to the whole U.S.

population, the target population for most national surveys consists of noninstitutionalized civilians. The latter group excludes members of the armed services and individuals living in institutions, such as correctional facilities and nursing and convalescent homes. These groups are usually excluded because of technical and logistical problems.

It is also important to understand the calendar period covered by the data collection system and the frequency with which the data are updated. Generally, the most current available data in the United States lags a year or two behind the present. This is because it takes researchers a long time to collect data, computerize the information, check it for errors, and conduct statistical and epidemiological analyses.

Every data collection system has some incomplete and inaccurate material. If data come from interview-based surveys, they are limited by the amount and type of information that a respondent can remember or is willing to report. For example, a person may not know detailed information on medical diagnoses and surgeries or may not want to report sensitive information on sexually transmitted diseases and prior induced abortions.

▶ Census of the U.S. Population

The U.S. Constitution requires that a **census**—that is, a complete count of the U.S. population—be taken every 10 years. The primary purpose of the census is to assign members of the House of Representatives to the states.[1] The decennial census of the population has been conducted since 1790, and a census of housing characteristics has been conducted since 1940. Permanently established in 1902, the U.S. Bureau of the Census currently oversees the population and housing census, compiles relevant statistics, and produces reports and computerized data files that are available to the public.

In recent years, the census has obtained information on certain characteristics (such as name, race, gender, age, and relationship of household members) from the entire population and information on additional characteristics (such as ancestry, income, mortgage, and size of housing unit) from a representative sample of persons. (About 17% of the U.S. population answers these additional questions.) The Census Bureau uses this approach to obtain the most comprehensive data possible while keeping costs reasonable. The complete population is surveyed on characteristics for which precise data are needed on small geographic areas. For example, accurate data on small areas are needed for congressional apportionments. On the other hand, samples are surveyed when estimates are sufficient for larger geographic areas, such as census tracts.

The Census Bureau tabulates complete count and sample population statistics for geographic areas in increasing size, from census tracts; to cities, counties, and metropolitan areas; to states; and to the entire nation. Information is also collected for Puerto Rico and other areas under U.S.

sovereignty. These population counts are crucial components of most public health indicators because they are typically used as the denominators of incidence and prevalence measures.

Although the census attempts to account for every person in the U.S. population, it is well known that some miscounting occurs. Although an evaluation of the 2010 Census found a small net overcounting (~0.01%) mainly from duplicate submissions, undercounting was observed for certain racial and ethnic groups, including Blacks (2.1%) and Hispanics (1.5%).[2]

▶ Vital Statistics

The National Vital Statistics System of the National Center for Health Statistics (NCHS) compiles and publishes data on births, deaths, marriages, divorces, and fetal deaths in the United States.[3] Registration offices in all 50 states, the District of Columbia, and New York City have provided information on births and deaths since 1933. Birth and death registration is considered virtually complete. Most states also provide marriage and divorce registration records.

Most birth and death certificates used in the 50 states correspond closely in content and organization to the standard certificate recommended by NCHS. Although some modifications are made to accommodate local needs, all certificates obtain a minimum amount of information on demographic characteristics. Examples of the standard live birth and death certificates appear in FIGURE 4-1 and FIGURE 4-2.

Public health data collected currently on birth certificates includes birth weight; gestational age; and adverse pediatric conditions, such as the presence of congenital malformations (birth defects), complications during pregnancy, and cigarette smoking. Birth certificates are completed by hospital personnel in consultation with parents. The medical professional who performs the delivery subsequently verifies the accuracy of the information. Certificates are then sent to the local health departments, which in turn send them to state health departments and then to the NCHS.

Death certificates collect information on "the chain of events—diseases, injuries, complications—that directly caused the death."[3] Thus, the certificate lists the immediate cause of death, any intermediate causes, and the underlying cause. For example, respiratory arrest may be the immediate cause of death, pneumonia the intermediate cause, and acquired immune deficiency syndrome (AIDS) the underlying cause of death. Other significant conditions contributing to the death may also be listed.

To generate national mortality statistics, "every death is attributed to one underlying condition, based on information reported on the death certificate and utilizing the international rules." These rules, now termed the International Classification of Diseases (ICD), were first developed

U.S. STANDARD CERTIFICATE OF LIVE BIRTH

LOCAL FILE NO.				BIRTH NUMBER:	

CHILD

1. CHILD'S NAME (First, Middle, Last, Suffix)			2. TIME OF BIRTH (24hr)	3. SEX	4. DATE OF BIRTH (Mo/Day/Yr)
5. FACILITY NAME (If not institution, give street and number)			6. CITY, TOWN, OR LOCATION OF BIRTH		7. COUNTY OF BIRTH

MOTHER

8a. MOTHER'S CURRENT LEGAL NAME (First, Middle, Last, Suffix)		8b. DATE OF BIRTH (Mo/Day/Yr)	
8c. MOTHER'S NAME PRIOR TO FIRST MARRIAGE (First, Middle, Last, Suffix)		8d. BIRTHPLACE (State, Territory, or Foreign Country)	
9a. RESIDENCE OF MOTHER-STATE	9b. COUNTY	9c. CITY, TOWN, OR LOCATION	
9d. STREET AND NUMBER		9e. APT. NO.	9f. ZIP CODE	9g. INSIDE CITY LIMITS? ☐ Yes ☐ No

FATHER

10a. FATHER'S CURRENT LEGAL NAME (First, Middle, Last, Suffix)	10b. DATE OF BIRTH (Mo/Day/Yr)	10c. BIRTHPLACE (State, Territory, or Foreign Country)

CERTIFIER

11. CERTIFIER'S NAME: _____ TITLE: ☐ MD ☐ DO ☐ HOSPITAL ADMIN. ☐ CNM/CM ☐ OTHER MIDWIFE ☐ OTHER (Specify)_____	12. DATE CERTIFIED ___/___/___ MM DD YYYY	3. DATE FILED BY REGISTRAR ___/___/___ MM DD YYYY

INFORMATION FOR ADMINISTRATIVE USE

MOTHER

14. MOTHER'S MAILING ADDRESS: ☐ Same as residence, or: State: City, Town, or Location:
Street & Number: Apartment No.:   Zip Code:
15. MOTHER MARRIED? (At birth, conception, or any time between) ☐ Yes ☐ No If No, Has Paternity Acknowledgment Been Signed in the Hospital? ☐ Yes ☐ No	16. SOCIAL SECURITY NUMBER REQUESTED For Child? ☐ Yes ☐ No	17. FACILITY ID. (NPI)
18. MOTHER'S SOCIAL SECURITY NUMBER:		19. FATHER'S SOCIAL SECURITY NUMBER:

INFORMATION FOR MEDICAL AND HEALTH PURPOSES ONLY

MOTHER

20. MOTHER'S EDUCATION (Check the box that best describes the highest degree or level of school completed at the time of delivery) ☐ 8th grade or less ☐ 9th–12th grade, no diploma ☐ High school graduate or GED completed ☐ Some college credit but no degree ☐ Associate degree (e.g., AA, AS) ☐ Bachelor's degree (e.g., BA, AB, BS) ☐ Master's degree (e.g., MA, MS, MEng, MEd, MSW, MBA) ☐ Doctorate (e.g., PhD, EdD) or Professional degree (e.g., MD, DDS, DVM, LLB, JD)	21. MOTHER OF HISPANIC ORIGIN? (Check the box that best describes whether the mother is Spanish/Hispanic/Latina. Check the "No" box if mother is not Spanish/Hispanic/Latina) ☐ No, not Spanish/Hispanic/Latina ☐ Yes, Mexican, Mexican American, Chicana ☐ Yes, Puerto Rican ☐ Yes, Cuban ☐ Yes, other Spanish/Hispanic/Latina (Specify)_____	22. MOTHER'S RACE (Check one or more races to indicate what the mother considers herself to be) ☐ White ☐ Black or African American ☐ American Indian or Alaska Native (Name of the enrolled or principal tribe)____ ☐ Asian Indian ☐ Chinese ☐ Filipino ☐ Japanese ☐ Korean ☐ Vietnamese ☐ Other Asian (Specify)_____ ☐ Native Hawaiian ☐ Guamanian or Chamorro ☐ Samoan ☐ Other Pacific Islander (Specify)_____ ☐ Other (Specify)_____

FATHER

23. FATHER'S EDUCATION (Check the box that best describes the highest degree or level of school completed at the time of delivery) ☐ 8th grade or less ☐ 9th–12th grade, no diploma ☐ High school graduate or GED completed ☐ Some college credit but no degree ☐ Associate degree (e.g., AA, AS) ☐ Bachelor's degree (e.g., BA, AB, BS) ☐ Master's degree (e.g., MA, MS, MEng, MEd, MSW, MBA) ☐ Doctorate (e.g., PhD, EdD) or Professional degree (e.g., MD, DDS, DVM, LLB, JD)	24. FATHER OF HISPANIC ORIGIN? (Check the box that best describes whether the father is Spanish/Hispanic/Latino. Check the "No" box if father is not Spanish/Hispanic/Latino) ☐ No, not Spanish/Hispanic/Latino ☐ Yes, Mexican, Mexican American, Chicano ☐ Yes, Puerto Rican ☐ Yes, Cuban ☐ Yes, other Spanish/Hispanic/Latino (Specify)_____	25. FATHER'S RACE (Check one or more races to indicate what the father considers himself to be) ☐ White ☐ Black or African American ☐ American Indian or Alaska Native (Name of the enrolled or principal tribe)____ ☐ Asian Indian ☐ Chinese ☐ Filipino ☐ Japanese ☐ Korean ☐ Vietnamese ☐ Other Asian (Specify)_____ ☐ Native Hawaiian ☐ Guamanian or Chamorro ☐ Samoan ☐ Other Pacific Islander (Specify)_____ ☐ Other (Specify)_____

Mother's Name _____   Mother's Medical Record No. _____

26. PLACE WHERE BIRTH OCCURRED (Check one) ☐ Hospital ☐ Freestanding birthing center ☐ Home birth: Planned to deliver at home? ☐ Yes ☐ No ☐ Clinic/Doctor's office ☐ OTHER (Specify)_____	27. ATTENDANT'S NAME, TITLE, AND NPI NAME: _____ NPI:____ TITLE: ☐ MD ☐ DO ☐ CNM/CM ☐ OTHER MIDWIFE ☐ Other (Specify) _____	28. MOTHER TRANSFERRED FOR MATERNAL MEDICAL OR FETAL INDICATIONS FOR DELIVERY? ☐ Yes ☐ No IF YES, ENTER NAME OF FACILITY MOTHER TRANSFERRED FROM: _____

REV. 11/2003

FIGURE 4-1 Sample of U.S. Standard Certificate of Live Birth.

MOTHER	29a. DATE OF FIRST PRENATAL CARE VISIT M M / D D / Y Y Y Y ☐ No Prenatal Care	29b. DATE OF LAST PRENATAL CARE VISIT M M / D D / Y Y Y Y	30. TOTAL NUMBER OF PRENATAL VISITS FOR THIS PREGNANCY _____ (If none, enter "0".)

31. MOTHER'S HEIGHT _____ (feet/inches)	32. MOTHER'S PREPREGNANCY WEIGHT _____ (pounds)	33. MOTHER'S WEIGHT AT DELIVERY _____ (pounds)	34. DID MOTHER GET WIC FOOD FOR HERSELF DURING THIS PREGNANCY? ☐ YES ☐ NO

35. NUMBER OF PREVIOUS LIVE BIRTHS (Do not include this child)	36. NUMBER OF OTHER PREGNANCY OUTCOMES (spontaneous or induced losses or ectopic pregnancies)	37. CIGARETTE SMOKING BEFORE AND DURING PREGNANCY For each time period, enter either the number of cigarettes or the number of packs of cigarettes smoked. IF NONE, ENTER "0". Average number of cigarettes or packs of cigarettes smoked per day.	38. PRINCIPAL SOURCE OF PAYMENT FOR THIS DELIVERY
			☐ Private Insurance

				# of cigarettes	# of packs	
35a. Now Living Number _____ ☐ None	35b. Now Dead Number _____ ☐ None	36a. Other Outcomes Number ____ ☐ None	Three Months Before Pregnancy	_____ OR	_____	☐ Medicaid ☐ Self-pay ☐ Other (Specify) _____
			First Three Months of Pregnancy	_____ OR	_____	
			Second Three Months of Pregnancy	_____ OR	_____	
			Third Trimester of Pregnancy	_____ OR	_____	

35c. DATE OF LAST LIVE BIRTH M M / Y Y Y Y	36b. DATE OF LAST OTHER PREGNANCY OUTCOME M M / Y Y Y Y	39. DATE LAST NORMAL MENSES BEGAN M M / D D / Y Y Y Y	40. MOTHER'S MEDICAL RECORD NUMBER

MEDICAL AND HEALTH INFORMATION	41. RISK FACTORS IN THIS PREGNANCY (Check all that apply) Diabetes ☐ Prepregnancy (Diagnosis prior to this pregnancy) ☐ Gestational (Diagnosis in this pregnancy) Hypertension ☐ Prepregnancy (Chronic) ☐ Gestational (PIH, preeclampsia) ☐ Eclampsia ☐ Previous preterm birth ☐ Other previous poor pregnancy outcome (Includes perinatal death, small for gestational age/ intrauterine growth restricted birth) ☐ Pregnancy resulted from infertility treatment— If yes, check all that apply: ☐ Fertility-enhancing drugs, artificial insemination or intrauterine insemination ☐ Assisted reproductive technology (e.g., in vitro fertilization (IVF), gamete intrafallopian transfer (GIFT)) ☐ Mother had a previous cesarean delivery. If yes, how many _____ ☐ None of the above 42. INFECTIONS PRESENT AND/OR TREATED DURING THIS PREGNANCY (Check all that apply) ☐ Gonorrhea ☐ Hepatitis B ☐ Syphilis ☐ Hepatitis C ☐ Chlamydia ☐ None of the above	43. OBSTETRIC PROCEDURES (Check all that apply) ☐ Cervical cerclage ☐ Tocolysis External cephalic version: ☐ Successful ☐ Failed ☐ None of the above 44. ONSET OF LABOR (Check all that apply) ☐ Premature Rupture of the Membranes (prolonged, ≥ 12 hrs.) ☐ Precipitous Labor (< 3 hrs.) ☐ Prolonged Labor (≥ 20 hrs.) ☐ None of the above 45. CHARACTERISTICS OF LABOR AND DELIVERY (Check all that apply) ☐ Induction of labor ☐ Augmentation of labor ☐ Non-vertex presentation ☐ Steroids (glucocorticoids) for fetal lung maturation received by the mother prior to delivery ☐ Antibiotics received by the mother during labor ☐ Clinical chorioamnionitis diagnosed during labor or maternal temperature ≥ 38°C (100.4°F) ☐ Moderate/heavy meconium staining of the amniotic fluid ☐ Fetal intolerance of labor such that one or more of the following actions was taken: in-utero resuscitative measures, further fetal assessment, or operative delivery ☐ Epidural or spinal anesthesia during labor ☐ None of the above	46. METHOD OF DELIVERY A. Was delivery with forceps attempted but unsuccessful? ☐ Yes ☐ No B. Was delivery with vacuum extraction attempted but unsuccessful? ☐ Yes ☐ No C. Fetal presentation at birth ☐ Cephalic ☐ Breech ☐ Other D. Final route and method of delivery (Check one) ☐ Vaginal/Spontaneous ☐ Vaginal/Forceps ☐ Vaginal/Vacuum ☐ Cesarean If cesarean, was a trial of labor attempted? ☐ Yes ☐ No 47. MATERNAL MORBIDITY (Check all that apply) (Complications associated with labor and delivery) ☐ Maternal transfusion ☐ Third- or fourth-degree perineal laceration ☐ Ruptured uterus ☐ Unplanned hysterectomy ☐ Admission to intensive care unit ☐ Unplanned operating room procedure following delivery ☐ None of the above

NEWBORN INFORMATION

NEWBORN	48. NEWBORN MEDICAL RECORD NUMBER:
	
	49. BIRTHWEIGHT (grams preferred, specify unit)
	_____ ☐ grams ☐ lb/oz
	
	50. OBSTETRIC ESTIMATE OF GESTATION: _____ (completed weeks)
	
	51. APGAR SCORE:
	Score at 5 minutes: _____
	If 5 minute score is less than 6,
	Score at 10 minutes: _____
	
	52. PLURALITY—Single, Twin, Triplet, etc. (Specify) _____
	
	53. IF NOT SINGLE BIRTH—Born First, Second, Third, etc. (Specify) _____
		54. ABNORMAL CONDITIONS OF THE NEWBORN (Check all that apply)
		☐ Assisted ventilation required immediately following delivery
		☐ Assisted ventilation required for more than 6 hours
		☐ NICU admission
		☐ Newborn given surfactant replacement therapy
		☐ Antibiotics received by the newborn for suspected neonatal sepsis
		☐ Seizure or serious neurologic dysfunction
		☐ Significant birth injury (skeletal fracture[s], peripheral nerve injury, and/or soft tissue/solid organ hemorrhage that requires intervention)
		☐ None of the above
			55. CONGENITAL ANOMALIES OF THE NEWBORN (Check all that apply)
			☐ Anencephaly
			☐ Meningomyelocele/Spina bifida
			☐ Cyanotic congenital heart disease
			☐ Congenital diaphragmatic hernia
			☐ Omphalocele
			☐ Gastroschisis
			☐ Limb reduction defect (excluding congenital amputation and dwarfing syndromes)
			☐ Cleft Lip with or without Cleft Palate
			☐ Cleft Palate alone
			☐ Down Syndrome
			  ☐ Karyotype confirmed
			  ☐ Karyotype pending
			☐ Suspected chromosomal disorder
			  ☐ Karyotype confirmed
			  ☐ Karyotype pending
			☐ Hypospadias
			☐ None of the anomalies listed above

56. WAS INFANT TRANSFERRED WITHIN 24 HOURS OF DELIVERY? ☐ Yes ☐ No IF YES, NAME OF FACILITY INFANT TRANSFERRED TO: _____	57. IS INFANT LIVING AT TIME OF REPORT? ☐ Yes ☐ No ☐ Infant transferred, status unknown	58. IS INFANT BEING BREASTFED AT DISCHARGE? ☐ Yes ☐ No

REV. 11/2003

Mother's Name _____
Mother's Medical Record No. _____

NOTE: This recommended standard birth certificate is the result of an extensive evaluation process. Information on the process and resulting recommendations as well as plans for future activities is available on the Internet at: http://www.cdc.gov/nchs/vital_certs_rev.htm.

FIGURE 4-1 Continued Sample of U.S. Standard Certificate of Live Birth.

NAME OF DECEDENT
For use by physician or institution

To Be Completed/Verified By:
FUNERAL DIRECTOR

To Be Completed By:
MEDICAL CERTIFIER

To Be Completed By:
FUNERAL DIRECTOR

U.S. STANDARD CERTIFICATE OF DEATH

LOCAL FILE NO.   STATE FILE NO.

| 1. DECEDENT'S LEGAL NAME (Include AKA's if any) (First, Middle, Last) | | 2. SEX | 3. SOCIAL SECURITY NUMBER |

| 4a. AGE—Last Birthday (Years) | 4b. UNDER 1 YEAR | | 4c. UNDER 1 DAY | | 5. DATE OF BIRTH (Mo/Day/Yr) | 6. BIRTHPLACE (City and State or Foreign Country) |
| | Months | Days | Hours | Minutes | | |

| 7a. RESIDENCE-STATE | 7b. COUNTY | | 7c. CITY OR TOWN |

| 7d. STREET AND NUMBER | | 7e. APT. NO. | 7f. ZIP CODE | 7g. INSIDE CITY LIMITS ☐ Yes ☐ No |

| 8. EVER IN U.S. ARMED FORCES? ☐ Yes ☐ No | 9. MARITAL STATUS AT TIME OF DEATH ☐ Married ☐ Married, but separated ☐ Widowed ☐ Divorced ☐ Never Married ☐ Unknown | 10. SURVIVING SPOUSE'S NAME (If wife, give name prior to first marriage) |

| 11. FATHER'S NAME (First, Middle, Last) | 12. MOTHER'S NAME PRIOR TO FIRST MARRIAGE (First, Middle, Last) |

| 13a. INFORMANT'S NAME | 13b. RELATIONSHIP TO DECEDENT | 13c. MAILING ADDRESS (Street and Number, City, State, Zip Code) |

14. PLACE OF DEATH (Check only one: see instructions)

| IF DEATH OCCURRED IN A HOSPITAL: ☐ Inpatient ☐ Emergency Room/Outpatient ☐ Dead on Arrival | IF DEATH OCCURRED SOMEWHERE OTHER THAN A HOSPITAL: ☐ Hospice facility ☐ Nursing home/Long term care facility ☐ Decedent's home |

| 15. FACILITY NAME (If not institution, give street and number) | 16. CITY OR TOWN, STATE, AND ZIP CODE | 17. COUNTY OF DEATH |

| 18. METHOD OF DISPOSITION: ☐ Burial ☐ Cremation ☐ Donation ☐ Entombment ☐ Removal from State ☐ Other (Specify): _____ |

| 19. PLACE OF DISPOSITION (Name of cemetery, crematory, other place) |

| 20. LOCATION-CITY, TOWN, AND STATE | 21. NAME AND COMPLETE ADDRESS OF FUNERAL FACILITY |

| 22. SIGNATURE OF FUNERAL SERVICE LICENSEE OR OTHER AGENT | 23. LICENSE NUMBER (Of Licensee) |

| ITEMS 24–28 MUST BE COMPLETED BY PERSON WHO PRONOUNCES OR CERTIFIES DEATH | 24. DATE PRONOUNCED DEAD (Mo/Day/Yr) | 25. TIME PRONOUNCED DEAD |

| 26. SIGNATURE OF PERSON PRONOUNCING DEATH (Only when applicable) | 27. LICENSE NUMBER | 28. DATE SIGNED (Mo/Day/Yr) |

| 29. ACTUAL OR PRESUMED DATE OF DEATH (Mo/Day/Yr) (Spell Month) | 30. ACTUAL OR PRESUMED TIME OF DEATH | 31. WAS MEDICAL EXAMINER OR CORONER CONTACTED? ☐ Yes ☐ No |

CAUSE OF DEATH (See instructions and examples)

32. PART I. Enter the chain of events—diseases, injuries, or complications—that directly caused the death. DO NOT enter terminal events such as cardiac arrest, respiratory arrest, or ventricular fibrillation without showing the etiology. DO NOT ABBREVIATE. Enter only one cause on a line. Add additional lines if necessary.

Approximate interval: Onset to death

IMMEDIATE CAUSE (Final disease or condition resulting in death)--------->   a. _____

Sequentially list conditions, if any, leading to the cause listed on line a.   b. _____   Due to (or as a consequence of):

Enter the **UNDERLYING CAUSE** (disease or injury that initiated the events resulting in death) **LAST**   c. _____   Due to (or as a consequence of):

    d. _____   Due to (or as a consequence of):

PART II. Enter other significant conditions contributing to death but not resulting in the underlying cause given in PART I.

| 33. WAS AN AUTOPSY PERFORMED? ☐ Yes ☐ No |
| 34. WERE AUTOPSY FINDINGS AVAILABLE TO COMPLETE THE CAUSE OF DEATH? ☐ Yes ☐ No |

| 35. DID TOBACCO USE CONTRIBUTE TO DEATH? ☐ Yes ☐ No ☐ Probably ☐ Unknown | 36. IF FEMALE: ☐ Not pregnant within past year ☐ Not pregnant, but pregnant within 42 days of death ☐ Unknown if pregnant within the past year ☐ Pregnant at time of death ☐ Not pregnant, but pregnant 43 days to 1 year before death | 37. MANNER OF DEATH ☐ Natural ☐ Homicide ☐ Accident ☐ Pending Investigation ☐ Suicide ☐ Could not be determined |

| 38. DATE OF INJURY (Mo/Day/Yr) (Spell Month) | 39. TIME OF INJURY | 40. PLACE OF INJURY (e.g., Decedent's home; construction site; restaurant; wooded area) | 41. INJURY AT WORK? ☐ Yes ☐ No |

| 42. LOCATION OF INJURY: State: ___ Street & Number: ___ | City or Town: ___ Apartment No.: ___ | Zip Code: ___ |

| 43. DESCRIBE HOW INJURY OCCURRED: | 44. IF TRANSPORTATION INJURY, SPECIFY: ☐ Driver/Operator ☐ Passenger ☐ Pedestrian ☐ Other (Specify) |

| 45. CERTIFIER (Check only one): ☐ Certifying physician—To the best of my knowledge, death occurred due to the cause(s) and manner stated. ☐ Pronouncing and Certifying physician—To the best of my knowledge, death occurred at the time, date, and place, and due to the cause(s) and manner stated. | ☐ Medical examiner/Coroner—On the basis of examination, and/or investigation, in my opinion, death occurred at the time, date, and place, and due to the cause(s) and manner stated. Signature of certifier: _____ |

| 46. NAME, ADDRESS, AND ZIP CODE OF PERSON COMPLETING CAUSE OF DEATH (Item 32) |

| 47. TITLE OF CERTIFIER | 48. LICENSE NUMBER | 49. DATE CERTIFIED (Mo/Day/Yr) | 50. FOR REGISTRAR ONLY—DATE FILED (Mo/Day/Yr) |

| 51. DECEDENT'S EDUCATION (Check the box that best describes the highest degree or level of school completed at the time of death) ☐ 8th grade or less ☐ 9th–12th grade; no diploma ☐ High school graduate or GED completed ☐ Some college credit, but no degree ☐ Associate degree (e.g., AA, AS) ☐ Bachelor's degree (e.g., BA, AB, BS) ☐ Master's degree (e.g., MA, MS, MEng, MEd, MSW, MBA) ☐ Doctorate (e.g., PhD, EdD) or Professional degree (e.g., MD, DDS, DVM, LLB, JD) | 52. DECEDENT OF HISPANIC ORIGIN? (Check the box that best describes whether the decedent is Spanish/Hispanic/Latino. Check the "No" box if decedent is not Spanish/Hispanic/Latino) ☐ No, not Spanish/Hispanic/Latino ☐ Yes, Mexican, Mexican American, Chicano ☐ Yes, Puerto Rican ☐ Yes, Cuban ☐ Yes, other Spanish/Hispanic/Latino (Specify) _____ | 53. DECEDENT'S RACE (Check one or more races to indicate what the decedent considered himself or herself to be) ☐ White ☐ Black or African American ☐ American Indian or Alaska Native (Name of the enrolled or principal tribe) ____ ☐ Asian Indian ☐ Chinese ☐ Filipino ☐ Japanese ☐ Korean ☐ Vietnamese ☐ Other Asian (Specify) ____ ☐ Native Hawaiian ☐ Guamanian or Chamorro ☐ Samoan ☐ Other Pacific Islander (Specify) ____ ☐ Other (Specify) ____ |

| 54. DECEDENT'S USUAL OCCUPATION (Indicate type of work done during most of working life. DO NOT USE RETIRED) | 55. KIND OF BUSINESS/INDUSTRY |

FIGURE 4-2 Sample of U.S. Standard Certificate of Death.

Cause-of-death—Background, Examples, and Common Problems
Accurate cause of death information is important
•to the public health community in evaluating and improving the health of all citizens, and
•often to the family, now and in the future, and to the person settling the decedent's estate.

The cause-of-death section consists of two parts. **Part I** is for reporting a chain of events leading directly to death, with the **immediate cause** of death (the final disease, injury, or complication directly causing death) on line a and the **underlying cause** of death (the disease or injury that initiated the chain of events that led directly and inevitably to death) on the lowest used line. **Part II** is for reporting all other significant diseases, conditions, or injuries that contributed to death but which did not result in the underlying cause of death given in Part I. **The cause-of-death information should be YOUR best medical OPINION.** A condition can be listed as "probable" even if it has not been definitively diagnosed.

Examples of properly completed medical certifications:

CAUSE OF DEATH (See instructions and examples)	Approximate interval:
32. PART I. Enter the <u>chain of events</u>—diseases, injuries, or complications—that directly caused the death. DO NOT enter terminal events such as cardiac arrest, respiratory arrest, or ventricular fibrillation without showing the etiology. DO NOT ABBREVIATE. Enter only one cause on a line. Add additional lines if necessary.	Onset to death
IMMEDIATE CAUSE (Final disease or condition ------> resulting in death) a. Rupture of myocardium	Minutes
Due to (or as a consequence of):	
Sequentially list conditions, if any, leading to the cause listed on line a. b. Acute myocardial infarction	6 days
Due to (or as a consequence of):	
Enter the **UNDERLYING CAUSE** c. Coronary artery thrombosis	5 years
(disease or injury that initiated the Due to (or as a consequence of):	
events resulting in death) **LAST** d. Atherosclerotic coronary artery disease	7 years

PART II. Enter other <u>significant conditions contributing to death</u> but not resulting in the underlying cause given in PART I.	33. WAS AN AUTOPSY PERFORMED? ■ Yes ☐ No
Diabetes, Chronic obstructive pulmonary disease, smoking	34. WERE AUTOPSY FINDINGS AVAILABLE TO COMPLETE THE CAUSE OF DEATH? ■ Yes ☐ No

35. DID TOBACCO USE CONTRIBUTE TO DEATH?	36. IF FEMALE:	37. MANNER OF DEATH
■ Yes ☐ Probably ☐ No ☐ Unknown	■ Not pregnant within past year ☐ Not pregnant, but pregnant within 42 days of death ☐ Not pregnant, but pregnant ☐ Unknown if pregnant within the past year 43 days to 1 year before death ☐ Pregnant at time of death	■ Natural ☐ Homicide ☐ Accident ☐ Pending Investigation ☐ Suicide ☐ Could not be determined

CAUSE OF DEATH (See instructions and examples)	Approximate interval:
32. PART I. Enter the *chain of events*—diseases, injuries, or complications—that directly caused the death. DO NOT enter terminal events such as cardiac arrest, respiratory arrest, or ventricular fibrillation without showing the etiology. DO NOT ABBREVIATE. Enter only one cause on a line. Add additional lines if necessary.	Onset to death
IMMEDIATE CAUSE (Final disease or condition ------> resulting in death) a. Aspiration pneumonia	2 Days
Due to (or as a consequence of):	
Sequentially list conditions, if any, leading to the cause listed on line a. b. Complications of coma	7 weeks
Due to (or as a consequence of):	
Enter the **UNDERLYING CAUSE** c. Blunt force injuries	7 weeks
(disease or injury that initiated the Due to (or as a consequence of):	
events resulting in death) **LAST** d. Motor vehicle accident	7 weeks

PART II. Enter other *significant conditions contributing to death* but not resulting in the underlying cause given in PART I.	33. WAS AN AUTOPSY PERFORMED? ■ Yes ☐ No
	34. WERE AUTOPSY FINDINGS AVAILABLE TO COMPLETE THE CAUSE OF DEATH? ■ Yes ☐ No

35. DID TOBACCO USE CONTRIBUTE TO DEATH?	36. IF FEMALE:	37. MANNER OF DEATH
☐ Yes ☐ Probably ■ No ☐ Unknown	☐ Not pregnant within past year ☐ Not pregnant, but pregnant within 42 days of death ☐ Not pregnant, but pregnant ☐ Unknown if pregnant within the past year 43 days to 1 year before death ☐ Pregnant at time of death	☐ Natural ☐ Homicide ■ Accident ☐ Pending Investigation ☐ Suicide ☐ Could not be determined

38. DATE OF INJURY (Mo/Day/Yr) (Spell Month) August 15, 2003	39. TIME OF INJURY Approx. 2320	40. PLACE OF INJURY (e.g., Decedent's home; construction site; restaurant; wooded area) road side near state highway	41. INJURY AT WORK? ☐ Yes ■ No

42. LOCATION OF INJURY: State: Missouri   City or Town: near Alexandria
Street & Number: Mile marker 17 on state route 46a   Apartment No.:   Zip Code:

43. DESCRIBE HOW INJURY OCCURRED: Decedent driver of van, ran off road into tree	44. IF TRANSPORTATION INJURY, SPECIFY: ■ Driver/Operator ☐ Passenger ☐ Pedestrian ☐ Other (Specify) _____

FIGURE 4-2 Continued Sample of U.S. Standard Certificate of Death.

in 1900 and have been revised about every 10 years by the World Health Organization. The 10th revision of the ICD has been used to classify mortality information for statistical purposes since 1999, and the 11th revision is being released in 2018.

Any time that the ICD is revised, a number of artifactual changes in the mortality statistics typically occur. Some revisions have led to small changes, and others have resulted in large ones. For example, male and female breast cancer used to be grouped together but now are classified separately. Because male breast cancer is so rare, comprising less than 1% of all breast cancers,[4] it is unlikely that this change made much of a difference in breast cancer mortality data. On the other hand, a large increase in Alzheimer's disease deaths is attributed in part to changes in the ICD classification of this disease.[5] Most of the increase is from diagnoses previously considered as presenile dementia being reclassified as Alzheimer's disease.

Death record information in the United States has been computerized at a national level since 1979.[6] The National Death Index is administered by the NCHS. Epidemiologists often use this data source to determine whether study subjects have died. It is necessary to write to individual state offices to acquire copies of death certificates for information on cause of death.

National data on fetal deaths are kept separately by the NCHS. These data have been reported in the United States and District of Columbia since 1982.[7] However, fetal death reporting depends on state requirements; most states require reporting deaths that occur at 20 or more weeks of gestational age. Because most pregnancy losses occur earlier in gestation, the reported data represent only a small proportion of pregnancy losses.

▶ National Survey of Family Growth

The purpose of this survey is to "provide reliable national data on marriage, divorce, contraception, infertility, and the health of women and infants in the United States," including information on sexual activity, marriage, contraception, sterilization, infertility, breastfeeding, pregnancy loss, low birth weight, use of medical care for infertility, family planning, and prenatal care.[8] To date, nine surveys have been conducted from 1973 to 2015.

Over time, the National Survey of Family Growth (NSFG) has expanded in scope and coverage. For example, women who have never been married were excluded from the first two surveys but were included in the later ones. Men were included for the first time in the 2002 survey. The 2013–2015 survey was based on a national sample of 10,205 men and women aged 15 to 44 years from the noninstitutionalized population of all 50 states. Statistical weighting procedures were applied to produce estimates for the entire country. In-person interviews were conducted by trained interviewers. Questions for women focused on their ability to become pregnant, pregnancy history, use of contraceptives, family planning, infertility services, breastfeeding, maternity leave, childcare, and adoption. Questions for men also focused on their reproductive health, including nonmarital childbearing and child support. In 2016, the 2013–2015 NSFG data files, including information from over 10,000 interviews along with code books and relevant documentation, were released for public use.

▶ National Health Interview Survey

Mandated by the National Health Survey Act of 1956, the National Health Interview Survey (NHIS) is currently the principal source of information on the health of the civilian noninstitutionalized population of the United States.[9] Administered on a yearly basis since 1957, the NHIS provides data on major health problems, including incidence of acute illnesses and injuries, prevalence of chronic conditions and impairments, and utilization of health services. The data are used to monitor trends in illness and disability and to track progress toward achieving national health objectives.

NHIS uses a stratified, multistage sampling scheme to select a sample of households that form a representative sample of the target population. Each year, approximately 39,000 households, including approximately 97,200 people, are selected for interview. Participation is voluntary, but more than 90% of eligible households respond each year. Nonresponse stems mainly from refusal or the inability to find eligible individuals in a household. Survey results are statistically weighted and adjusted for nonresponse to produce national estimates.

Personal interviews are conducted by the permanent interviewer staff from the Bureau of the Census. All adult household members aged 17 years and older who are home at the time of the survey are invited to participate and respond for themselves. A responsible adult aged 18 and older also responds for adults who are not at home and for children. Every year, basic demographic and health information is collected on age; race; gender; educational level; family income; and acute and chronic conditions and associated disability days, physician visits, and hospital stays. Supplemental data collection on special health topics varies from year to year.

▶ National Health and Nutrition Examination Survey

Since 1960, NCHS has conducted the National Health and Nutrition Examination Survey (NHANES) to gather information on the health and diet of the U.S. population.[10] Participants are selected using a census-based stratified random sample. The survey includes both a home interview and health tests done in a mobile examination center. The current NHANES, the eighth in this series of surveys, was started in 1999 and will continually survey 15 locations throughout the United States and enroll 5,000 people each year.

▶ Behavioral Risk Factor Surveillance System

The Behavioral Risk Factor Surveillance System is a telephone health survey that was established in 1984 with 15 states and is now conducted in all 50 states, the District of Columbia, and three U.S. territories.[11] The purpose of this state-based survey is to monitor a wide variety of health risk behaviors that are related to chronic disease, injuries, and death, including use of screening and preventive services, smoking, alcohol use, physical activities, fruit and vegetable consumption, seat belt use, and weight control. Participants are adults from randomly selected households. About 400,000 interviews are conducted annually, making it one of the largest continuous telephone surveys in the world.

▶ National Health Care Surveys

The National Health Care Surveys provide information on the use and quality of health care and the effect of medical technology in a wide variety of settings, including hospital inpatient and outpatient departments, emergency rooms, hospices, home health agencies, and medical professionals' offices.[12] The following paragraphs describe the component surveys.

The National Hospital Discharge Survey (NHDS) was a national probability survey that was conducted annually from 1965 to 2010. Its purpose was to collect information, including data on diagnoses, procedures, length of stay, and characteristics of inpatients discharged from nonfederal short-stay hospitals in the United States.

The National Hospital Ambulatory Medical Care Survey (NHAMCS) began in 1992 to collect information on the utilization and provision of ambulatory services in hospital emergency and outpatient departments. The annual survey is based on a national sample of visits to the emergency and outpatient departments of noninstitutional general and short-stay hospitals in all 50 states and the District of Columbia. A random sample of visits during a randomly assigned 4-week period is chosen from randomly selected facilities. Data are collected on patient demographics, diagnostic and screening services, therapeutic and preventive services, surgical procedures, and facility characteristics.

In 2012, the National Hospital Care Survey (NHCS) began incorporating data formerly collected from the NHDS, emergency department and outpatient department data collected by the NHAMCS, and substance-involved visit data previously collected by the Drug Abuse Warning Network (DAWN). Its purpose is to describe national patterns of healthcare delivery across treatment settings using a new sample of hospitals and a sample of freestanding ambulatory surgery centers. It will also be possible to link these survey data to outside data sources, such as the National Death Index, to obtain a more complete picture of patient care.[13]

The National Ambulatory Medical Care Survey (NAMCS), which has been conducted since 1973, collects information on the provision and use of ambulatory medical services in the United States. The survey is based on a sample of visits to non–federally employed office-based physicians who are primarily engaged in direct patient care. Specialists, such as anesthesiologists, pathologists, and radiologists, are excluded. Data are collected from the physician, not the patient. Each physician is randomly assigned to a 1-week reporting period. Information is obtained on demographic characteristics of patients and services provided for a random sample of visits during the reporting period.

In 2012, NCHS initiated the National Study of Long-Term Care Providers (NSLTCP), a biennial study of adult day services centers, residential care communities, nursing homes, home health agencies, and hospice agencies. NSLTCP uses administrative data for the nursing home sector obtained from the Centers for Medicare and Medicaid Services (CMS) to monitor trends in the supply, provision, and use of the major sectors of paid, regulated long-term care services.[14]

▶ National Notifiable Diseases Surveillance System

Managed by the Centers for Disease Control and Prevention (CDC) and the Council of State and Territorial Epidemiologists, the National Notifiable Diseases Surveillance System (NNDSS) collects weekly provisional data and compiles annual summaries on the occurrence of more than 60 notifiable diseases throughout the United States.[15] The CDC's *Morbidity and Mortality Weekly Report* (*MMWR*)[16] defines a notifiable disease as "one for which regular, frequent and timely information regarding individual cases is considered necessary for the prevention and control of the disease." Nationally notifiable conditions in 2017 included human immunodeficiency virus (HIV) infection, botulism, gonorrhea, all forms of hepatitis, malaria, plague, human and animal rabies, syphilis, toxic shock syndrome, elevated blood lead levels, severe acute respiratory syndrome (SARS), and Zika virus disease and infection. Reports of notifiable diseases are sent to the CDC voluntarily by the 50 states, New York City, the District of Columbia, and five U.S. territories. Completeness of reporting depends on the disease and local notification practices. *Morbidity and Mortality Weekly Report* publishes weekly reports and annual summaries of these diseases.

▶ Surveillance of HIV Infection

Since 1985, the CDC has collected information on the occurrence of HIV cases from all 50 states; the District of Columbia; and U.S. dependencies, possessions, and independent associated countries (such as Puerto Rico).[17] The HIV surveillance case definitions have been modified several times to improve the accuracy of reporting. Every change in definition has led to artifactual changes in incidence estimates. The stages of HIV infection in the 2014 case definition are based on age-specific CD4 lymphocyte counts or percentages of total lymphocytes. The definition includes three categories of HIV infection increasing in severity from stage 1 through stage 3 (AIDS) based on CD4 T lymphocyte count; an unknown stage and a stage 0, where a negative test result occurs within 6 months before the first positive HIV test result, also are included. For every person meeting the HIV case definition, data are gathered on demographic characteristics, exposure category (such as injecting drug users and men who have sex with men), AIDS-defining conditions (such as Kaposi's sarcoma and *Pneumocystis carinii* pneumonia), and diagnosis date.

▶ Reproductive Health Statistics

The CDC Division of Reproductive Health (DRH) monitors maternal and infant mortality and collects data on maternal and infant morbidity, adverse behaviors during pregnancy, and long-term consequences of pregnancy.[18] The major surveillance systems in the division are outlined below.

The Pregnancy Risk Assessment Monitoring System (PRAMS) was developed in 1987 to collect data on maternal attitudes and experiences before, during, and shortly after pregnancy. PRAMS surveillance currently covers about 83% of all U.S. births. The PRAMS questionnaire is revised periodically. With each revision or new phase of the questionnaire, some of the questions change. Although most indicators can be compared across phases, it is often easier to analyze data within a single phase. Eight phases of the study have been conducted since 1988.[19]

The National Assisted Reproductive Technology Surveillance System (NASS) collects data from all 440 clinics in the United States that provide services to patients seeking to overcome infertility. NASS collects data on patient demographics, patient obstetrical and medical history, parental infertility diagnosis, clinical parameters of the Assisted Reproductive Technology (ART) procedure, and information regarding resultant pregnancies and births. Data are cycle specific, and data from women who undergo multiple cycles in one year are unlinked.[20]

The Pregnancy Mortality Surveillance System (PMSS) collects information from 52 reporting areas (50 states, New York City, and Washington, DC). Copies of death certificates for all women who died during pregnancy or within 1 year of pregnancy and copies of the matching birth or fetal death certificates are reviewed by the CDC.[21]

CDC also collaborated with organizations to develop the Sudden Unexpected Infant Death (SUID) Case Registry, which seeks to improve population-based SUID surveillance in 16 states and 2 jurisdictions. Reports are generated from these systems on a routine ongoing basis.[22]

Since 1969, the CDC has maintained a surveillance system to document the number and characteristics of women obtaining abortions, monitor unintended pregnancies, and assist in the effort to eliminate preventable morbidity and mortality associated with abortions.[23] The CDC receives annual reports on the number and characteristics of women obtaining legal abortions from centralized state reporting systems, hospitals, and other medical facilities in almost all states, the District of Columbia, and New York City. Data are collected on the type of abortion procedure; the number of weeks' gestation when the abortion was performed; and the patient's age, race, and marital status. The Alan Guttmacher Institute, the research and development division of the Planned Parenthood Federation of America, Inc., also conducts annual surveys of abortion providers, including hospitals, nonhospital clinics, and physicians.

▶ National Immunization Survey

Several surveys, including the National Immunization Survey, currently collect information on the immunization coverage of children in the United States.[24] The National Immunization Survey began in 1994 as a continuing survey to provide estimates of vaccination coverage among children aged 19 to 35 months in 78 geographic areas designated as "Immunization Action Plan areas." These areas consist of the 50 states, the District of Columbia, and 27 large urban areas. Vaccinations included in the survey are diphtheria and tetanus toxoids, acellular pertussis vaccine, poliovirus vaccine, measles–mumps–rubella vaccine, hepatitis B vaccine, and influenza vaccine. The survey is administered to households via random digit dialing as well as vaccination providers. The latter are identified by parents who respond to the household survey.

In addition to children aged 19 to 35 months, vaccination data are also available for kindergarten-aged children. Each school year, states and local areas report the estimated number of children attending kindergarten who have received vaccinations recommended or required by their state or who have received an exemption to one or more required vaccinations. Teenage vaccination data are also available for local areas, states, and the nation from the National Immunization Survey-Teen (NIS-Teen). These vaccinations include human papillomavirus, whooping cough, and meningococcal vaccines.

The National Health Interview Survey[9] and the Behavioral Risk Factor Surveillance System,[11] described earlier, also collect information on immunizations among U.S. children and adults. Vaccinations included in the adult surveys include influenza, pneumococcal, whooping cough, and shingles vaccines.

▶ Survey of Occupational Injuries and Illnesses

Since 1972, the Department of Labor has gathered annual data on occupational injuries and illnesses among employees in the private sector.[25] Data are collected from a national sample of approximately 230,000 establishments representing the total private economy (except for mines and railroads). Self-employed individuals; small farm employees; and local, state, and federal government employees are excluded. Typically, about 95% of selected employers respond to the survey.

The survey data are based on records of injuries and illnesses that employers are required to maintain under the federal Occupational Safety and Health Act.[25] An occupational illness is defined as any abnormal condition or disorder, other than one resulting from an occupational injury, caused by exposure to factors associated with employment. It includes acute and chronic illnesses or diseases which may be caused by inhalation, absorption, ingestion, or direct contact.[25]

In addition, an occupational injury is defined as "any injury, such as a cut, fracture, sprain, amputation, and so forth, which results from a work-related event or from a single instantaneous exposure in the work environment."[25]

▶ National Survey on Drug Use and Health

Since 1971, the National Survey on Drug Use and Health (NSDUH) has obtained information on mental health issues, illicit drug use, alcohol use, and substance use disorders (SUDs).[26] The survey includes civilian, noninstitutionalized individuals living in all 50 states and aged 12 years and older and does not include homeless people not in shelters. In the 2015 survey, screening was completed at 132,210 addresses, and 68,073 completed interviews were obtained, including 16,955 interviews from adolescents aged 12 to 17 and 51,118 interviews from adults aged 18 or older. Recent changes in the survey instrument make it difficult to assess trends over time.

▶ Air Quality System

The federal Clean Air Act of 1970 requires the Environmental Protection Agency (EPA) to collect data on the levels of certain ambient air pollutants because they pose serious threats to public health.[27] These pollutants include particulate matter less than 10 microns in size, lead, carbon monoxide, sulfur dioxide, nitrogen dioxide, reactive volatile organic compounds, and ozone. Currently, more than 4,000 monitoring sites, located mainly in highly populated urban areas, provide data that are used to determine whether a particular geographic area complies with the National Ambient Air Quality Standards. These standards include an adequate margin of safety that protects even the most sensitive members of the population (such as asthmatics) and define a maximum concentration level for each pollutant that cannot be exceeded during a prescribed time period. The monitors send hourly or daily measurements of pollutant concentrations to EPA's Air Quality System (AQS) database.[28] It has every measured value the EPA has collected via the national ambient air monitoring program.

▶ Surveillance, Epidemiology and End Results Program

Mandated by the National Cancer Act, the Surveillance, Epidemiology and End Results (SEER) program has collected data on the prevention, diagnosis, and treatment of cancer in the United States since 1973.[29] In particular, the SEER program monitors trends in the incidence, mortality, and survival of about 40 types of cancer according to geographic and demographic characteristics.

Currently, SEER statistics are based on 18 population-based registries, including Connecticut, Hawaii, Iowa, New Mexico, Utah, California, Kentucky, Louisiana, New Jersey, Detroit, Atlanta, Seattle-Puget Sound, and selected counties and populations in Georgia, Arizona, and Alaska. The populations living in these areas cover about 30% of the U.S. population.

Reporting systems have been set up in each region to gather data on all newly diagnosed cancer cases among area residents. Information is gathered from a variety of sources, including medical records, death certificates, laboratories, and radiotherapy units, to ensure complete ascertainment of the cancer cases. Data are gathered on the cancer patients' demographic characteristics, primary cancer site (e.g., the lung), method of diagnostic confirmation (such as a pathology report), severity of the disease, and first mode of therapy. Patients are actively followed to provide survival information.

▶ Birth Defects Surveillance and Research Programs

From 1970 through 1994, the CDC operated the Birth Defects Monitoring Program (BDMP), the first national system for monitoring occurrence of congenital malformations.[30] The system was launched in part in response to the epidemic of limb reduction defects among children whose mothers had taken the sedative thalidomide during pregnancy in the 1960s.

While it was operating, BDMP was the largest single source of uniformly collected data on birth defects in the country. Collected data include dates of birth and discharge, diagnoses and surgical procedures, gender, race, and birth weight. BDMP data were reviewed quarterly to determine whether the prevalence of a birth defect had increased. If increases were identified, investigators explored both real and artifactual explanations, sometimes by conducting more detailed studies.

In 1998, Congress passed the Birth Defects Prevention Act, which authorized the CDC to (1) collect, analyze, and make available data on birth defects; (2) operate regional centers for applied epidemiological research on the prevention of birth defects; and (3) educate the public about the prevention of birth defects.[31] To date, nine Centers for Birth Defects Research have been established to accomplish this mission in Arkansas, California, Iowa, Massachusetts, New York, North Carolina, and Utah. The CDC also operates its own research center in Atlanta, Georgia, and provides funding to 14 additional states to help improve their birth defects surveillance activities.

▶ *Health, United States*

The publication *Health, United States* is one of the most comprehensive sources of information on the current health status of the U.S. population.[32] Published yearly, the report compiles information from various branches of the CDC (including the National Center for Health Statistics; the National Center for HIV, STD, and TB Prevention; and the Epidemiology Program Office), the Substance Abuse and Mental Health Services Administration, the National Institutes of Health (including the National Cancer Institute), and the Bureau of the Census. A compilation of data from these and other sources, this publication includes the most recent data on mortality, morbidity, health behaviors, reproductive health, healthcare access and utilization, and substance use. Each edition of *Health, United States* focuses on a major health topic. The 2015 edition included a special feature on racial and ethnic health disparities.

▶ *Demographic Yearbook*

Since 1948, the Statistical Office of the United Nations has compiled official demographic statistics from countries throughout the world for its annual *Demographic Yearbook*.[33] Currently, data are collected from over 230 countries and areas of the world on population size, distribution, and growth; births; deaths (including fetal, infant, and maternal mortality); and marriages and divorces. Because the *Demographic Yearbook* is intended for a broad audience, health data are reprinted for the World Health Statistics (described in the following section) to make them more readily accessible to medical and public health professionals. Because definitions of health events vary from country to country and some countries provide incomplete or inaccurate vital statistics and population data, the *Demographic Yearbook* data should be interpreted carefully.

▶ *World Health Statistics*

The World Health Organization (WHO) has reported international morbidity and mortality data since 1951.[34] Its most recent statistics are presented in *World Health Statistics 2016* and describe health indicators among WHO's 194 Member States. The data in these reports can be obtained from the WHO's Global Health Observatory (GHO), which provides access to country data and statistics with a focus on comparable estimates. Available data include mortality and burden of disease, health systems, environmental health, noncommunicable diseases, infectious diseases, health equity, and violence and injuries.[35]

▶ Cancer Incidence on Five Continents

Since the 1960s, WHO's International Agency for Research on Cancer (IARC) has collected data on cancer incidence and mortality from many countries around the world.[36] Most of the registries rely on medical records, laboratory records, and death certificates as their data sources. All registries record the cancer case's name, address, gender, and cancer site. Most registries also collect information on age or date of birth, occupation, and the method of cancer diagnosis. The IARC processes the submitted data, assessing its quality, completeness, and comparability. The IARC publishes the information every few years in a monograph titled *Cancer Incidence on Five Continents*. The latest volume presents cancer incidence data from 68 countries, 290 cancer registries, and 424 populations. A main goal of the monograph is to allow comparisons of incidence across populations and over time that will lead to the formulation of hypotheses about the causes of cancer. Data should be interpreted carefully given variations between cancer registries, including variations in populations, the methods used to collect data on new cases, and the sources of data accessed.

▶ Other Resources

A number of additional sources of information are collected by state and local health departments.

- *State cancer registries:* In addition to the SEER cancer registries, almost all U.S. states currently have population-based cancer registries. For example, the Massachusetts Cancer Registry began operation in 1982 and uses a system of hospital-based tumor registrars to collect data on cancer incidence. Compilation of these data has enabled the Massachusetts registry to monitor trends in cancer incidence over time and according to demographic characteristics, such as age, gender, race, and geographic area.[37]
- *Internet resources:* Numerous data sources are available through the Internet. Because the quality of information on the Internet is often unknown, it is best to rely on only resources from the U.S. government and other reliable sources. For example, the home page for the National Center for Health Statistics is located at www.cdc.gov/nchs/index.htm.
- *Wide-Ranging Online Data for Epidemiologic Research (WONDER):* This computerized information system provides online access to a wide variety of epidemiological and public health datasets.[38] WONDER has data and documentation for many of the data sources

listed in this chapter and allows the user to access both published documents and public use datasets about mortality, cancer incidence, HIV, behavioral risk factors, diabetes, births, and census data. WONDER can be accessed through the Internet at wonder.cdc.gov.

- *Data.gov:* Under the terms of the 2013 Federal Open Data Policy, newly generated government data are required to be made available in open, machine-readable formats and ensure privacy and security. Data.gov is managed and hosted by the U.S. General Services Administration, Technology Transformation Service, and it provides data, tools, and resources to conduct research, develop Web and mobile applications, and design data visualizations.[39] Data.gov does not host data directly but rather aggregates metadata about open data resources in one centralized location. Both data.gov and healthdata.gov offer datasets, tools, and applications related to health and health care.

Summary

Many sources of information are readily available on a wide variety of health-related states and events, including diseases, injuries, disabilities, and death among individuals living in the United States and around the world. The types and sources of information described in this chapter are summarized in **TABLE 4-1**. When interpreting data from these sources, it is important to consider (1) the population about which the information was obtained, (2) the calendar period that was covered, and (3) the level of missing and inaccurate data. It is also important to know about any changes in data collection methods that may have created artifactual changes in the frequency of disease.

TABLE 4-1 Sources of Public Health Data

Type of information	Source of information
Population size and characteristics	U.S. Census, Bureau of Census, Department of Commerce
Births	National Vital Statistics System, National Center for Health Statistics
Deaths	National Vital Statistics System, National Death Index, National Center for Health Statistics
Fetal deaths	Fetal Death Data, National Center for Health Statistics
Childbearing, adoption, maternal and child health, family planning	National Survey of Family Growth, National Center for Health Statistics

Major health problems and utilization of health services	National Health Interview Survey, National Center for Health Statistics
Indicators of nutrition and health	National Health and Nutrition Examination Survey, National Center for Health Statistics
Use and quality of health care in a wide variety of settings	National Health Care Survey, National Center for Health Statistics
Notifiable diseases	National Notifiable Diseases Surveillance System, Centers for Disease Control and Prevention
HIV	HIV Surveillance, Centers for Disease Control and Prevention
Cancer incidence, mortality, and survival	Surveillance, Epidemiology and End Results Program; National Cancer Institute; state cancer registries
Birth defects	Birth Defects Surveillance, Center for Birth Defects Research and Prevention, Centers for Disease Control and Prevention
Reproductive health	Pregnancy Risk Assessment Monitoring System; Pregnancy Mortality Surveillance System; National Assisted Reproductive Technology Surveillance System; Sudden Unexpected Infant Death (SUID) Case Registry; Abortion Surveillance System, Centers for Disease Control and Prevention; Alan Guttmaker Institute; Planned Parenthood Federation of America
Immunizations	National Immunization Survey; National Health Interview Survey; Behaviorial Risk Factor Surveillance System; National Center for Health Statistics, Centers for Disease Control and Prevention
Occupational health	Survey of Occupational Injuries and Illnesses, U.S. Department of Labor
Behaviors affecting health	Behavioral Risk Factor Surveillance System, Centers for Disease Control and Prevention
Alcohol, cigarette, drug use, and mental health	National Survey on Drug Use and Health, Substance Abuse and Mental Health Services Administration
Air pollutant levels	Air Quality System, Environmental Protection Agency

References

1. *Congressional Apportionment: 2010 Census Briefs.* census.gov. http://www.census.gov/prod/cen2010 /briefs/c2010br-08.pdf.IssuedNovember2011.Accessed April 2017.

2. *Census Coverage Measurement Estimation Report: Summary of Estimates of Coverage for Persons in the United States.* census.gov. https://www.census.gov /coverage_measurement/pdfs/g01.pdf. Published May 22, 2012. Accessed December 2017.

3. National Vital Statistics System. cdc.gov. http://www .cdc.gov/nchs/nvss/index.htm. Accessed April 2017.

4. Sasco AJ, Lowenfels AB, Pasker-de Jong J. Review article: epidemiology of male breast cancer: a meta-analysis of published case-control studies and discussion of selected aetiological factors. *Int J Cancer* 1993;53(4):538-549.

5. Anderson RN, Miniño AM, Hoyert DL, Rosenberg HM. Comparability of cause of death between ICD-9 and ICD-10: preliminary estimates. *Natl Vital Stat Rep.* 2001;49(2):1-32.

6. Bernier RH, Watson VM, Nowell A, et al. (eds.). *Episource: A Guide to Resources in Epidemiology.* 2nd ed. Roswell, GA: The Epidemiology Monitor; 1998.

7. MacDorman MF, Kirmeyer S. Fetal and perinatal mortality, United States, 2005. *Natl Vital Stat Rep.* 2009;57(8):1-19.

8. National Survey of Family Growth. cdc.gov. http:// www.cdc.gov/nchs/nsfg.htm. Accessed April 2017.

9. National Health Interview Survey (NHIS). cdc.gov. http://www.cdc.gov/nchs/nhis/about_nhis.htm. Accessed April 2017.

10. National Health and Nutrition Examination Survey. cdc.gov. http://www.cdc.gov/nchs/nhanes/index.htm. Accessed April 2017.

11. Behavioral Risk Factor Surveillance System. cdc.gov. http://www.cdc.gov/brfss. Accessed April 2017.

12. National Health Care Surveys. cdc.gov. http://www .cdc.gov/nchs/dhcs/index.htm. Accessed April 2017.

13. National Hospital Care Survey. cdc.gov. https://www .cdc.gov/nchs/nhcs/index.htm. Accessed April 2017.

14. National Study of Long-Term Care Providers. cdc.gov. https://www.cdc.gov/nchs/nsltcp/index.htm.Accessed April 2017.

15. National Notifiable Diseases Surveillance System (NNDSS). cdc.gov. http://www.cdc.gov/nndss. Accessed April 2017.

16. Summary of Notifiable Infectious Diseases and Conditions—United States, 2014. cdc.gov. *MMWR.* 2016;63(54). https://www.cdc.gov/mmwr/volumes /63/wr/mm6354a1.htm?s_cid=mm6354a1_w. Accessed April 2017.

17. HIV/AIDS Surveillance Report: Diagnoses of HIV Infection in the United States and Dependent Areas, 2015. cdc.gov. https://www.cdc.gov/hiv/pdf/library /reports/surveillance/cdc-hiv-surveillance-report -2015-vol-27.pdf. Published November 2016. Accessed April 2017.

18. Reproductive Health: Data and Statistics. cdc.gov. https://www.cdc.gov/reproductivehealth/data_stats /index.htm. Accessed April 2017.

19. Pregnancy Risk Assessment Monitoring System (PRAMS). cdc.gov. https://www.cdc.gov/prams/index .htm. Accessed April 2017.

20. Assisted Reproductive Technology (ART): National ART Surveillance. cdc.gov. https://www.cdc.gov/art /nass/index.html. Accessed April 2017.

21. Pregnancy Mortality Surveillance System. cdc.gov. https://www.cdc.gov/reproductivehealth /maternalinfanthealth/pmss.html. Accessed April 2017.

22. SUID and SDY Case Registries. cdc.gov. https://www .cdc.gov/sids/caseregistry.htm. Accessed April 2017.

23. Abortion Surveillance System. cdc.gov. https://www .cdc.gov/reproductivehealth/data_stats/abortion .htm. Accessed April 2017.

24. VaxView. cdc.gov. https://www.cdc.gov/vaccines /vaxview/index.html. Accessed April 2017.

25. Handbook of Methods. bls.gov. http://www.bls.gov /opub/hom/homch9.htm. Accessed April 2017.

26. Key Substance Use and Mental Health Indicators in the United States: Results from the 2015 National Survey on Drug Use and Health. samhsa.gov. https://www .samhsa.gov/data/sites/default/files/NSDUH-FFR1 -2015/NSDUH-FFR1-2015/NSDUH-FFR1-2015.pdf. Accessed April 2017.

27. The Aerometric Information Retrieval System (AIRS) Data System—The National Repository for EPA Air Pollution Data. gcmd.nasa.gov. https://gcmd.nasa.gov /records/GCMD_AIRS_EPA.html. Accessed April 2017.

28. Air Data: Air Quality Data Collected at Outdoor Monitors Across the US. epa.gov. https://www.epa.gov /outdoor-air-quality-data. Accessed April 2017.

29. Howlader N, Noone AM, Krapcho M, Miller D, Bishop K, Kosary CL, et al. (eds). *SEER Cancer Statistics Review, 1975–2014.* cancer.gov. https://seer .cancer.gov/csr/1975_2014/. Published April 2017. Accessed April 2017.

30. Edmonds LD, Layde PM, James LM, Flynt JW, Erickson JD, Oakley GP. Congenital malformations surveillance: two American systems. *Int J Epidemiol.* 1981;10:247-252.

31. Birth Defects. cdc.gov. http://www.cdc.gov/ncbddd /birthdefects/research.html. Accessed April 2017.

32. National Center for Health Statistics. *Health, United States, 2010, With Special Feature on Racial and Ethnic Health Disparities.* Hyattsville, MD: Government Printing Office; 2016.

33. Statistics Division—Demographic and Social Statistics. *Demographic Yearbook*; 2016:66. un.org. https://unstats.un.org/unsd/demographic/products/dyb/dyb2015.htm. Accessed April 2017.

34. *World Health Statistics 2016: Monitoring Health for the SDGs*. World Health Organization. http://www.who.int/gho/publications/world_health_statistics/2016/en/. Accessed April 2017.

35. Global Health Observatory (GHO) data. who.int. http://www.who.int/gho/en/. Accessed April 2017.

36. Forman D, Bray F, Brewster DH, Gombe Mbalawa C, Kohler B, Piñeros M, et al. (eds.). *Cancer Incidence in Five Continents*. Vol. X. Lyon: International Agency for Research on Cancer; 2014. http://www.iarc.fr/en/publications/pdfs-online/epi/sp164. Accessed June 8, 2018.

37. National Program of Cancer Registries (NPCR). cdc.gov. https://www.cdc.gov/cancer/npcr/. Accessed April 2017.

38. CDC WONDER. cdc.gov. http://wonder.cdc.gov. Accessed April 2017.

39. The home of the U.S. Government's open data. data.gov. https://www.data.gov/. Accessed April 2017.

Chapter Questions

1. Undercounting in the U.S. Census could affect the accuracy of which of the following epidemiological activities?
   a. Assessing the prevalence of a disease in the U.S. population
   b. Assessing the incidence of a disease in the U.S. population
   c. Comparing the occurrence of disease in different segments of the U.S. population
   d. All of the above

2. Over the period 2002–2012, the Centers for Disease Control and Prevention estimated that the prevalence of autism spectrum disorder in the United States increased by 121% from 6.6 to 14.6 per 1,000 children. Among the possible explanations for this marked increase are
   a. The incidence of the disorder truly increased
   b. Awareness of the disorder increased and therefore previously unrecognized cases were more likely to be identified and diagnosed
   c. Both A and B

3. In 2012, the American Psychiatric Association proposed that the definition of autism spectrum disorder be narrowed. Under their new definition, a person needs to exhibit three deficits in social interaction and at least two repetitive behaviors. This is a much stricter standard than previously used. Assuming no changes in diagnosis and reporting, what effect would having a stricter disease definition have on the incidence of this disorder?
   a. The incidence would increase
   b. The incidence would decrease
   c. The incidence would remain the same

4. The United Nations collects data on infant mortality from over 230 countries around the world for its annual *Demographic Yearbook*. The *Yearbook* defines infant mortality as infant deaths of liveborn infants under 1 year of age. List two reasons why it is difficult to make accurate comparisons of infant mortality rates across so many diverse countries.

CHAPTER 5

Descriptive Epidemiology

▶ Introduction

Epidemiology is defined as the study of the distribution and determinants of disease frequency in human populations and the application of this study to control health problems.[1(p1),2(p95)] Distribution of disease is the domain of **descriptive epidemiology**, which involves the analysis of disease patterns according to the characteristics of person, place, and time. In other words, epidemiologists seek answers to the questions: Who is getting the disease? Where is it occurring? and How is it changing over time? Variations in disease occurrence by these three characteristics provide useful information for understanding the health status of a population; formulating hypotheses about the causes of disease; and planning, implementing, and evaluating public health programs to control and prevent adverse health events. This chapter describes the components and uses of descriptive epidemiology and then provides examples of analyses of the patterns of death and three important diseases in the United States.

▶ **Person**

Personal characteristics that are usually available for descriptive epidemiology include age, gender, race and ethnic group, socioeconomic status, occupation, religion, and marital status. These attributes can be associated with major variations in disease occurrence. Age is probably the most important among them because it is associated with striking changes in disease rates. The frequency of most diseases increases with age. For example, the prevalence of hypertension among adults in the period from 2011 to 2014 increased steadily with age from 7.3% of 18 to 39 year olds to 64.9% of those age 60 and older.[3] On the other hand, the incidence of some diseases declines with age. For example, pertussis (also known as whooping cough) occurs predominantly in childhood, particularly among young children.[4(pp449-454)]

Why does disease occurrence vary dramatically with age? The answer is complicated because an individual's numerical age reflects both the aging process and that person's experiences. The latter includes the accumulation of harmful exposures as well as protective factors. For example, the prevalence of habits such as alcohol consumption increases with age (at least from 12 through 34 years of age)[5(p213)] as does the prevalence of protective characteristics such as immunity to infectious diseases.

Sex is another personal characteristic associated with variations in disease occurrence. Certain diseases are more common among men and others are more prevalent among women. A striking example of this type of variation is breast cancer, a disease for which less than 1% of cases occur among men and more than 99% occur among women.[6] The opposite is seen with HIV infection in the United States, for which women accounted for only 19% of HIV diagnoses in 2015.[7] Possible reasons for variations in disease rates between sexes include differences in (1) hormone levels (e.g., female hormones may protect women against heart disease); (2) habits, such as the use of tobacco, alcohol, and drugs (which are more common among men); (3) sexual practices (e.g., anal intercourse, a risk factor for HIV transmission, is most commonly practiced among men who have sex with men); and (4) occupational exposures (e.g., men are more likely than women to hold jobs involving exposure to toxic exposures).[8]

Race and ethnicity also have a profound influence on disease patterns and can be particularly difficult to measure. The U.S. Census currently distinguishes between more than 12 racial groups, including White, Black, American Indian or Alaskan Native, Asian Indian, Chinese, Filipino, Japanese, Korean, Vietnamese, Native Hawaiian, Samoan, and Gaumanian or Chamorro.[9] The Census also identifies persons of Hispanic, Latino, or Spanish origin independent of racial category. In the 2010 U.S. Census, "Some Other Race" represented the third largest race group primarily because almost half of Hispanic or Latino respondents do not identify within any of the racial categories as defined in the U.S. Census.[9,10]

Rates for many diseases in the United States are higher among minority groups, particularly Black people. For example, diabetes is nearly twice as high among Black and Mexican people as among Whites. In addition, infants born to Black women are more than two times as likely to die before their first birthdays compared to those born to White women.[11] These racial health disparities stem from complex histories of racial discrimination and dispossession coupled with differences in socioeconomic status, health practices, psychosocial stress and resources, environmental exposures, and access to health care. Because many of these factors are highly correlated, it is often difficult for epidemiologists to tease apart their contributions.

Socioeconomic status is also a prominent characteristic by which diseases vary. Commonly used measures of socioeconomic status include educational level, income, and occupation. The sinking of the *Titanic* is a historic example of health disparities between the poor and wealthy. Death rates among passengers of low socioeconomic status were twice as high as those among passengers of high socioeconomic status because the small supply of life jackets was preferentially given to wealthy passengers, particularly wealthy women and children.[12]

Today, large disparities for almost all measures of health exist between people from low and high socioeconomic groups. For example, **life expectancy** is strongly related to income levels. A recent analysis found that, at the age of 40, the gap in life expectancy between individuals in the top and bottom 1% of the income distribution in the United States is 15 years for men and 10 years for women.[13] The relationship between income and health is complex because income is related to race, nutrition, risk factors such as smoking and alcohol use, environmental and occupational exposures, and access to and use of healthcare services.

Religious affiliation also influences disease rates. Like most of the personal characteristics described thus far, religion represents a mixture of factors, including genetic, environmental, cultural, and behavioral factors. For example, Tay-Sachs disease, a degenerative disease of the brain and nervous system, is associated with a genetic mutation that is present mainly among Jewish people of Eastern European decent.[14(pp347-350)] On the other hand, the likely reason for the 2.9% fewer cases of cancer among male Mormons and the 7.9% fewer cases among female Mormons is their prohibition against cigarette smoking and alcohol consumption as well as different sexual and reproductive patterns.[15]

It is not surprising that occupation influences disease patterns because potent and sustained exposures to harmful substances can occur on some jobs.[16(pp94-98)] One of the earliest associations between an occupation and disease was observed almost 200 years ago by Dr. Percivall Pott, who noted that London chimney sweeps had a high rate of scrotal cancer. It was only many years later that the constituents of soot, called polycyclic aromatic hydrocarbons, were found to cause cancer in laboratory animals. Today, we know that the patterns of numerous diseases vary by occupation. For example, people with jobs in aluminum production, boot and shoe manufacturing, coal gasification, furniture making, iron and steel founding, rubber manufacturing, and nickel refining are known to have higher rates of cancer than the general population.

Finally, marital status is known to have an important effect on the patterns of disease and death. For example, death rates are higher among people who are unmarried than for those who are married and living with their spouses.[17] The increased rates of death are greatest among those who never married, particularly never-married men. Data such as these suggest that the psychological and economic support associated with marriage exerts a protective effect against certain adverse health events, especially for men.[18,19] Alternatively, it is possible that the characteristics that lead a person to marry may be responsible for this protection.[20]

▶ Place

Place can be defined in terms of geopolitical units, such as countries or states, or in terms of natural geographic features, such as mountains or rivers. The characteristics of place encompass numerous aspects of the environment, including the physical environment (such as climate, water, and air), biological environment (such as flora and fauna), and social environment (such as cultural traditions). For example, malaria occurs in parts of the world where all these facets of the environment are conducive to the life cycle of the *Anopheles* mosquito, the vector that carries disease from one host to another.[21] Physical conditions that are necessary for the development and survival of the mosquito include a favorable temperature (20°C to 30°C is optimal), adequate humidity, moderate rainfall, and the presence of standing or gently flowing water. Biological factors beneficial to the mosquito include plants that can collect small pools of water. Social factors that encourage transmission of the disease include the proximity of homes to mosquito breeding sites, housing construction that facilitates mosquito entry, and certain occupations that increase a person's exposure to mosquitos, such as those involving outdoor work at night.

The scale of geographic comparisons can range from a global scale, in which rates are compared between continents and countries; to a regional scale, in which regions, states, and cities are compared; and to a local scale, in which neighborhoods are examined. Regardless of the scale that is used, striking geographic patterns of infectious and noninfectious diseases are often observed. For example, almost all cases of malaria are limited to Africa south of the Sahara Desert, central and southeast Asia, eastern Asia, and Central and South America (see **FIGURE 5-1**).

Rates of chronic diseases, such as cancer, also show tremendous worldwide variation (see **TABLE 5-1**). For example, rates of liver cancer among males are 9 times higher in Eastern Asia than rates in South-Central Asia.[22] Epidemiologists hypothesize that higher rates of hepatitis infection in Eastern Asia account for this particular difference.[23]

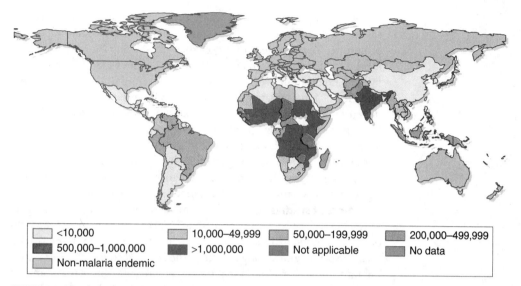

FIGURE 5-1 Number of malaria reported confirmed cases, 2014.

Reproduced from the World Health Organization. Malaria: number of reported cases (confirmed by slide examination or rapid diagnostic test): 2014. http://gamapserver.who.int/gho/interactive_charts/malaria /cases/atlas.html. Accessed September 2017.

TABLE 5-1 International Range of Cancer Incidence					
Cancer site	**Area with high rate**	**Rate***	**Area with low rate**	**Rate***	**Ratio (high to low)**
Males					
Liver	Eastern Asia	31.9	South-Central Asia	3.7	8.6
Stomach	Eastern Asia	35.4	Western Africa	3.3	10.7
Bladder	Southern Europe	21.8	Western Africa	2.1	10.4
Females					
Cervix	Eastern Africa	42.7	Western Asia	4.4	9.7
Lung	Northern America	33.8	Middle Africa	0.8	42.3
Breast	Western Europe	96.0	Middle Africa	26.8	3.6

*Rate per 100,000 population. The rates were age adjusted to eliminate the differences in rates caused by differences in the age composition of the underlying population.

Reproduced from the World Health Organization. Malaria: number of reported cases (confirmed by slide examination or rapid diagnostic test): 2014. http://gamapserver.who.int/gho/interactive_charts/malaria/cases/atlas.html. Accessed September 2017.

An example of disease variation on a regional scale is the apparent east-to-west gradient in semen quality across the Nordic-Baltic area of Europe. The adjusted total sperm counts among Finnish, Estonian, Danish, and Norwegian men are 185, 174, 144, and 133 million, respectively.[24] A common protocol was used to examine the men who were considered "representative of the normal population of young men," and therefore the researchers concluded that the gradient was real.

An example of neighborhood variation in disease occurrence is the distribution of childhood lead poisoning within the city of Boston. The prevalence of childhood lead poisoning was been highest in certain areas of the city. Historically, the residences in these areas contained lead-based paint, and the surrounding soil had high levels of lead contamination.

Migrant studies are one of the ways that epidemiologists investigate the effect of place on disease occurrence. These studies compare the rates of disease among natives of a homeland to rates among immigrants (and their offspring) and among natives of the adopted country. For example, migrant studies have found that the rate of prostate cancer is low among Japanese in Japan, intermediate among Japanese immigrants to Hawaii, and high among Hawaiian Whites.[25(pp185-187)] Recent data comparing breast cancer incidence rates among Japanese women living in the United States to Japanese women living in Japan show a similar increase toward rates approaching that of White women in the United States.[26] If the rate of disease among migrants approaches that of the host country, epidemiologists hypothesize that environmental factors may cause the disease. In the case of prostate cancer, those environmental factors may include the adoption of the dietary patterns of the host country, such as higher consumption of animal fat. For breast cancer, it may include changes in reproductive factors, such as age at first birth and age at menopause.

▶ Time

Analysis of the changes in disease and death rates over calendar time provides epidemiologists with useful information for causal research and public health planning and evaluation. The scale of time that is examined depends on the disease and can range from decades or years to months, weeks, days, or hours. For example, the age-adjusted death rate from Alzheimer's disease has increased 25% among women from 2005 to 2015.[5] Over the same period, there has been a dramatic decline in deaths from stroke. Both of these are examples of long-term trends.

Short-term trends are commonly examined for infectious diseases. For example, the famous 1976 outbreak of Legionnaires' disease at a Philadelphia convention occurred over a 1-month period.[27] Short-term trends are also relevant for noninfectious diseases that follow climatic changes, such as heat waves, hurricanes, and pollution episodes. For example, the 4-day 1952 smog disaster in London was associated with an increase in cardiovascular and respiratory deaths, particularly among the elderly.[28] More recently, temporal elevations in air pollution levels in Philadelphia were associated with concomitant increases in death rates from chronic obstructive pulmonary disease, pneumonia, heart disease, and stroke.[28,29]

Other types of temporal changes include periodic or regular fluctuations occurring on an annual, weekly, or even daily basis. Seasonal variations in disease frequency are the most common type of periodic fluctuations. For example, influenza peaks every winter season, and Lyme disease crests in late spring and summer.[4(pp363-367)] Regarding weekly and diurnal variations, studies have found that heart attacks occur most frequently on weekends and Mondays and in the morning and afternoon.[30-32]

What can we infer from time trends? First, they may result from concomitant changes in exposure to causal agents and/or susceptibility to the disease. However, it is also possible that temporal changes in disease and death rates result from parallel fluctuations in diagnostic capabilities, disease definition or reporting methods, the accuracy of the enumeration of the denominator population, or age distribution of the population. For example, the increased prevalence of birth defects of the heart in the late 1990s stemmed in part from the use of sophisticated ultrasounds that could detect theretofore undiagnosed cases.[33] In addition, when examining mortality rates over time, epidemiologists must consider the influence of improvements in treatment that increase survival. How do we know which factor or factors are responsible for a particular time trend? Information gathering and detailed analysis of all possible explanations provide useful clues, but in many cases the answers are never learned.

▶ Disease Clusters and Epidemics

Disease Clusters in Place and Time

A **disease cluster** is defined as an "aggregation of relatively uncommon events or disease in space and/or time in amounts that are believed or perceived to be greater than could be expected by chance."[2(p47)] Thus, the hallmark of a cluster is the occurrence of cases of disease close together in space (spatial clustering), time (temporal clustering), or both space and time (spatio-temporal clustering).

A well-known historical disease cluster is known as "eleven blue men."[34(pp1-13)] Here, 11 indigents were found ill or unconscious in a single neighborhood of New York City over the course of a single day. This finding would not have prompted much concern on the part of health authorities were it not for the unusual blue color of the men's skin. Given this peculiar symptom, the investigating epidemiologist easily identified the condition as methemoglobinemia, which results from the ingestion of sodium nitrite. This disease is so rare that the occurrence of 11 cases is far more than that expected by chance. A follow-up investigation found that a local cafeteria where all the men had eaten had mistakenly put sodium nitrite instead of sodium chloride in its salt shakers.

More recently, a cluster of leukemia cases occurred in Woburn, Massachusetts, over an 11-year period.[35] Two of the eight wells supplying drinking water to the town were discovered to be contaminated with several chlorinated organic chemicals. Follow-up investigations confirmed that the cluster was real and found that the individuals with leukemia were more likely than others to live in homes that received water from the two contaminated wells.

Epidemiologists have varying opinions about the usefulness of investigating the causes of disease clusters because follow-up investigations often fail to produce fruitful results and they consume time and resources.[36,37] Successful disease cluster investigations are rare because good information on exposure to the responsible agent is often unavailable.[37] This is particularly true for diseases that have a long induction period in which the likely cause (such as contaminated air or water) may have long since disappeared. Characteristics of clusters that are more likely to produce useful results are those involving diseases with a few unique and well-understood causes, a sufficient number of cases, and an environmentally persistent and measurable agent.

Outbreaks and Epidemics

Analysis of disease occurrence by person, place, and time is used to determine whether an **outbreak** or **epidemic** is occurring. A disease outbreak is the occurrence of cases of disease in excess of what would normally be expected in a given area or among a specific group of people.[38] Outbreaks are synonymous with epidemics, though the former often describes a localized as opposed to a widespread epidemic.[39] Additionally, though infectious disease outbreaks are most common, outbreaks may also be from noninfectious causes. Determining what is "in excess of normal" varies by disease, season, and area, and there is no hard-and-fast rule for defining an outbreak. As an example, the World Health Organization (WHO) defines the occurrence of three or more confirmed measles cases in a population of 100,000 in a month as a confirmed outbreak in the United States.[40] Alternatively, for influenza, the U.S. Centers for Disease Control and Prevention (CDC) calculates the typical proportion of pneumonia and influenza deaths during a season and defines an epidemic as an increase of 1.645 standard deviations above this typical level.[41]

Outbreak investigations are an essential and challenging activity of epidemiologists that helps identify the source of ongoing outbreaks and prevent new ones. Even if an outbreak is over by the time an investigation begins, it is still valuable for developing strategies to prevent future ones.

Outbreaks are often recognized by a clinician or clinical laboratory worker who notices an unusual disease or a sudden increase in a disease and alerts public health officials. Increasingly, Internet surveillance has contributed to the early identification of disease outbreaks, including searches of global media sources such as news wires. The WHO Global Outbreak Alert and Response Network relies on these data for day-to-day surveillance activities. According to the WHO, more than 60% of initial outbreak reports come from unofficial sources and require verification.[42] The usefulness of these aggregator networks was demonstrated in 2002 when Health Canada's Global Public Health Intelligence Network identified the outbreak of severe acute respiratory syndrome (SARS) in Guangdong Province, China, more than 2 months before the WHO released details on the new disease.[43]

The general approach to conducting an outbreak investigation is described below. After initial recognition of an outbreak, a thorough investigation includes (1) formulating case definitions, (2) conducting case confirmation, (3) establishing the background rate of disease and finding cases, (4) examining the descriptive epidemiology of the outbreak cases, (5) generating and testing hypotheses about the causes of the outbreak, (6) collecting and testing environmental samples, (7) implementing control measures, and (8) interacting with the press and public to disseminate information.[44,45]

Case definition and confirmation: In many outbreak investigations, multiple case definitions are used. For example, cases from an outbreak of gastroenteritis caused by *Salmonella* infection may be defined using a culture-confirmed infection with *Salmonella* for the laboratory case definition and new onset of diarrhea for the clinical case definition.[44] For an emergent disease with an unknown range of clinical manifestations, however, defining a case may be more complicated. Often, establishing a case definition is a fine balance between crafting a simple definition and ensuring there are enough cases available for the investigation while also maintaining strict enough exclusion criteria to reduce the chance of including cases of unrelated illness as outbreak-related cases. For example, the WHO uses the following criteria for defining a case of measles. A clinically confirmed case is (1) any person with fever and a nonvesicular rash and either a cough, runny nose, or conjunctivitis or (2) any person in whom the clinician suspects measles because of his or her exposure history. (For example, the person may be a close contact of a confirmed measles case.) In addition, a laboratory-confirmed case is a person with a positive blood test for measles-specific antibodies.[40] Of course, one would have the most confidence in the accuracy of cases defined by both clinical and laboratory criteria. In many outbreaks, case confirmation is also necessary given certain clinical findings may be from laboratory error. Case confirmation usually comprises detailed medical record review and discussion with healthcare providers, especially when a new disease appears to be emerging.

Finding cases and background rate: Another essential element of outbreak investigation involves finding all cases in a given population (based on the case definition) over a specific time period before the outbreak began and using these cases to establish a background rate. This analysis should prove that the number of cases is truly in excess of what might be expected based on the historical level of disease and can also help to define the geographic and temporal scope of the outbreak. Substantial effort is often required in outbreaks of new diseases to determine whether cases have gone unrecognized. An outbreak can also be difficult to identify when there are fluctuations in patient care-seeking behavior and access to care, provider referral patterns and test-ordering practices, diagnostic tests used by laboratories, and the prevalence of underlying immunosuppressive conditions or other characteristics of the population.

Descriptive epidemiology: These case finding and background rate generation exercises all contribute to the descriptive epidemiologic features of the outbreak. Investigators can plot an "epidemic curve," with date or time of illness onset among cases along the *x*-axis and number of cases along the *y*-axis. From an epidemic curve, investigators may be able to discern the distribution of cases over time, an outbreak's magnitude, pattern of spread, and most likely time of exposure.[45(pp436-442)]

The shape of an outbreak curve can also be used to make inferences about an outbreak's most likely mode of transmission. In a *point source outbreak*, persons are exposed over a brief time to the same source, such as a single meal or an event. The number of cases rises rapidly to a peak and falls gradually. The majority of cases occur within one incubation period, that is, the time interval between infection and clinical onset of the disease (see **FIGURE 5-2**). On the other hand, in a *continuous common source outbreak*, persons are exposed to the same source but exposure is prolonged over a period of days, weeks, or longer. The epidemic curve rises gradually and might plateau. It eventually falls off when the exposure ends (see Figure 5-2). Finally, in a *propagated outbreak*, there is no common source because the outbreak spreads from person to person. The epidemic graph will cycle through progressively taller peaks that are often one incubation period apart (see Figure 5-2).

Generating and testing hypotheses: Extrapolations from the epidemic curve and examination of the characteristics of cases often lead investigators to the next step in the investigation process: generating ideas about the cause of the outbreak. Generating these ideas is challenging when the cause of an outbreak is entirely unknown and even in those instances when the cause seems relatively obvious. In 2014 for instance, 864 foodborne disease outbreaks were recorded by the CDC. These outbreaks resulted in 13,246 illnesses and 21 deaths, but a single cause was confirmed in only 53% of outbreaks.[46] A literature review can provide background for what is already known about a particular disease, but it is not always helpful in investigating new diseases or unsuspected sources of exposure. When a literature review and the descriptive epidemiology do not give rise to a definitive source or route of exposure, open-ended interviews of cases can be useful.

If the initial investigation finds no association between hypothesized source and risk of disease, several steps may be taken. First, it is essential to consider whether the number of cases was large enough to find an association. Second, the accuracy of the available information

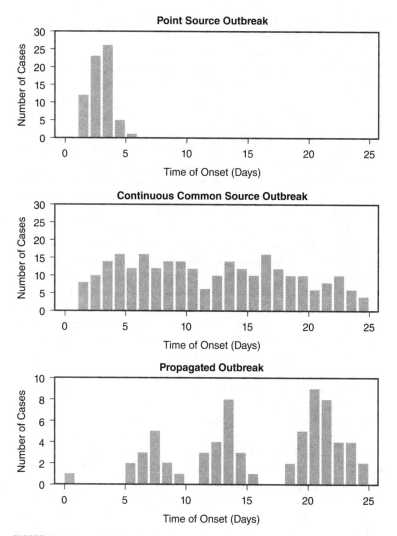

FIGURE 5-2 Types of outbreak curves.

concerning the exposures should be carefully considered. For example, generally, it is quite difficult to remember every food eaten in a day, especially when that day is several weeks past. Finally, it is possible the true source of the outbreak was not investigated.

Environmental and/or laboratory investigation: When environmental exposures, such as contaminated food or water, are found to be the cause of an outbreak, laboratory testing of environmental samples is the ideal next step. The epidemiological, environmental, and laboratory arms of an investigation complement one another, and often environmental and laboratory testing confirm the source of an outbreak. In many cases, however, it may be too late to collect such samples. For example, if the cause of an outbreak is contaminated food, the food source may no longer be available, or if interventions have already been implemented to alter the environment, samples will be of little use. Even if an environmental sample is obtained, many laboratory tools are not sensitive enough to detect a contaminant or, in the case of a new disease or exposure, laboratory methods or tests for the cause may not yet exist.[47(pp463-464)]

Control measures: Outbreak investigations require the timely implementation of appropriate control and prevention measures to minimize further disease. Control measures are usually directed against one or more segments in the path from the exposure source to cases of disease that are amenable to intervention. For example, a product recall or processing plant shutdown after a foodborne outbreak targets the source of illness, bed nets block mosquitos carrying malaria from biting susceptible people, and flu vaccinations aim to increase a person's defenses against illness.

The timing and nature of implementing such measures are complex. Although results of the epidemiological investigation should guide implementation of control measures, waiting for these results can delay prevention of exposure to a suspected source, making it difficult to defend from a public health perspective. Conversely, acting too quickly and harshly is also problematic considering control measures may have a negative effect on a given food product or restaurant, in the case of foodborne illnesses, or on the lives of individuals who may be unnecessarily quarantined in the case of infectious diseases. If an outbreak investigation is premised on incorrect information, there may also be damaging legal implications. Therefore, control measure implementation is often a balancing act between timely interventions to prevent further spread of disease and deferring action until accurate information regarding the source of disease is available.

Dissemination of information: Finally, media attention and public concern often become part of outbreak investigations, and dissemination of information to the public is critical. Sometimes, the media learn about incidents and reports on events as they unfold and before much is known about the disease or source of exposure. For example, in 2008, the Public Health Agency of Canada coordinated communication of a national response to an incident involving passengers on a train in northern Ontario. One death, one medical evacuation, and influenza-like illnesses had occurred on board the train, and the media reported the events live on television. It turned out that three unrelated health events had occurred, none of which posed an active public health threat.[43] Even though media reports can be inaccurate, media outlets are a powerful means of sharing information about an investigation with the public and disseminating timely information about control measures.

▶ Ebola Outbreak and Its Investigation

The Ebola virus outbreaks in Central and West Africa have been among the most devastating infectious disease outbreaks in recent times. Following, we describe the course of these outbreaks and the response of the public health and medical communities. You will see that, even in the most difficult circumstances, investigators used the epidemiological principles described previously to identify the cause and mode of transmission and implement control measures.

Nzara, South Sudan, 1976: In 1976, the first Ebola virus outbreaks occurred in two remote villages in Central Africa, one in what is now Nzara, South Sudan (formerly Sudan), and the other in Yambuku, Democratic Republic of Congo (formerly Zaire).[48-50] The first cases occurred in Nzara, where cotton factory workers were affected with an unknown and fatal disease. Though the early symptoms of Ebola virus are nonspecific—fever, muscle pain, severe headache, weakness, diarrhea, vomiting, and abdominal pain—later stages of the disease are unique and often dramatic. Internal bleeding may cause broken capillaries, which appear as a raised rash, and organ failure. The worst cases cause individuals to vomit blood, have bloody diarrhea, and bleed from their nose and mouth.[48,49]

In August 1976, one of the first cases was transferred to the district hospital of Maridi. Within 4 weeks, one-third of the 220 staff at the hospital had acquired infection and 41 died.[48,51] At this time, the mode of transmission of this disease was unknown, and therefore no effective form of infection control was utilized. Before the disease was recognized, most wards of the hospital had hemorrhaging Ebola patients with no protective measures in place, and at the height of the epidemic, the hospital was in chaos. After the adoption of protective clothing, the number of cases declined in early October. A considerable increase in the number of cases was observed in late October and early November after protective clothing supplies ran out. By the time a WHO investigative team arrived in late October, there were almost no patients left in the Maridi district hospital, and very few nurses were reporting for duty. It was readily apparent to the community that the hospital was a prime source of the outbreak.[48]

The first step for the WHO and Sudanese outbreak investigators was to develop a case definition. The late-stage presentation of most cases was clinically unique; therefore, a case definition based on clinical signs or merely on the hospital physician's judgment was deemed sufficient. Moreover, the causative agent of the disease was still unknown, and therefore a laboratory-confirmed case definition was not feasible. Thus, investigators developed the following case definition: any person "(1) having fever and headache lasting for at least 2 days with diarrhea or vomiting or chest pain; or (2) diagnosed by a physician in a hospital."[48]

Given the sudden onset, rapid transmission, and deleterious effects of the disease, control measures were immediately necessary and implemented before a thorough epidemiological investigation was conducted. The disease affected those in very close contact with patients with active disease, and therefore it was safe to postulate that the illness was infectious and spread by direct contact from person to person. Contact tracing was used to identify cases, leading to isolation of cases. Contact tracing involves finding everyone who has close contact with infected individuals and watching for signs of sickness for a given period of time. If any of these contacts shows symptoms of the disease, they are isolated and cared for. Then, the process is repeated by tracing the contacts' contacts.[52] While in isolation, patients were cared for by hospital staff who had had the infection and had now fully recovered. Protective clothing and careful training regarding the use of protective clothing and its subsequent decontamination were provided.

A surveillance team of 30 individuals was dispatched to visit every home in Maridi to find active cases. Each case was reported to Sudanese officials, and an ambulance was sent to the house. Patients were persuaded to enter the isolation wards at the hospital, though some refused. In addition to tracing all active cases of infection, the surveillance teams sought out recovered cases, who were approached regarding the possibility of obtaining immune plasma. Within 3 weeks, blood samples had been obtained from 51 recovered individuals.

The high mortality rate and alarmingly high rate of infection among Maridi hospital staff left medical staff understandably reluctant to carry out any postmortem examinations. Two limited postmortem exams were carried out by WHO investigation team members, and tissues were removed for study. By the end of the outbreak in October, there were 284 cases and 151 deaths.[48]

Yambuku, Zaire, 1976: One month after the initial case presented with signs of infection in Sudan, a similar disease became apparent roughly 500 miles southwest of Maridi in Yambuku, Zaire. The first case in Zaire is believed to have been a 44-year-old teacher who sought treatment for what was thought to be malaria at Yambuku Mission Hospital on August 26, 1976. At least nine other cases occurred during the first week of September, all among people who had received treatment for other diseases at the outpatient clinic at the mission hospital.[49]

Two Zairean doctors who traveled to the Bumba region, the main epidemic area in northwest Zaire, containing Yambuku, diagnosed the illness as yellow fever. However, in addition to high fever, headache, and vomiting, the patients began to suffer violent hemorrhagic symptoms, including extensive bleeding from the anal passage, nose, and mouth, symptoms quite unusual in yellow fever. With shocking rapidity, 11 of the 17 hospital workers died, and the hospital was forced to close on September 30. Specimens were collected and sent out to labs across the world, and within several weeks, three external labs discovered the new illness was similar to Marburg virus. In fact, one of the labs tested samples from the outbreak in Sudan, meaning three labs independently identified the same new virus that was the probable cause of two simultaneous, deadly epidemics.

In mid-October, an International Commission was formed in Zaire by the Minister of Health to investigate the cause, clinical manifestations, and epidemiology of the new disease and to advise and assist with control measures. Implementation of several control measures occurred promptly within the outbreak investigation timeline, and the entire Bumba Zone was quarantined in early October, just 2 days after the hospital closure. The quarantine was put into place so early largely because of the fear caused by such a grisly and devastating disease. The first visit by a commission subgroup to Yambuku almost did not occur because terrified pilots, having heard stories of birds dropping out of the sky, sick with fever, and of human bodies being found by the roadsides, at first refused to fly the team to the closest airfield in Bumba. Once they arrived in Yambuku, the team found the nuns of the mission and hospital had posted a sign around the guesthouse where they were sleeping that warned "anybody who passes this fence will die."[53(p38)] They also found no effective communication between the isolated city of Yambuku and the capital city of Kinshasa. The mission hospital had little electricity, no diesel fuel, no functional laboratory, and no protective clothing for staff. A report from the International Commission described the members' work as being carried out "under circumstances which at times seemed to us those of a small war."[49] Applying the same case definition as used in Sudan, in just over a week, the team found a disconcerting number of cases and deaths from the disease across at least 20 villages.

The next step was for the investigative team to determine how the virus was moving from person to person—by air, in food, by direct contact, or spread by insects. The team members mapped out the number of infections in each village, piecing together data from their notes and interviews, and they were able to discern two key elements linking almost every victim of the epidemic. First, people were becoming ill after attending funerals. Second, the outbreak was closely related to areas served by the mission hospital, with nearly every early case having attended the outpatient clinic a few days before becoming symptomatic. The team drew epidemic curves showing the number of cases by location, age, and gender and found that more women, particularly those between the ages of 18 and 25, were likely to have the disease.[53(pp48-49)] It turned out that many of the women in this age group were pregnant and had attended an antenatal clinic at the hospital. This provided an important clue as to the mode of transmission.

Pregnant women in Yambuku attended the mission hospital where nuns administered vitamin shots reusing infected needles. If transmission occurred through blood or bodily fluids, this explanation was compatible with cases becoming ill after attending to their deceased relatives. As part of the funeral ritual, cadavers were thoroughly cleaned, often by family members working bare-handed. The bodies of Ebola victims were usually covered in blood, feces, and vomit, and therefore any direct contact, such as washing or preparation of the deceased without protection, was a serious risk. Though it was difficult, investigators tried to convince locals not to attend to their diseased relatives. After this first visit, the Commission determined that mobilization of all available resources was necessary to cope with such a major threat.

The case definitions used for any future surveillance visits to Zairean villages were different from the definition created in Sudan. First, the team discovered that syringes used in the clinic were likely causes of the spread in Yambuku. Second, given the later timeline, researchers had already isolated the virus, and thus a lab-confirmed case definition could be utilized. Investigators therefore developed the following case definitions:

> A *probable case* of Ebola haemorrhagic fever was a person living in the epidemic area who died after one or more days with two or more of the following symptoms and signs: headache, fever, abdominal pain, nausea and/or vomiting, and bleeding. The patient must have, within the three preceding weeks, received an injection or had contact with a probable or a proven case, the illness not having been otherwise diagnosed on clinical grounds. A *proven case* was a person from whom Ebola virus was isolated or demonstrated by electron microscopy or who had an indirect fluorescent antibody (IFA) titre of at least 1:64 to Ebola virus within three weeks after onset of symptoms.[49]
>
> Reprinted from World Health Organization. Ebola haemorrhagic fever in Zaire, 1976. *Bull WHO*. 1978;56:271-293.

Equipped with these new definitions, two mobile teams were airlifted to the region between Sudan and the Bumba Zone to search for recent and active cases and to identify commercial trade routes and human travel patterns between the Bumba Zone and southern Sudan, where the other outbreak was occurring. Additionally, a more structured study that retrospectively compared sick and healthy individuals was conducted to identify contributing factors to the spread of disease. Ten surveillance teams were trained and provided with standard forms, a written schedule, and detailed maps. Teams contacted the village chief and enlisted support for a house-to-house survey, and suspect cases were provided medicine and isolated in the village. Investigators wore protective gear, consisting of gloves; a gown; and a full-face respirator, which was nearly impossible to wear in the midday heat, causing wearers to often swap it out for goggles and a paper surgical mask. Barriers were erected along roads and paths to restrict entry to and exit from affected villages.[53(pp44-45)]

The surveillance teams visited 550 villages and interviewed about 238,000 individuals. A team of physicians also traveled through the same villages to follow up with suspect cases and take blood samples from recovered cases. In 85 of 288 cases where the means of transmission was determined, the only significant risk factor investigators found between cases and matched family and village controls was receipt of one or more injections at the hospital. Other factors, such as previous case contact; exposure to food, water, hospital buildings, or domestic and wild animals; or travel within 3 months prior to onset, were not associated with this type of transmission. Therefore, the closure of Yambuku Mission Hospital was likely the most important single occurrence in the eventual termination of the outbreak.

Investigators also tested healthy individuals for Ebola antibodies to assess the extent of Ebola infection in the area to establish whether some people had already contracted the infection but had either shown no symptoms or survived them. The method for measuring Ebola antibodies was imperfect, but investigators found at least 2.5% of people in contact with fatal cases had such antibodies, suggesting they experienced either asymptomatic or undiagnosed infection and survived it. Because the mode of transmission was unknown, investigators also tested mosquitos, bed bugs, wild rodents, and bats in villages. No virus was recovered from these animals.

Between September 1 and October 24, 1976, investigators documented 318 probable and confirmed cases of Ebola and 280 deaths, an alarming fatality rate of 88%. After a final village check by surveillance teams in mid-December, 6 weeks after the last death from Ebola, the International Commission advised lifting the quarantine in the Bumba Zone, and the International Commission was disbanded in January 1977.[49] The commission recommended that the government of Zaire maintain active national surveillance for acute haemorrhagic disease and institute procedures for clinical isolation and the use of protective clothing for medical personnel. Investigators also recommended a national campaign to inform health personnel of the proper methods for sterilizing syringes and needles and for staff to reconsider the need for injections when oral medication was available.[49]

West Africa, 2014–2016: Nearly 40 years later, the 2014–2016 West Africa epidemic was the largest and most complex outbreak to date. The first cases were recorded in Guinea in December 2013, and the disease spread to neighboring Liberia and Sierra Leone, reaching 950 confirmed cases per week at the height of the outbreak.[54] Case isolation methods no longer worked in 2014 when the virus reached crowded capital cities, where it spread like wildfire and dead bodies piled up in the streets. By the time the WHO terminated the emergency status of the outbreak, almost 29,000 suspected cases and over 11,000 deaths were reported, more than in all previous outbreaks combined.[55]

Unlike in the 1976 Ebola outbreaks, global media coverage was a significant component of outbreak investigation in 2014. In fact, the West Africa outbreak raised concerns about risk communication to the public. In early 2014, a team of Doctors Without Borders had to temporarily stop work at an isolation ward in Guinea because the medical personnel were falsely accused of having brought the virus to the country.[56] Early communications used to alert the population about this new and dangerous disease were focused on its severity and fatality. In West Africa, this backfired because people thought there was no survival from Ebola. Sick people did not attend treatment centers because they preferred to die at home.[57] In the United States, media hysteria led to disproportionate concern in relation to the very low risk of contracting Ebola.[58,59] Finally, the 2014 outbreak also exposed the insufficient amount of personal protective equipment available to be able to provide adequate protection for healthcare workers, patients, and others during an outbreak.

In 2015, the WHO, the Guinean Health Ministry, and Norway's Institute of Public Health began a 2-year trial of an experimental Ebola vaccine in Guinea. In the midst of a massive public health crisis, international and local health organizations had to design a study that they could carry out in unstable, sometimes remote regions, while producing useful data about safety and efficacy. By the time testing could start in mid-2015, isolation and treatment of the sick in tent hospitals had made Ebola cases so rare that researchers had to switch to ring vaccination around the few cases they could find. Once a confirmed case was found, researchers contacted everyone in the circle of family, friends, neighbors, and caregivers around the victim, and about half of these groups were offered vaccine.[60] In December 2016, the WHO announced that the vaccine appeared to offer protection from the strain of Ebola responsible for the West Africa outbreak. Even before receiving approval from any regulatory authority, 300,000 doses were already stockpiled.[61]

▶ Uses of Descriptive Epidemiology

In addition to determining whether an outbreak has occurred, there are several other purposes for describing disease occurrence by person, place, and time (see **TABLE 5-2**). Scientists examine the distribution of disease to search for clues about causes of disease and to generate specific hypotheses about these causal relationships. Public health administrators and planners examine these patterns to establish priorities and to plan and evaluate the effectiveness of clinical and public health programs.

▶ Generating Hypotheses About Causal Relationships

Exactly what is a hypothesis? According to the *American Heritage Dictionary*, a **hypothesis** is "a tentative explanation for an observation, phenomenon, or scientific problem that can be tested by further

TABLE 5-2 Elements and Uses of Descriptive Epidemiology	
Elements	Person (age, sex, race, religion, socioeconomic class) Place (country, state, city, neighborhood) Time (year, season, month, week, day, hour)
Uses	Assessing the health status of a population Generating hypotheses about causal factors Planning and evaluating public health programs

investigation."[62(p866)] Thus, a hypothesis is usually a specific statement that attempts to explain certain observations. The process of generating hypotheses is a creative endeavor that combines these observations with biomedical information, often from other fields such as genetics, biochemistry, physiology, and toxicology. For example, an epidemiologist might hypothesize that the high incidence of stomach cancer in Japan is caused by the higher consumption of salts. High salt concentration destroys the mucosal barrier in the gastric system, causing inflammation and cell damage. This may enhance the effect of carcinogens found in foods.[63]

Although epidemiologists do not follow a rigid set of steps to generate a hypothesis, they often rely on several types of comparisons during the process. First, investigators often compare groups with very different disease rates and try to identify different characteristics that may account for the disparate rates. For example, the differences in infant mortality rates according to race may be explained in part by documented racial differences in access to prenatal care.[11] Second, researchers often look for common characteristics that link the affected groups. For example, increased death rates from the cancer non-Hodgkin's lymphoma have been observed among diverse occupational groups, including agricultural workers, rubber workers, chemists, and dry cleaners. Solvents are the single exposure that all of these occupations have in common.[64(pp170-174)] Third, when examining changes in disease rates over time or from place to place, epidemiologists search for concomitant variation of a likely causal factor. For example, the large increase in lung cancer deaths among men from 1930 to 1990 was attributed to the increased prevalence of cigarette smoking over the same time period.[65] The increase in lung cancer deaths among women trails behind that of men (it started in 1960) because women adopted cigarette smoking later than men. Fourth, it is helpful to look for analogies with other better-known diseases. For example, at the beginning of the HIV/AIDS epidemic, researchers noted that many of its descriptive features resembled those of hepatitis B, a virally transmitted disease.[66(p103)] These features included "characteristics associated with a sexually active life style," such as a history of sexually transmitted diseases and large numbers of nonsteady sexual partners and percutaneous needle exposures.[66(p103)] Thus, these similarities led investigators to postulate a viral etiology of AIDS early in the epidemic.

▸ Public Health Planning and Evaluation

Public health administrators and planners use descriptive epidemiology to establish priorities, allocate resources, and plan and evaluate the effectiveness of programs. On a national level, the U.S. Department of Health and Human Services has used descriptive data to provide baseline estimates and plan goals and objectives for *Healthy People 2020*, a comprehensive plan to improve the nation's health and health awareness by 2020. The plan has four overarching goals: to increase the quality and years of healthy life, eliminate health disparities, create healthy environments, and promote healthy living.[67] These goals are supported by specific objectives in 42 focus areas, including access to quality health services; cancer; diabetes; environmental health; family planning; health communication; HIV; maternal, infant, and child health; medical product safety; physical activity and fitness; sexually transmitted diseases; substance abuse; tobacco use; and food safety. The plan uses "leading health indicators" to illustrate individual behaviors, physical and social environmental factors, and health system issues that significantly affect the health of individuals and communities.

▶ Example: Patterns of Mortality in the United States According to Age

To illustrate the main elements and uses of descriptive epidemiology, this section describes the pattern of mortality in the United States according to age.

Demographic Characteristics of the U.S. Population

First, it is necessary to present background demographic characteristics of the U.S. population.

Size

The U.S. Census Bureau estimates a total resident population of 323,127,513 individuals in the United States as of July 1, 2016, representing a 4.7% increase since the 2010 Census.[68] Officials anticipate that population growth will continue slowly for the foreseeable future. Population growth stems from both a "natural increase" (wherein the number of births exceeds the number of deaths) and immigration from other countries.

Gender Ratio

According to 2015 Census estimates, the U.S. population was 50.8% female, for an overall gender ratio of 96.9 males for every 100 females.[69] The gender ratio varies with age. There are more males than females (105 males for every 100 females) among individuals younger than 18 years of age and fewer males than females (95 males for every 100 females) among those 18 years and older. There are only 78 men for every 100 women among individuals age 65 years and older.

Age Structure

The median (or the midpoint) age of the U.S. population has increased steadily over time, rising from 30 years in 1980 to 37.6 years in 2015.[69] This increase reflects the "aging of the population." That is, the proportion of U.S. adults, particularly elderly adults, has grown over time. In 1980, adults age 65 years and older formed 11.3% of the population; by 2015, they formed 14.1% (see TABLE 5-3). The median age is expected to continue to increase because the elderly population is growing at a faster rate than is the population as a whole.

Race

According to 2016 Census estimates, the U.S. population is predominantly White (76.9%) and not of Hispanic origin (82.2%) (see FIGURE 5-3).[68] However, many racial and ethnic groups are represented, with people identifying as Black making up a large portion of the population and

TABLE 5-3 Age Distribution of U.S. Resident Population, 1980 and 2015

Age (in years)	1980		2015	
	Number (in thousands)	Percentage	Number (in thousands)	Percentage
14 and younger	51,290	22.6	61,094	19.3
15–24	42,487	18.8	43,959	13.8
25–34	37,082	16.4	42,882	13.5
35–44	25,635	11.3	40,652	12.8
45–54	22,800	10.1	43,896	13.9
55–64	21,703	9.6	39,418	12.4
65–74	15,581	6.9	25,135	7.9
75–84	7,729	3.4	13,542	4.3
85 and older	2,240	1.0	5,939	1.9

Data from ACS Demographic and Housing Estimates, 2011-2015, American Community Survey 5-Year Estimates. census.gov. https://factfinder.census .gov/faces/tableservices/jsf/pages/productview.xhtml?src=bkmk. Accessed October 2017; Kramarow E, Lentzer H, Rooks R, Weeks J, Saydah S. *Health and Aging Chartbook: Health, United States, 1999.* Hyattsville, MD: National Center for Health Statistics; 1999.

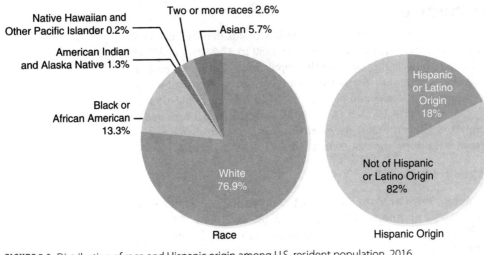

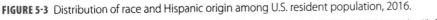

FIGURE 5-3 Distribution of race and Hispanic origin among U.S. resident population, 2016.

Data from Annual Estimates of the Resident Population by Sex, Race, and Hispanic Origin for the United States, States, and Counties: April 1, 2010 to July 1, 2016. census.gov. https://factfinder.census.gov/faces /tableservices/jsf/pages/productview.xhtml?src=bkmk. Released June 2017. Accessed September 2017.

Mexicans predominating among people of Hispanic origin. The racial and ethnic diversity of the U.S. population is expected to increase in the coming years.

Natality

The number of live births occurring in the United States peaked at 4.3 million in 2007 and has since declined to about 3.9 million in 2015.[70] In the United States, the birth rate has declined in women under age 30, increased for women age 30–44, and remained the same for those over 45 years of age.

The teen birth rate for the United States in 2015 was 22.3 births per 1,000 females age 15–19, falling 46% since 2007, the most recent high, and 64% since 1991, a long-term high.[70] The birth rate for women in their 20s has also fallen to 76.8 births per 1,000 women age 20–24 and 104.3 births per 1,000 women age 25–29. The birth rate was 101.5 births per 1,000 women age 30–34 and 51.8 births per 1,000 women age 35–39 in 2015, the highest rates since 1964 and 1962, respectively. The birth rate of women age 40–44 has risen over the past 3 decades to 11.0 births per 1,000 women in 2015 (see **FIGURE 5-4**).

Life Expectancy

Life expectancy—that is, the average number of years of life remaining to a person at a given age—has increased substantially over time.[5(p16)] In the United States, the average life expectancy in 1950 was 68.2 years at birth and 13.9 years at age 65. Comparable figures for 2015 were 78.8 and 19.4 years,

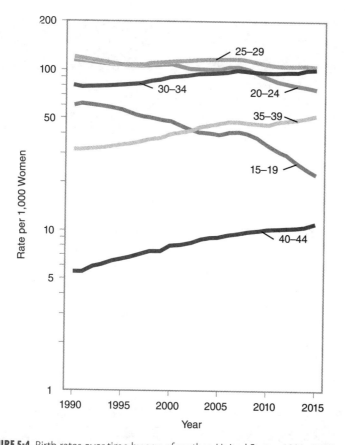

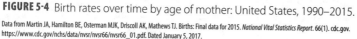

FIGURE 5-4 Birth rates over time by age of mother: United States, 1990–2015.

Data from Martin JA, Hamilton BE, Osterman MJK, Driscoll AK, Mathews TJ. Births: Final data for 2015. *National Vital Statistics Report*. 66(1). cdc.gov. https://www.cdc.gov/nchs/data/nvsr/nvsr66/nvsr66_01.pdf. Dated January 5, 2017.

respectively (see **TABLE 5-4**).[5(p116)] For as long as U.S. mortality data have been collected, life expectancy has been higher for women than men and higher for Whites than Blacks. In 2015, White women had the highest life expectancy (81.3 years), and Black men had the lowest (72.2 years).

According to the WHO, the United States ranked 34th in life expectancy at birth for males and 33rd for females in 2015. Switzerland and Japan ranked first for males and females, respectively, and Sierra Leone ranked last for both males and females (81.3 and 86.8 years, respectively, for top-ranked countries and 49.3 years and 50.8 years, respectively, for the bottom-ranked country).[71]

▶ Overall Pattern of Mortality

More than 2.7 million deaths occurred in the United States in 2015.[5(p128)] More than half (51%) of these deaths could be attributed to three causes: heart disease, cancer, and chronic respiratory disease (see **TABLE 5-5**).

TABLE 5-4 Life Expectancy at Birth and at 65 Years of Age According to Race and Gender: United States, 2015

Race	Gender	Remaining life expectancy in years	
		At birth	At 65 years
All races	Both genders	78.8	19.4
	Male	76.3	18.0
	Female	81.2	20.6
White	Both genders	79.0	19.4
	Male	76.6	18.0
	Female	81.3	20.5
Black	Both genders	75.5	18.2
	Male	72.2	16.4
	Female	78.5	19.7

Data from National Center for Health Statistics. *Health, United States, 2016: With Chartbook on Long-term Trends in Health*. Hyattsville, MD; 2017.

TABLE 5-5 Leading Causes of Death: Number and Percentage of Deaths in the U.S. Population, 2015

Rank	Cause of death	Number of deaths	Percentage of total deaths
1	Heart diseases	633,842	23.4%
2	Cancer	595,930	22.0%
3	Chronic lower respiratory diseases	155,041	5.7%
4	Unintentional injuries	146,571	5.4%
5	Cerebrovascular diseases	140,323	5.2%
6	Alzheimer's disease	110,561	4.1%
7	Diabetes	79,535	2.9%
8	Influenza and pneumonia	57,062	2.1%
9	Kidney diseases	49,959	1.8%
10	Suicide	44,193	1.6%

National Center for Health Statistics. *Health, United States, 2016: With Chartbook on Long-term Trends in Health*. Hyattsville, MD; 2017.

These three diseases were the leading causes among White females. However, chronic respiratory disease was supplanted by unintentional injuries for White and Black males and cerebrovascular disease for Black women as the third-leading cause of death. Leading sites for cancer deaths were the lung, prostate, and colon–rectum among men and lung, breast, and colon–rectum among women (see **TABLE 5-6**).[6] Other important causes of death for both men and women were Alzheimer's disease, diabetes, infectious diseases (including pneumonia and influenza), and kidney diseases.[5(p107)]

Mortality Rates by Age

In the U.S. population, there is a J-shaped relationship between age and the rate of death (see **FIGURE 5-5**).[5(p134)] That is, mortality rates are

TABLE 5-6 Death Rates for the Five Leading Cancer Sites for Males and Females, United States, 2010–2014

Gender and cancer site	Death rates*
Males	
Lung and bronchus	55.9
Prostate	20.1
Colon and rectum	17.7
Pancreas	12.6
Liver and intrahepatic bile duct	9.2
Females	
Lung and bronchus	36.3
Breast	21.2
Colon and rectum	12.4
Pancreas	9.5
Ovary	7.4

*Rates are per 100,000 and age adjusted to the 2000 U.S. standard.

Data from Howlader N, Noone AM, Krapcho M, Miller D, Bishop K, Kosary CL, et al. (eds). *SEER Cancer Statistics Review, 1975-2014*. cancer.gov. https://seer.cancer.gov/csr/1975_2014. Published April 2017. Accessed April 2017.

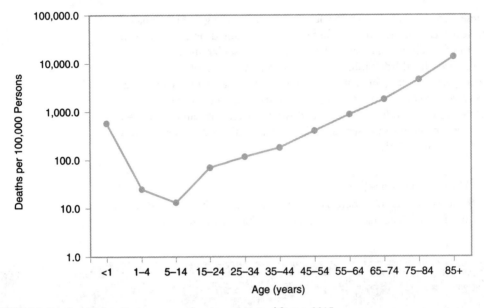

FIGURE 5-5 Death rates for all causes according to age: United States, 2015.

Data from National Center for Health Statistics. *Health, United States, 2016, With Chartbook on Long-term Trends in Health.* Hyattsville, MD; 2017.

relatively high during the first year of life. They decline until age 14 and then increase thereafter with age. Because age is such an important determinant of death, the remainder of this section describes the rates and important causes of death for each age group.

Infants (Less than 1 Year of Age)

The infant mortality rate is considered a sensitive indicator of the overall health of a population. In 2015, the leading causes of infant deaths were congenital malformations, short gestation and/or low birth weight, and sudden infant death syndrome (SIDS), accounting for 45% of the infant deaths that occurred.[5(p132)] Although U.S. rates have declined over time (from 12.9 to 5.9 per 1,000 live births over the period from 1980 to 2015), there is a great disparity between racial and ethnic groups (see **FIGURE 5-6**). For example, during this period, the rate among Black people was consistently more than twice that of White people. When compared to similar developed countries, the United States had one of the highest infant mortality rates in 2015, ranking 32nd among the 35 Organisation for Economic Cooperation and Development (OECD) countries, behind most European countries as well as Canada, Japan, Korea, Israel, Australia, and New Zealand.[72]

Children (1 to 14 Years of Age)

In 2015, major causes of death among children 1 to 14 years old were unintentional injuries, malignant neoplasms, congenital anomalies,

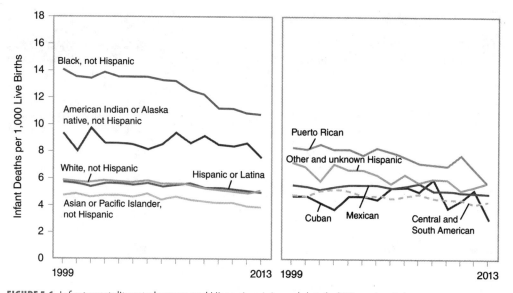

FIGURE 5-6 Infant mortality rate by race and Hispanic origin and detailed Hispanic origin of mother: United States, 1999–2013.

Reprinted from National Center for Health Statistics. *Health United States, 2015, With Special Feature on Racial and Ethnic Health Disparities.* Hyattsville, MD; 2016.

and homicides.[5(p132)] Motor vehicle accidents caused the greatest number of deaths ascribed to unintentional injuries. Although deaths from motor vehicle accidents have dropped over time, they have generally been higher among males than females and higher among Blacks than Whites. Although this disparity has been decreasing over time, there was an increase in the rates of death caused by motor vehicle accidents among Black children between 2010 and 2015, whereas death rates in White children continued to decline (see **TABLE 5-7**).

Adolescents and Young Adults (15 to 24 Years of Age)

In 2015, unintentional injuries were the most common cause of death among adolescents and young adults, accounting for over 40% of the deaths in this age group.[5(p132)] Again, most of these deaths resulted from motor vehicle accidents.

Other common causes of death in 2015 included suicides (18% of deaths) and homicides (16% of deaths). These two causes of death have exhibited large increases over time in this age group. From 1950 to 2015, deaths caused by homicide increased from 5.8 to 13.1 per 100,000, and those caused by suicide rose from 4.5 to 12.5 per 100,000 population. White males in this age group have experienced the largest rise in suicide death rates from 1950 to 2015, increasing from 6.6 to 20.9 per 100,000 population. Both White and Black people have experienced increases in homicides since 1950, but rates among Black men and women have been consistently higher than rates among Whites (see **TABLE 5-8**). Black men had about 10 times the homicide rate of White men in this age

TABLE 5-7 Death Rates for Motor Vehicle Accidents over Time Among Children 1–14 Years of Age, by Race and Gender

Year	All races	Males		Females	
		White	Black	White	Black
1970	10.5	12.5	16.3	7.5	10.2
1980	8.2	9.8	11.4	6.2	6.3
1990	6.0	6.6	8.9	4.8	5.3
2000	4.3	4.8	5.5	3.7	3.9
2010	2.3	2.7	3.0	2.1	2.0
2015	2.2	2.5	3.2	1.8	2.6

Data from National Center for Health Statistics. *Health, United States, 2016: With Chartbook on Long-term Trends in Health*. Hyattsville, MD; 2017.

TABLE 5-8 Death Rates for Homicides Among White and Black Males, 15–24 Years of Age

Year	White males	Black males
1950	3.2	53.8
1960	5.0	43.2
1970	7.6	98.3
1980	15.1	82.6
1990	15.2	137.1
2000	9.9	85.3
2010	8.2	71.0
2015	7.3	74.9

Data from National Center for Health Statistics. *Health, United States, 2016: With Chartbook on Long-term Trends in Health*. Hyattsville, MD; 2017.

group in 2015 (74.9 versus 7.3, respectively, per 100,000). Black females had higher rates than White females (7.5 versus 1.9, respectively, per 100,000), but homicide rates for females have always been much lower than those among males.[5(pp161-164)]

Adults (25 to 64 Years of Age)

In 2015, the three leading causes of death among adults 25 to 44 years old were unintentional injuries (30% of deaths), cancer (12% of deaths), and heart disease (11% of deaths).[5(p133)] Among adults age 45 to 64, cancer ranked first (30% of deaths), heart disease ranked second (21% of deaths), and unintentional injuries was a distant third (8% of deaths).

From 1975 to 1990, the overall age-adjusted death rate for all types of cancer increased, followed by periods of stability and decline during 1990 to 2000, and finally a steady decline during 2000 to 2015. During the period from 1975 to 2015, greater declines in age-adjusted heart disease than cancer mortality have narrowed the gap between heart disease and cancer deaths. Since 1994, mortality rates have increased for some types of cancer, including liver, thyroid, esophagus, lung and bronchus (in females), testis, and uterus. On the other hand, they have decreased for many other types of cancer, including prostate, cervix, stomach, breast, colon and rectum, lung and bronchus (for males), and leukemia.

Deaths caused by heart disease have also declined substantially over time among U.S. adult men and women.[3] Men experience higher mortality rates from heart disease than women at all ages. For example, in 2015, male mortality rates from heart disease were 2.4 times the rate among women aged 55 to 64 years (see **FIGURE 5-7**).

Elderly Adults (65 Years of Age and Older)

As one would expect, the elderly population experiences the highest mortality rates of all age groups.[5(p134)] In 2015, the leading causes of death in this age group were heart disease (25% of deaths), cancer (21%), and chronic lower respiratory diseases (7%). However, death rates have declined considerably over time among all elderly adults. For example, from 1950 through 2015, death rates for all causes have declined by 56% among men and women age 65 to 74, by 51% among those age 75–84, and by 32% among those age 85 and over.

Strengths and Limitations of Mortality Data

There are many advantages to using mortality data to learn about the health status of a population. First, because this information is completely reported for the entire country, it can be used to study fatal illnesses on a national, state, city, or neighborhood level. Second, the National Center for Health Statistics conducts extensive and ongoing analysis of deaths

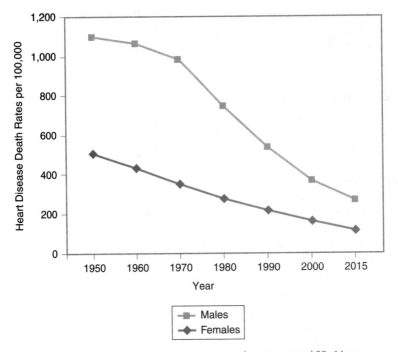

FIGURE 5-7 Heart disease death rates over time among men and women, aged 55–64 years.

Data from National Center for Health Statistics. *Health United States, 2016, With Chartbook on Long-term Trends in Health*. Hyattsville, MD; 2017.

and produces readily available statistics for public health practitioners. Third, death rates provide information on the ultimate effect of a disease.

As previously described, numerous patterns are evident in the U.S. mortality data. For example,

- Life expectancy has increased over time, is higher for women than men, and is higher for White compared to Black people.
- Death rates increase from adolescence onward.
- Leading causes of death vary among age groups (unintentional injuries predominate among the young, and chronic diseases predominate among adults and the elderly).
- Many cause-specific death rates—particularly those from motor vehicle accidents and homicides—are higher among Black than White people.
- Many cause-specific death rates—particularly those from heart disease and lung cancer—are higher among males than females.

Although mortality patterns such as these provide useful information for etiologic research and public health planning and administration, mortality data also have important limitations. First, information about the cause of death may be inaccurate because it is sometimes difficult for physicians to assign a single underlying cause of death, particularly when numerous conditions are present or when insufficient clinical, laboratory, and autopsy data are available. Second, mortality data are inadequate for examining nonfatal diseases. Thus, they give an incomplete picture of the health status of a population. This is particularly true for children and young adults, whose mortality rates are low. Even among older and elderly adults, nonfatal conditions, such as arthritis and visual and hearing impairments, are of great concern because of their significant effect on daily living.

▶ Examples: Three Important Causes of Morbidity in the United States

The remainder of this chapter focuses on three important causes of morbidity in the United States: childhood lead poisoning, HIV/AIDS, and breast cancer. Studying the patterns of these diseases in terms of person, place, and time can help us understand their causes and preventions.

Background and Descriptive Epidemiology of Childhood Lead Poisoning

Childhood lead poisoning is considered "one of the worst environmental threats to children in the United States."[73] Very high blood lead levels can lead to convulsions, coma, and even death; moderately elevated levels can adversely affect the brain, kidney, and blood-forming tissues. In fact, no safe blood lead levels in children have been identified. Even blood lead levels at or below 5 µg/dL have been associated with permanent neurological damage and behavioral disorders.[74-77]

According to one expert, lead poisoning threatens the health of our nation's children because "lead has subtly become an intrinsic part of our contemporary ways of life."[78(pp43-45)] A naturally occurring element in the Earth's crust, lead's unique properties of softness, malleability, and imperviousness have made it "one of the most useful metals in the industrial world."[78(p44)] Lead has been used in storage batteries, sewer and water pipes, roofing materials, solder for food cans and electronic equipment, containers for corrosive liquids, and gasoline. It has also been used to enhance the durability and brightness of paint. Dutch Boy paint advertisements from the 1930s encouraged consumers to purchase lead-based paint because "it lasts."[79]

The National Health and Nutrition Examination Surveys (NHANES) and state and local surveillance programs serve as the primary data sources on the descriptive epidemiology of elevated blood lead levels among U.S. children.[74] The following sections provide information on how children's blood lead levels have changed over time, what characteristics are associated with elevated levels, and what areas of the United States are most affected.

Person

The prevalence of elevated blood lead levels among young children rises sharply with age, peaking at 18–24 months.[74] Young children are at increased risk because their bodies are growing rapidly; they have a less developed blood–brain barrier than adults; and they tend to put their hands and other objects in their mouth, sometimes causing them to ingest lead. Non-Hispanic Blacks have the highest proportion of elevated levels, as do those with low family income (see **TABLE 5-9**).

Place

Elevated blood lead levels are significantly lower among children living in the West, but there is no significant difference in average blood lead levels among children living in the South, Midwest, and Northeast regions of

TABLE 5-9 Percentage of Children Aged 1–2 Years with Blood Lead Levels ≥ 5 µg/dL, by Sex, Race, and Income-to-Poverty Ratio—National Health and Nutrition Examination Survey, United States, 2007–2010

Characteristic	Percent
Sex	
Male	3.1
Female	3.2
Race/ethnicity	
Black, non-Hispanic	7.7
Mexican-American	1.6
White, non-Hispanic	3.2
*Income-to-poverty ratio**	
< 1.3	6.0
≥ 1.3	0.5

*Income-to-poverty ratios represent the ratio of family or unrelated individual income to their appropriate poverty threshold.

Data from Raymond J, Wheeler W, Brown MJ. Lead Screening and Prevalence of Blood Lead Levels in Children Aged 1–2 Years—Child Blood Lead Surveillance System, United States, 2002–2010; National Health and Nutrition Examination Survey, United States, 1999–2010. *MMWR.* 2014;63(02):36–42. https://www.cdc.gov /mmwr/preview/mmwrhtml/su6302a6.htm.

the United States.[80] A large number of children with elevated levels live in areas with a high prevalence of housing units built before 1950, when paint had a high lead content. In 2014, of 30 states (plus the District of Columbia and New York City) that reported data to the CDC, Pennsylvania, Illinois, and Ohio reported the highest number of newly identified cases of blood lead levels $\geq$ 10 µg/dL among children less than 5 years old.[80]

Time

Elevated blood lead levels among children 1 to 5 years old have declined dramatically over the years as documented by the periodic NHANES.[81] The largest reduction in children's blood lead levels was seen between NHANES II in 1976–1980 and the first phase of NHANES III (1988–1991), when the prevalence of blood lead levels $\geq$ 10 µg/dL decreased from 88.2% to 8.9%. During the second phase of NHANES III (1991–1994), this prevalence decreased further to 4.4%. Beginning in 2012, the CDC defined elevated blood lead levels among children as $\geq$ 5 µg/dL. Using this definition of elevated blood lead levels, from 1988–1994 to 2007–2014, the percentage of children 1–5 years old with blood lead levels $\geq$ 5 µg/dL declined from 25.6% to 1.9%[81] (see **FIGURE 5-8**). According

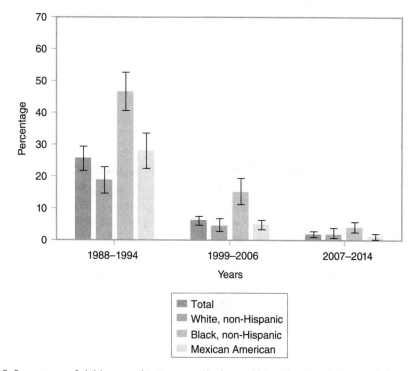

FIGURE 5-8 Percentage of children aged 1–5 years with elevated blood lead levels, by race/ethnicity, United States, 1988–1994, 1999–2006, and 2007–2014.

to the CDC's 2015 national surveillance data, of almost 2.5 million children under the age of 6 with blood lead level testing, 11,681 (0.5%) had a confirmed blood lead level ≥ 10 µg/dL, and almost 80,000 children (3.3%) had a confirmed blood lead level ≥ 5 µg/dL.[82]

Discussion

The dramatic reduction in children's blood lead levels has been hailed as "one of the most remarkable public health achievements"[73] and is the result of concerted governmental action over several decades, including the removal of lead from gasoline for automobiles, the phaseout of cans with lead-soldered seams, and the recent effort to remove residential lead-based paint in U.S. homes.

Nevertheless, the *Healthy People 2010* goal of eliminating blood lead levels > 10 mg/dL was not achieved. As noted earlier, thousands of children continue to be identified with elevated blood lead levels. An infamous crisis occurred in 2014, when cost-cutting measures in Flint, Michigan, resulted in lead contamination of the water supply. The city switched its water source from the Detroit Water Authority to the Flint Water System, and according to a class-action lawsuit, the state Department of Environmental Quality did not treat the Flint River water with an anticorrosive agent, a violation of federal law. Because the water was not properly treated, lead from aging water pipes began leaching into the Flint water supply.[83] This exposure pathway is particularly harmful for children because they drink and absorb more water per unit of body weight than adults do.[84] Successful accomplishment of the goal of eliminating blood lead levels > 10 mg/dL for 2020 will require even more intensified efforts to identify remaining lead hazards and children at risk for lead exposure.[67]

Background and Descriptive Epidemiology of HIV/AIDS

The HIV/AIDS epidemic officially started in the United States in 1981 when several cases of *Pneumocystis carinii* pneumonia and Kaposi's sarcoma (a rare cancer of the blood vessels) were reported among previously healthy, young gay men living in New York and California.[85,86] These cases were notable because *Pneumocystis carinii* pneumonia had previously occurred only among immunocompromised individuals, and Kaposi's sarcoma had occurred mainly among elderly men. In the early days, the CDC did not have an official name for the disease, but the term "acquired immune deficiency syndrome" (AIDS) was introduced in July 1982. A year after scientists identified AIDS, they discovered HIV, the retrovirus that causes AIDS, though the virus was not officially named HIV until 1986.[87]

Today, the official definition of HIV/AIDS includes three categories of HIV infection increasing in severity from stage 0 through stage 3 (AIDS) based on CD4 T lymphocyte count.[7(pp12-13)] There is no cure for HIV, but there is treatment called antiretroviral therapy (ART) that enables most people living with the virus to live a long and healthy life.[87] In the absence of ART, the virus generally progresses at a rate that varies considerably between individuals. Data on the occurrence of HIV/AIDS in the United States come from the Division of HIV/AIDS Prevention, National Center for HIV/AIDS, Viral Hepatitis, STD, and TB Prevention at the CDC.

Incidence and Mortality

At the end of 2014, an estimated 1.1 million adults and adolescents and over 11,000 children under the age of 13 were living with HIV in the United States.[88] The CDC divides annual HIV incidence statistics into two distinct categories. *HIV infections* are the estimated number of new infections (HIV incidence) that occurred in a particular year, regardless of when those infections were diagnosed, whereas *HIV diagnoses* are the number of people who received a diagnosis of HIV in a given year. This distinction is important because a person may be infected long before the year of HIV diagnosis. In 2014, there were an estimated 37,600 new HIV infections in the United States. Over 40,000 people received an HIV diagnosis in 2014, representing an HIV diagnosis rate of 12.6 per 100,000 population. Of these cases, over 99% were diagnosed among adults and adolescents, and less than 1% were diagnosed among children less than 13 years of age. In 2014, 6,721 deaths were attributed directly to HIV, but over 15,000 people with diagnosed HIV infection died, representing a death rate of 4.7 per 100,000.[7(p64)]

Time

In 2014, an estimated 40,000 HIV diagnoses represented a 19% decline since 2005 in annual diagnoses nationwide. Currently known modes of HIV transmission include homosexual and heterosexual intercourse, injection with nonsterile needles, transplantation of infected tissue, transfusion of blood and clotting factors, and transmission from an infected mother to child.[89(p89)] The most marked declines in HIV diagnoses from 2005 to 2014 occurred among people who inject drugs (63%) and heterosexuals (35%). Among women, diagnoses declined 40%, from 12,499 in 2005 to 7,533 in 2014. Among men, diagnoses decreased by 11% over the 10-year period, from 36,296 to 32,185. This smaller reduction is mainly from diagnoses among men who have sex with men (MSM), which increased by about 6% over the 10-year period (see **FIGURE 5-9**).[90]

Place

Data on the global occurrence of HIV come from the WHO. At the end of 2016, some 36.7 million people, including 2.1 million children under the age of 15, were estimated to be living with HIV.[91] Worldwide,

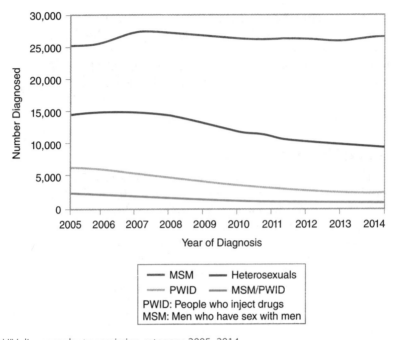

FIGURE 5-9 HIV diagnoses by transmission category, 2005–2014.

Reprinted from Trends in U.S. HIV Diagnoses, 2005-2014. cdc.gov. https://www.cdc.gov/nchhstp/newsroom/docs/factsheets/HIV-Data-Trends-Fact-Sheet-508.pdf. Accessed October 2017.

an estimated 1.8 million people became newly infected with HIV in 2016, an 18% decline from 2.2 million in 2010. The highest number of people living with HIV was in sub-Saharan Africa as well as South and Southeast Asia, but the highest prevalence of HIV as a percentage of total people in a given region was in sub-Saharan Africa and the Americas (see **FIGURE 5-10**). Several African countries have a particularly high number of people living with HIV. Adult HIV prevalence exceeds 20% in Swaziland, Lesotho, and Botswana.[92]

In the United States, there is considerable geographic variation in the annual rate of HIV diagnoses.[7(p99)] In 2015, the lowest rates were in New Hampshire, Vermont, Montana, and Idaho (1.9 to 2.8 per 100,000). The highest rates were in the District of Columbia (66.1 per 100,000), Louisiana (29.2 per 100,000), and Georgia (28.3 per 100,000) (see **FIGURE 5-11**). Metropolitan areas with 500,000 or more people had the highest rates of diagnosis. The metropolitan areas with the highest HIV diagnosis rates in the United States were Miami, Florida, and Baton Rouge, Louisiana.[7(p109)]

HIV diagnosis rates (per 100,000 people) in 2015 were highest in the South (16.8), followed by the Northeast (11.6), the West (9.8), and the Midwest (7.6). Although Southern states are home to 37% of the U.S. population, they accounted for 50% of estimated infections in 2014. Looking among those living with HIV in the United States, people in the South are also less likely to be aware of their infection than those in other U.S. regions. Nationally, 87% of Americans living with HIV knew their

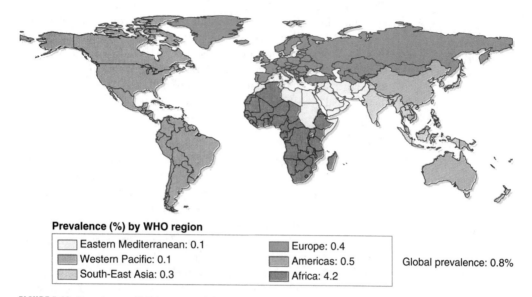

Prevalence (%) by WHO region

Eastern Mediterranean: 0.1		Europe: 0.4	
Western Pacific: 0.1		Americas: 0.5	Global prevalence: 0.8%
South-East Asia: 0.3		Africa: 4.2	

FIGURE 5-10 Prevalence of HIV among adults aged 15–49, 2016, by WHO region.

Reprinted from World Health Organization. Global Health Observatory (GHO) data: HIV/AIDS. http://www.who.int/gho/hiv/en/. Accessed October 2017.

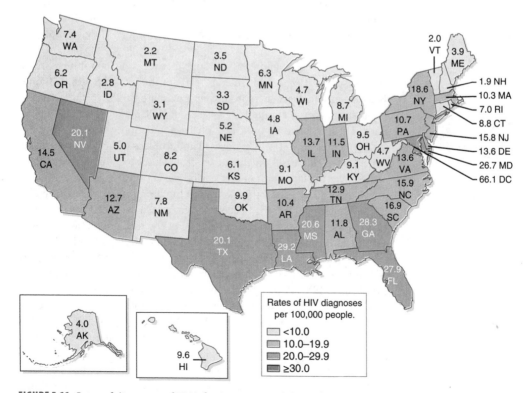

FIGURE 5-11 Rates of diagnoses of HIV infection among adults and adolescents, 2015, United States.

Reprinted from Centers for Disease Control and Prevention. HIV in the United States by Geographic Distribution. Statistics Center. https://www.cdc.gov/hiv/statistics/overview/geographicdistribution
.html. Accessed October 2017.

HIV status in 2012—but of the 15 states below 85%, one-third were states in the South. Southern states also have much worse outcomes for people living with HIV. One goal of the National HIV/AIDS Strategy for the United States is to reduce the death rate among people living with HIV to 21.7 per 1,000 individuals by 2015. Seven of the 10 states that had not met the goal by 2012 were in the South.[90]

Person

In the United States, advances in HIV research, prevention, and treatment have helped to decrease the number of HIV infections through perinatal transmission by more than 90% since the early 1990s. The risk of a pregnant woman transmitting HIV to her unborn child is 1% or less.[93] Therefore, the age distribution of HIV diagnoses reflects the primary modes of HIV transmission in the United States, through anal or vaginal sex or by sharing drug-use equipment with an infected person. Of about 40,000 people who received an HIV diagnosis in 2015, less than 1% were children under 13 years of age, 4% were age 13–19, 37% were age 20–29, 24% were age 30–39, 17% were age 40–49, 12% were age 50–59, and 5% were age 60 and over.[7(p18)] Youth and young adults 13 to 24 years old are a particularly vulnerable group. They account for 22% of all new HIV diagnoses in the United States, yet they are the least likely age group to be linked to care and have a suppressed viral load (low level of virus in the body).[88]

Across all racial and ethnic groups, Black people continue to be the most disproportionately affected by HIV in the United States. Although Black men and women represent approximately 12% of the total U.S. population, they accounted for 44% of all HIV diagnoses in 2014. Similarly, Latinos make up only 17% of the population, yet they accounted for 23% of all new HIV diagnoses. Though Blacks, Whites, and Latinos experienced decreases in diagnoses from 2005 to 2014, declines have stalled over the latter half of that period for Latinos.[90]

Gay, bisexual, and other MSM are the group most affected by HIV in the United States. MSM accounted for nearly 67% of HIV diagnoses in 2014 but make up approximately 2% of the U.S. population. Though diagnoses among MSM overall increased slightly from 2005–2014, trends over the decade varied considerably by race and ethnicity. Diagnoses rose 24% for Latino MSM, increased 22% for Black MSM, and declined 18% for White MSM. Although the number of diagnoses has been rather small among Asian American MSM, there were concerning increases over the same time period (see **FIGURE 5-12**).

Across these various subgroups, the steepest increases occurred among young Black and Latino MSM age 13–24, who both experienced increases of about 87% from 2005–2014. HIV testing remained stable or increased among the groups experiencing declines in diagnoses, and HIV testing remained stable among Latino gay and bisexual men during this period. Researchers therefore believe the decreases in diagnoses also

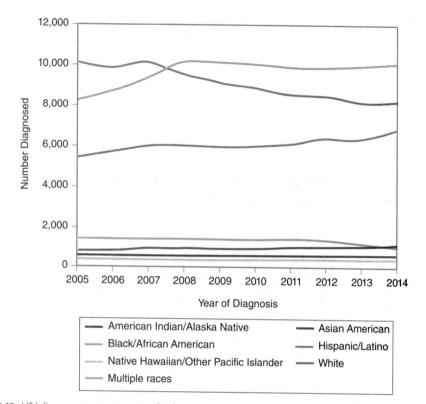

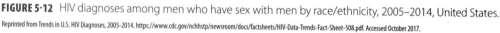

FIGURE 5-12 HIV diagnoses among men who have sex with men by race/ethnicity, 2005–2014, United States.

Reprinted from Trends in U.S. HIV Diagnoses, 2005-2014. https://www.cdc.gov/nchhstp/newsroom/docs/factsheets/HIV-Data-Trends-Fact-Sheet-508.pdf. Accessed October 2017.

reflect a decline in new infections and the increases in HIV diagnoses among Latino MSM suggest infections are likely increasing in this group.[90]

Discussion

HIV surveillance data are used to track the spread of the epidemic and to plan and evaluate prevention and treatment programs.[7] For example, several areas of the United States have implemented needle-exchange programs among people who inject drugs (PWID) in which possibly infected needles are exchanged for new ones. An analysis found that PWID who participated in New York City syringe-exchange programs were about 70% less likely to become infected with HIV than PWID who did not participate.[94] Although HIV infections fell from 2005–2014 among PWID, this progress may be threatened by the nation's opioid epidemic.

As another example, the use of antiretroviral therapy as primary prevention among high-risk uninfected individuals and as treatment of HIV-infected individuals (which has the added benefit of making them less infectious) has been found to be highly effective in reducing HIV transmission. Several studies (including tens of thousands of sexual encounters) have found no HIV transmissions to an HIV-negative partner occurred when the HIV-positive person was virally suppressed. These were both heterosexual and homosexual sexual encounters without the use of condoms or pre-exposure prophylaxis (PrEP), a drug that people at high risk for HIV take daily to lower their chances of getting infected.[95-98] The CDC has therefore stated that people who take ART daily as prescribed and are able to maintain a suppressed viral load "have effectively no risk" of transmitting HIV to their sexual partner.[99]

Background and Descriptive Epidemiology of Breast Cancer Among Women

Breast cancer is an abnormal growth in a woman's mammary gland that is characterized by a tendency to invade the surrounding tissues and spread to new locations. The most common types of breast cancer arise in the lining of the ducts or in the lobules of the breast. Like other types of cancer, a malignancy of the breast is thought to develop through a multistep process known as carcinogenesis.[100] The first step in this process, called initiation, involves DNA damage and genetic changes. Initiation is followed by numerous promotion steps that help the cancerous cells grow and establish a blood supply. Growth continues until the cancer is detected by a screening test (such as a mammogram) or produces physical symptoms (such as a lump or nipple discharge). Often, many years of unapparent disease elapse between initiation and the cancer diagnosis. For breast cancer, this period may be anywhere from 7 to 30 years.[101-103]

The best available epidemiological data on breast cancer in the United States come from the National Cancer Institute's Surveillance, Epidemiology and End Results (SEER) program.

Incidence and Mortality

Approximately 236,968 cases of female breast cancer were diagnosed in 2014, making it the most commonly diagnosed cancer among women in the United States for all racial and ethnic groups.[6] The estimated lifetime risk (the lifetime cumulative incidence) of breast cancer for women is currently 12.41%. From 2007 through 2013, about 62% of all women diagnosed with breast cancer were diagnosed with localized disease (no sign of the cancer in the lymph nodes), 31% were diagnosed with regional disease (some evidence of lymph node involvement), and 6% were diagnosed with distant disease (evidence of cancer spread to organs, such as the lungs and bone). The stage was unknown for the remaining 2% of women diagnosed with breast cancer.

From 2007 to 2013, the average 5-year relative survival rate among women diagnosed with breast cancer was 89.7%. The relative survival rate is defined as the ratio of the observed survival rate for a group with cancer to the expected rate among a similar group without cancer. As expected, women diagnosed with localized disease had much better survival (98.9%) than those diagnosed with regional (85.2%) and distant disease (26.9%).

Although the 5-year survival data are encouraging, they represent only the short-term consequences of the disease. The ultimate effect of breast cancer can be assessed solely by examining mortality rates. With an age-adjusted mortality rate of 21.2 per 100,000 women during 2010–2014, breast cancer ranked second only to lung cancer among female cancer deaths.

Time

Age-adjusted incidence rate of breast cancer among all women increased from 105.0 per 100,000 women in 1975 to 130.6 per 100,000 women in 2014.[6] This increase was quite steep during the 1980s but has attenuated in recent years for Black women and has stabilized for White women (see **FIGURE 5-13**). Since 1975, mortality rates have fallen by 37% among White women and only 5% among Black women.[6] These mortality trends vary by age at diagnosis. Among White women, mortality rates declined by 56% among those under the age of 50 years but only by 32% for those age 50 and older. Among Black women, mortality rates declined by 30% among those under the age of 50 years but increased by 4% among those age 50 and older.

Person

Many individual characteristics, such as age, race, socioeconomic level, and religion, are associated with the risk of breast cancer.[104] Breast cancer incidence rates rise sharply with age. The increase is very steep from age 40 through 79 years and then drops off (see **FIGURE 5-14**). Incidence rates are highest among White women, intermediate among Black and Hispanic women, and lowest among Asian and American Indian women. Rates are also higher among Jewish women and among women of high socioeconomic status. Various reproductive characteristics also influence a woman's risk of breast cancer.[105] For example, a younger age at menarche and older age at menopause are associated with a higher risk, and surgical removal of both ovaries is associated with a lower risk.

Place

Incidence rates are highest in North America, western and northern Europe, and Oceania, and lowest in Africa and Asia.[22] However, incidence rates in many African and Asian countries are currently increasing because of changes in reproductive patterns and other risk factors (see the following section) and increases in breast cancer awareness and screening mammography.

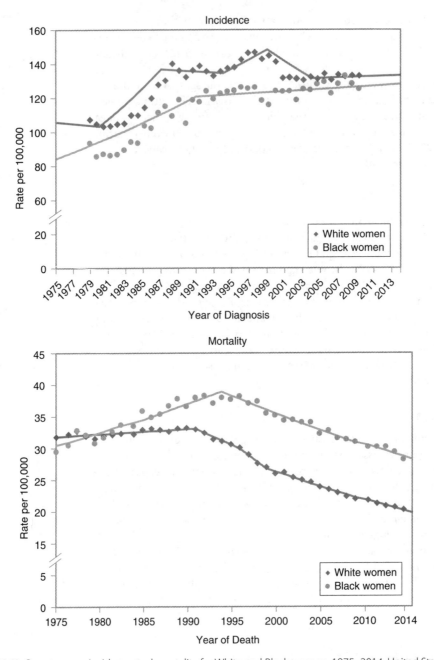

FIGURE 5-13 Breast cancer incidence and mortality for White and Black women, 1975–2014, United States.

Modified from Howlader N, Noone AM, Krapcho M, Miller D, Bishop K, Kosary CL, et al. (eds). *SEER Cancer Statistics Review, 1975-2014*. cancer.gov. https://seer.cancer.gov/csr/1975_2014/. Published April 2017. Accessed April 2017.

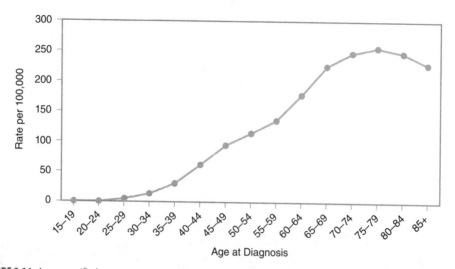

FIGURE 5-14 Age-specific breast cancer incidence rates, 2010–2014.

Data from Howlader N, Noone AM, Krapcho M, Miller D, Bishop K, Kosary CL, et al. (eds). *SEER Cancer Statistics Review, 1975-2014*. cancer.gov. https://seer.cancer.gov/csr/1975_2014/. Published April 2017. Accessed April 2017.

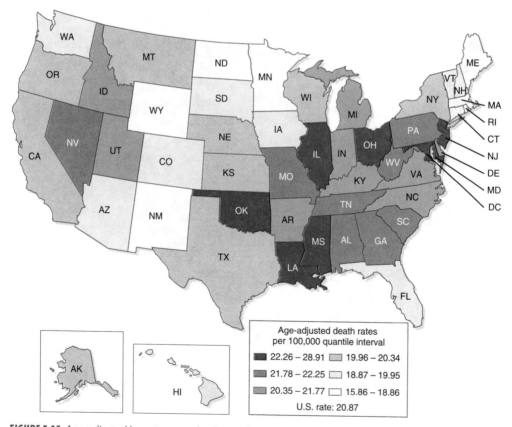

FIGURE 5-15 Age-adjusted breast cancer death rates by state, 2011–2015.

From Noone AM, Howlader N, Krapcho M, Miller D, Brest A, Yu M, Ruhl J, Tatalovich Z, Mariotto A, Lewis DR, Chen HS, Feuer EJ, Cronin KA (eds). SEER Cancer Statistics Review, 1975-2015, National Cancer Institute. Bethesda, MD, https://seer.cancer.gov/csr/1975_2015/, based on November 2017 SEER data submission, posted to the SEER web site, April 2018.

Death rates also vary dramatically within the United States (see **FIGURE 5-15**). They are highest in the District of Columbia, Louisiana, Mississippi, Oklahoma, and Ohio and lowest in Massachusetts, Connecticut, Maine, North Dakota, and Hawaii. These mortality rates are adjusted for age differences between the states, and so the geographic variation is, in part, due to differences in stage at diagnosis and access to care.

Discussion

Because the epidemiological data are so consistent, many of the characteristics described earlier are considered "established" risk factors for breast cancer[106] (see **TABLE 5-10**). Most of these characteristics also fit into the

TABLE 5-10 Risk Factors for Breast Cancer

Characteristic	High-risk group
Gender	Female
Age	Old
Country of birth	North America, western and northern Europe, Australia, and New Zealand
Place of residence in United States	Northeast, Pacific Coast
Mother, sister, or daughter with breast cancer	Yes
Personal history of breast cancer	Yes
Personal history of endometrium, ovary, or colon cancer	Yes
History of atypical hyperplasia or breast densities	Yes
Certain inherited genetic mutations	Yes
High doses of radiation to chest	Yes
Bone density (postmenopausal)	High
Socioeconomic status	High
Breast cancer at ≥ 35 years of age	White
Breast cancer at < 35 years of age	Black
Religion	Ashkenazi Jewish heritage
Reproductive history	No full-term pregnancies

Age at first full-term birth	> 30 years at first birth
History of breastfeeding	Never breastfed
Age at menarche and menopause	< 12 years at menarche and > 55 years at menopause
Endogenous estrogen or testosterone levels	High
Oral contraceptives	Recent use
Hormone replacement therapy	Recent and long-term use
Obesity (for postmenopausal breast cancer)	Yes
Alcohol consumption	Daily drinking
Height	Tall

Adapted from *Breast Cancer Facts and Figures 2017-2018*. cancer.org. https://www.cancer.org/content/dam/cancer-org/research/cancer-facts-and-statistics/breast-cancer-facts-and-figures/breast-cancer-facts-and-figures-2017-2018.pdf. Jemal A, Bray F, Center M, Ferlay J, Ward E, Forman D. Global cancer statistics. *CA Cancer J Clin*. 2011;62:169-190.

well-accepted hypothesis that circulating sex hormones, such as estrogen and andogen, play a crucial role in some types of breast cancer development.[107,108] For example, the low rates among women in Japan and other Asian countries can be accounted for by low serum levels of these hormones. Furthermore, the association with family history and Jewish religion may be partly explained by two gene alterations (BRCA1 and BRCA2) that predispose a woman to breast and ovarian cancer. These genetic alterations in BRCA1 and BRCA2 are extremely rare in the general population but occur slightly more often in certain ethnic or geographically isolated groups, such as those of Ashkenazi Jewish descent (about 2%).[109,110]

Unfortunately, the "established" risk factors cannot account for all cases of breast cancer, and many of these factors are not personally modifiable, such as age, family history, height, and age at menarche. Furthermore, many established risk factors for breast cancer are specifically associated with certain subtypes of breast cancer that express the estrogen receptor (ER+/luminal breast cancer); less is known about risk factors for ER− or basal-like breast cancers. Clearly, more research is needed to determine additional risk factors for breast cancer. For example, hypotheses have been postulated involving exposure to electromagnetic fields[111] and environmental estrogens.[112] The environmental estrogens, termed *xenoestrogens*, are a diverse group of chemicals, including pesticides, plasticizers, and detergents, that have been released into the environment in great quantities.[113] Although hypotheses about electromagnetic fields and xenoestrogens as risk factors for breast cancer are biologically plausible because exposure to these items is thought to influence a woman's estrogen levels, recently completed studies have found mixed results.[114-118] Further research on the correlation between specific environmental exposures during different critical windows of mammary gland development and breast cancer risk will be crucial.

Chemopreventive agents are drugs used to inhibit or delay cancer.[100] Tamoxifen and raloxifene are approved chemopreventive agents in healthy women at high risk for breast cancer.[119,120] Aromatase inhibitors are a class of drug undergoing clinical trials to examine whether they may also be helpful chemopreventive agents among high-risk postmenopausal women.[106] Aromatase inhibitors lower estrogen levels by stopping an enzyme in fat tissue from changing other hormones into estrogen. They lower estrogen levels in women whose ovaries are not making estrogen and thus are effective only in postmenopausal women. Currently, these drugs are approved to prevent only breast cancer recurrence, but early clinical trial results for prevention are promising.[121,122]

Although breast cancer cannot yet be prevented, survival may be improved through early diagnosis via clinical breast examination and mammography. For women at average risk of breast cancer, current guidelines from the American Cancer Society recommend that those 40 to 44 years of age have the option to begin annual mammography, those 45 to 54 years should undergo annual mammography, and those 55 years of age or older may transition to mammography every 2 years or continue with annual mammograms.[106] In contrast, the U.S. Preventive Services Task Force recommends that women age 40 up to 49 have the option to begin screening mammography every 2 years, and women age 50 to 74 should screen every 2 years. For women 75 and older, no recommendation is provided given current evidence is insufficient to assess the balance of benefits and harms of screening mammography in this group.[123] Descriptive data on screening mammography can be used to monitor the public response to these often confusing recommendations. In fact, use of mammography among women over 40 years of age more than doubled from 1987 through 2015.[5(p267)]

Summary

Descriptive epidemiology involves the analysis of disease patterns by person, place, and time. Personal characteristics include age, gender, race and ethnicity, and socioeconomic status. Place, which is usually defined in geopolitical units, such as countries, encompasses the physical environment (such as water and air), biological environment (such as flora and fauna), and social environment (such as cultural traditions). Time trends are examined for short- and long-term changes (ranging from days to decades) as well as cyclical fluctuations.

The principal reasons for describing disease rates by person, place, and time are (1) to assess the health status of a population, (2) to generate hypotheses about causal factors for disease, and (3) to plan and evaluate public health programs.

Descriptive analyses can also be used to identify disease clusters, outbreaks and epidemics. A disease cluster is the occurrence of cases of disease close together in space, time, or both space and time. A disease outbreak or epidemic is the occurrence of disease in excess of what would normally be expected. Even though the terms are synonymous, a disease outbreak often describes a localized rather than a widespread epidemic. The Ebola virus outbreaks in Africa have been among the most devastating infectious disease outbreaks in recent times.

The analysis of U.S. mortality rates by age reveals numerous patterns, including higher death rates from unintentional injuries among the young than among older individuals, higher death rates from motor vehicle accidents and homicides among Blacks than among Whites, and lower death rates from heart disease and lung cancer among females than among males. Although mortality data have many advantages, including complete reporting and easy access, they also have several disadvantages, including inaccurate information on cause of death and insufficient data on serious nonfatal diseases. Thus, epidemiologists rely on other data sources to learn about descriptive patterns of important fatal and nonfatal illnesses, such as childhood lead poisoning, HIV/AIDS, and breast cancer. For example, the NHANES, the primary data source on the descriptive epidemiology of childhood lead poisoning in the United States, reveals continuing racial disparities in children's blood lead levels, despite significant decreases in all groups over time. Similarly, descriptive statistics on HIV from the CDC and the WHO show a lower prevalence in the United States than in other parts of the world, especially in sub-Saharan Africa. In addition, breast cancer data from the National Cancer Institute's Surveillance, Epidemiology and End Results program indicate that breast cancer is the most commonly diagnosed cancer among U.S. women and that rates are highest among White women, women of high socioeconomic status, and women residing in the Northeast.

References

1. MacMahon B, Trichopoulos D. *Epidemiology: Principles and Methods*. 2nd ed. Boston, MA: Little, Brown and Co; 1996.
2. Porta M. *A Dictionary of Epidemiology*. 6th ed. New York, NY: Oxford University Press; 2014.
3. Yoon SS, Fryar CD, Carroll MD. Hypertension prevalence and control among adults: United States, 2011–2014. NCHS data brief, no 220. Hyattsville, MD: National Center for Health Statistics; 2015.
4. Heymann DL (ed.). *Control of Communicable Diseases Manual*. 20th ed. Washington, DC: American Public Health Association; 2015.
5. National Center for Health Statistics. *Health, United States, 2016, With Chartbook on Long-term Trends in Health*. Hyattsville, MD; 2017.
6. Howlader N, Noone AM, Krapcho M, Miller D, Bishop K, Kosary CL, et al. (eds). *SEER Cancer Statistics Review, 1975–2014*. cancer.gov. https://seer.cancer .gov/csr/1975_2014/. Published April 2017. Accessed April 2017.
7. HIV/AIDS Surveillance Report: Diagnoses of HIV Infection in the United States and Dependent Areas, 2015. cdc.gov. https://www.cdc.gov/hiv/pdf/library /reports/surveillance/cdc-hiv-surveillance

-report-2015-vol-27.pdf. Published November 2016. Accessed April 2017.

8. Olsson AC, Gustavsson P, Kromhout H, Peters S, Vermeulen R, Bruske I, et al. Exposure to diesel motor exhaust and lung cancer risk in a pooled analysis from case-control studies in Europe and Canada. *Am J Respir Crit Care Med.* 2011;183:941-948.

9. Humes K, Jones N, Ramirez R. *Overview of Race and Hispanic Origin: 2010.* census.gov. www.census.gov /prod/cen2010/briefs/c2010br-02.pdf. Issued March 2011. Accessed September 2017.

10. Ríos M, Romero F, Ramirez, R. *Race Reporting Among Hispanics: 2010.* census.gov. www.census .gov/population/www/documentation/twps0102 /twps0102.pdf. Issued March 2014. Accessed September 2017.

11. National Center for Health Statistics. *Health, United States, 2015, With Special Feature on Racial and Ethnic Health Disparities.* Hyattsville, MD: U.S. Government Printing Office; 2016.

12. Wade WC. *The Titanic: End of a Dream.* New York, NY: Rawson Wade; 1979.

13. Chetty R, Stepner M, Abraham S, Lin S, Scuderi B, Turner N, et al. The association between income and life expectancy in the United States, 2001–2014. *JAMA.* 2016;315:1750-1766.

14. Davis RL, Robertson DM (eds.). *Textbook of Neuropathology.* 2nd ed. Baltimore, MD: Williams and Wilkins; 1991.

15. Merrill RM, Lyon JL. Cancer incidence among Mormons and non-Mormons in Utah (United States), 1995–1999. *Prev Med.* 2005;40:535-541.

16. Blair A. Occupation. In: Harras A, Edwards BK, Blot WJ, Ries LAG (eds.). *Cancer Rates and Risks.* NIH pub no 96–691. Bethesda, MD: National Cancer Institute; 1996.

17. Kaplan RM, Kronick RG. Marital status and longevity in the United States population. *J Epidemiol Commun H.* 2006;60:760-765.

18. McIntosh JH, Berman K, Holliday FM, Byth K, Chapman R, Piper DW. Some factors associated with mortality in perforated peptic ulcer: a case-control study. *J Gastroen Hepatol.* 1996;11:82-87.

19. Ebrahim S, Wannamethee G, McCallum A, Walker M, Shaper AG. Marital status, change in marital status, and mortality in middle-aged British men. *Am J Epidemiol.* 1995;142:834-842.

20. Goldman N, Korenman S, Weinstein R. Marital status and health among the elderly. *Soc Sci Med.* 1995;40:1717-1730.

21. Cotter C, Sturrock HJ, Hsiang MS, Liu J, Phillips AA, Hwang J, et al. The changing epidemiology of malaria elimination: new strategies for new challenges. *Lancet.* 2013;382:900-911.

22. Torre LA, Bray F, Siegel RL, Ferlay J, Lortet-Tieulent J, Jemal A. Global cancer statistics, 2012. *CA Cancer J Clin.* 2015;65:87-108.

23. Bosch FX, Ribes J, Cleries R, Diaz M. Epidemiology of hepatocellular carcinoma. *Clin Liver Dis.* 2005;9:191–211.

24. Jorgensen N, Carlsen E, Nermoen I, et al. East-West gradient in semen quality in the Nordic-Baltic area: a study of men from the general population in Denmark, Norway, Estonia and Finland. *Hum Reprod.* 2002;17:2199-2208.

25. Hayes RB. Prostate. In: Harras A, Edwards BK, Blot WJ, Ries LAG (eds.). *Cancer Rates and Risks.* NIH pub no 96–691. Bethesda, MD: National Cancer Institute; 1996.

26. Katanoda K, Hori M. Incidence rate for breast cancer in Japanese in Japan and in the United States from the Cancer Incidence in Five Continents. *Jpn J Clin Oncol.* 2016;46:883.

27. Fraser DW, Tsai TR, Orenstein W, et al. and the Field Investigation Team. Legionnaires' disease: description of an epidemic of pneumonia. *New Engl J Med.* 1977;297:1189-1197.

28. Schwartz J. What are people dying of on high air pollution days? *Environ Res.* 1994;64:26-35.

29. Schwartz J, Dockery DW. Increased mortality in Philadelphia associated with daily air pollution concentrations. *Am Rev Respir Dis.* 1992;145:600-604.

30. Van der Palen J, Doggen CJ, Beaglehorn R. Variation in the time and day of onset of myocardial infarction and sudden death. *New Zealand Med J.* 1995;108:332-334.

31. Cohen MC, Rohtla KM, Lavery CE, Muller JE, Mittleman MA. Meta-analysis of the morning excess of acute myocardial infarction and sudden cardiac death. *Am J Cardio.* 1997;79:1512-1516.

32. Willich SN, Lowel H, Lewis M, Hormann A, Arntz HR, Keil U. Weekly variation of acute myocardial infarction. Increased Monday risk in the working population. *Circulation.* 1994;90:87-93.

33. Carvalho JS, Mavrides E, Shinebourne EA, Campbell S, Thilaganathan B. Improving the effectiveness of routine prenatal screening for major congenital heart defects. *Heart.* 2002;88:387-391.

34. Roueche B. *Eleven Blue Men and Other Narratives of Medical Detection.* New York, NY: Berkeley Publishing Co; 1953.

35. Lagakos S, Wessen B, Zelen M. An analysis of contaminated well water and health effects in Woburn, Massachusetts. *J Am Stat Assoc.* 1986; 81:583-595.

36. Rothman KJ. A sobering start for the cluster busters' conference. *Am J Epidemiol.* 1990;132:S6-S13.

37. Neutra RR. Counterpoint from a cluster buster. *Am J Epidemiol.* 1990;132:1-8.

38. Disease outbreaks. who.int. www.who.int/topics/disease_outbreaks/en/. Accessed February 20, 2017.

39. Outbreak. Epidemiology Glossary. cdc.gov. www.cdc.gov/reproductivehealth/data_stats/glossary.html#O. Updated January 21, 2015. Accessed February 23, 2017.

40. Response to Measles Outbreaks in Measles Mortality Reduction Settings: Immunization, Vaccines and Biologicals. NCBI.gov. www.ncbi.nlm.nih.gov/books/NBK143963/.

41. Overview of Influenza Surveillance in the United States. cdc.gov. www.cdc.gov/flu/weekly/overview.htm. Updated October 13, 2016. Accessed February 23, 2017.

42. Epidemic intelligence - systematic event detection. who.int. www.who.int/csr/alertresponse/epidemicintelligence/en. Accessed February 24, 2017.

43. *Responding to an Infectious Disease Outbreak: Progress Between SARS and Pandemic Influenza H1N1*. Public Health Agency Canada. www.phac-aspc.gc.ca/ep-mu/rido-iemi/index-eng.php. Updated April 11, 2012. Accessed March 2, 2017.

44. Reingold AL. Outbreak investigations: a perspective. *Emerg Infect Dis*. 1998;4:21-27.

45. Lesson 6: Investigating an outbreak. In: *Principles of Epidemiology in Public Health Practice*. 3rd ed. cdc.gov. www.cdc.gov/ophss/csels/dsepd/ss1978/ss1978.pdf. Updated May 2012. Accessed February 26, 2017.

46. *Surveillance for Foodborne Disease Outbreaks, United States, 2014: Annual Report*. cdc.gov. www.cdc.gov/foodsafety/pdfs/foodborne-outbreaks-annual-report-2014–508.pdf. Published 2016. Accessed February 19, 2017.

47. Lesson 6: Investigating an outbreak. In: *Principles of Epidemiology in Public Health Practice*. 3rd ed. cdc.gov. www.cdc.gov/ophss/csels/dsepd/ss1978/ss1978.pdf. Updated May 2012. Accessed February 26, 2017.

48. World Health Organization. Ebola haemorrhagic fever in Sudan, 1976. *Bull WHO*. 1978;56:247-270.

49. World Health Organization. Ebola haemorrhagic fever in Zaire, 1976. *Bull WHO*. 1978;56:271-293.

50. Brès P. The epidemic of Ebola haemorrhagic fever in Sudan and Zaire, 1976: introductory note. *Bull WHO*. 1978;56:245.

51. Shears P, O'Dempsey TJ. Ebola virus disease in Africa: epidemiology and nosocomial transmission. *J Hosp Infect*. 2015;90:1-9.

52. Frieden TR, Damon I, Bell BP, Kenyon T, Nichol S. Ebola 2014—new challenges, new global response and responsibility. *N Engl J Med*. 2014;371:1177-1180.

53. Piot P. *No Time to Lose: A Life in Pursuit of Deadly Viruses*. New York, NY: W. W. Norton & Co.; 2012.

54. World Health Organization. *Ebola Outbreak Monthly Update, November 2016*. www.afro.who.int/en/disease-outbreaks/outbreak-news/4790-ebola-outbreak-monthly-update-november-2015.html. Accessed March 5, 2017.

55. *Situation Report, 10 June 2016*. who.int. apps.who.int/iris/bitstream/10665/208883/1/ebolasitrep_10Jun2016_eng.pdf?ua=1. Accessed March 5, 2017.

56. Busting the myths about Ebola is crucial to stop the transmission of the disease in Guinea. who.int. who.int/features/2014/ebola-myths/en/. Published April 23, 2014. Accessed March 3, 2017.

57. Böl G. Risk communication in times of crisis: pitfalls and challenges in ensuring preparedness instead of hysterics. *EMBO Reports*. 2016;17:1-9.

58. Levi J, Segal L, Lieberman D, May K, St. Laurent R. *Outbreaks: Protecting Americans from Infectious Diseases, 2014*. healthyamericans.org. healthyamericans.org/assets/files/Final%20Outbreaks%202014%20Report.pdf. Accessed on March 6, 2017.

59. Halabi SF, Gostin LO, Crowley JS (eds.). *Global Management of Infectious Disease After Ebola*. Oxford, UK: Oxford University Press; 2017:26-27.

60. Henao-Restrepo A, Camacho A, Longini IM, Watson CH, Edmunds WH, Egger M, et al. Efficacy and effectiveness of an rVSV-vectored vaccine in preventing Ebola virus disease: final results from the Guinea ring vaccination, open-label, cluster-randomised trial (Ebola Ça Suffit!). *Lancet*. 2016;389:505-518.

61. Successful Ebola vaccine will be fast-tracked for use. *BBC News*. December 23, 2016. http://www.bbc.com/news/world-africa-38414060. Accessed March 24, 2017.

62. Pickett JP (exec. ed.). *The American Heritage Dictionary of the English Language*. 4th ed. Boston, MA: Houghton Mifflin Co.; 2000.

63. Tsugane S. Salt, salted food intake, and risk of gastric cancer: epidemiologic evidence. *Cancer Science*. 2005;96:1-6.

64. Zahm S. Non-Hodgkin's lymphoma. In: Harras A, Edwards BK, Blot WJ, Ries LAG (eds.). *Cancer Rates and Risks*. NIH pub no 96–691. Bethesda, MD: National Cancer Institute; 1996.

65. Escobedo LG, Peddicord JP. Smoking prevalence in U.S. birth cohorts: the influence of gender and education. *Am J Public Health*. 1996;86:231-236.

66. Alter MJ, Francis DP. Hepatitis B virus transmission between homosexual men: a model of the acquired immune deficiency syndrome (AIDS). In: Ma P, Armstrong D (eds.). *The Acquired Immune Deficiency Syndrome and Infections of Homosexual Men*. New York, NY: Yorke Medical Books; 1984.

67. *Healthy People 2020*. healthypeople.gov. http://www.healthypeople.gov/2020/topicsobjectives2020/default.aspx. Accessed September 2017.

68. Annual Estimates of the Resident Population by Sex, Race, and Hispanic Origin for the United States, States,

and Counties: April 1, 2010 to July 1, 2016. census.gov. https://factfinder.census.gov/faces/tableservices/jsf/pages/productview.xhtml?src=bkmk. Released June 2017. Accessed September 2017.

69. ACS Demographic and Housing Estimates, 2011–2015, American Community Survey 5-Year Estimates. census.gov. https://factfinder.census.gov/faces/tableservices/jsf/pages/productview.xhtml?src=bkmk. Accessed October 2017.

70. Martin JA, Hamilton BE, Osterman MJK, Driscoll AK, Mathews TJ. Births: Final data for 2015. *National Vital Statistics Report*. 66(1). cdc.gov. https://www.cdc.gov/nchs/data/nvsr/nvsr66/nvsr66_01.pdf. Dated January 5, 2017.

71. Life expectancy at birth (years), 2000–2015. who.int. http://gamapserver.who.int/gho/interactive_charts/mbd/life_expectancy/atlas.html. Accessed September 2017.

72. OECD Health Statistics 2017. oecd.org. http://www.oecd.org/health/health-data.htm. Accessed September 2017.

73. Goldman LR, Carra J. Childhood lead poisoning in 1994 [editorial]. *JAMA*. 1994;272:315-316.

74. Raymond J, Brown MJ. Childhood blood lead levels in children aged <5 years—United States, 2009–2014. *MMWR Surveill Summ*. 2017;66(No. SS-3):1-10.

75. **Gump BB**, Dykas MJ, MacKenzie JA, Dumas AK, Hruska B, Ewart CK, et al. Background lead and mercury exposures: psychological and behavioral problems in children. *Environ Res*. 2017;158:576-582.

76. Bellinger DC. Very low lead exposures and children's neurodevelopment. *Curr Opin Pediatr*. 2008;20:172-177.

77. Wani AL, Ara A, Usmani JA. Lead toxicity: a review. *Interdiscip Toxicol*. 2015;8:55-64.

78. Lin-Fu J. Historical perspective on health effects of lead. In: Mahaffey KR (ed.). *Dietary and Environmental Lead: Human Health Effects*. Amsterdam, Netherlands: Elsevier Science Publishers BV; 1985.

79. Rabin R. Warnings unheeded: a history of child lead poisoning. *Am J Public Health*. 1989;79:1668-1674.

80. **Scott L**, Nguyen L. Geographic region of residence and blood lead levels in US children: results of the National Health and Nutrition Examination Survey. *Int Arch Occup Environ Health*. 2011;84:513.

81. Centers for Disease Control and Prevention. QuickStats: Percentage of Children Aged 1–5 Years with Elevated Blood Lead Levels, by Race/Ethnicity—National Health and Nutrition Examination Survey, United States, 1988–1994, 1999–2006, and 2007–2014. *MMWR*. 2016;65:1089. https://www.cdc.gov/mmwr/volumes/65/wr/mm6539a9.htm.

82. Tested and Confirmed Elevated Blood Lead Levels by State, Year, and Blood Lead Level Group for Children <72 months of age. cdc.gov. https://www.cdc.gov/nceh/lead/data/national.htm. Updated October 28, 2016. Accessed September 2017.

83. Kennedy C, Yard E, Dignam T, Buchanan S, Condon S, Brown MJ, et al. Blood lead levels among children aged <6 years—Flint, Michigan, 2013–2016. *MMWR*. 2016;65. https://www.cdc.gov/mmwr/volumes/65/wr/mm6525e1.htm

84. Mushak P. Gastro-intestinal absorption of lead in children and adults: overview of biological and biophysico-chemical aspects. *Chem Speciation Bioavailability*. 1991;3:87-104.

85. Gottlieb MS, Schanker HM, Fan PT, Saxon A, Weisman JD, Pozalski I. *Pneumocystis* pneumonia—Los Angeles. *MMWR*. 1981;30:250-252.

86. Friedman-Kien A, Laubenstein L, Marmor M, et al. Kaposi's sarcoma and *Pneumocystis* pneumonia among homosexual men—New York City and California. *MMWR*. 1981;30:305-308.

87. Centers for Disease Control and Prevention. HIV Surveillance—United States, 1981–2008. *MMWR*. 2011;60:689-693. https://www.cdc.gov/mmwr/preview/mmwrhtml/mm6021a2.htm

88. HIV in the United States: At a Glance. cdc.gov. https://www.cdc.gov/hiv/statistics/overview/ataglance.html. Accessed September 2017.

89. Kaslow RA, Francis DP. Epidemiology: general considerations. In: Kaslow RA, Francis DP (eds.). *The Epidemiology of AIDS: Expression, Occurrence, and Control of Human Immunodeficiency Virus Type 1 Infection*. New York, NY: Oxford University Press; 1989.

90. Trends in U.S. HIV Diagnoses, 2005–2014. cdc.gov. https://www.cdc.gov/nchhstp/newsroom/docs/factsheets/HIV-Data-Trends-Fact-Sheet-508.pdf. Accessed October 2017.

91. Fact Sheet—World AIDS Day 2017. unaids.org. http://www.unaids.org/sites/default/files/media_asset/UNAIDS_FactSheet_en.pdf. Accessed October 2017.

92. *The World Factbook*. cia.gov. https://www.cia.gov/library/publications/the-world-factbook/index.html. Accessed October 2017.

93. European Collaborative Study. Mother-to-child transmission of HIV infection in the era of highly active antiretroviral therapy. *Clin Infect Dis*. 2005;40:458-465.

94. Des Jarlais DC, Marmor M, Paone D, Titus S, Shi Q, Perlis T, et al. HIV incidence among injecting drug users in New York City syringe-exchange programmes. *Lancet*. 1996;348:987-991.

95. Cohen MS, Chen YQ, McCauley MB, Gamble T, Hosseinipour MC, Kumarasamy N, et al. Prevention of HIV-1 infection with early antiretroviral therapy. *New Engl J Med*. 2011;365:493-505.

96. Grant RM, Lama JR, Anderson PL, McMahan V, Liu AY, Vargas L, et al. Preexposure chemoprophylaxis

for HIV prevention in men who have sex with men. *New Engl J Med.* 2010;363:2587-2599.

97. Rodger AJ, Cambiano V, Bruun T, Vernazza P, Collins S, van Lunzen J, et al. Sexual activity without condoms and risk of HIV transmission in serodifferent couples when the HIV-positive partner is using suppressive antiretroviral therapy. *JAMA.* 2016;316:1-11.

98. Bavinton B, Grinsztejn B, Phanuphak N, Jin F, Zablotska I, Prestage G, et al. HIV treatment prevents HIV transmission in male serodiscordant couples in Australia, Thailand and Brazil. 9th IAS Conference on HIV Science; July 23–26th, 2017; Paris, France (Abstract TUAC0506LB).

99. McCray E, Mermin J. Dear colleague: September 27, 2017. cdc.gov. https://www.cdc.gov/hiv/library/dcl /dcl/092717.html.

100. Greenwald P, Kelloff G, Burch-Whitman C, Kramer BS. Chemoprevention. *CA-Cancer J Clin.* 1995;45:31-49.

101. Schottenfeld D, Haas JF. Carcinogens in the workplace. *CA-Cancer J Clin.* 1979;29:144.

102. Aschengrau A, Paulu C, Ozonoff D. Tetrachloro-ethylene contaminated drinking water and risk of breast cancer. *Environ Health Persp.* 1998;106:947-953.

103. Petralia SA, Vena JE, Freudenheim JL, Dosemeci M, Michalek A, Goldberg MA, et al. Risk of premenopausal breast cancer in association with occupational exposure to polycyclic aromatic hydrocarbons and benzene. *Scandin J Work Envir Health.* 1999;25:215-221.

104. Rojas K, Stuckey A. Breast cancer epidemiology and risk factors. *Clin Obstet Gynecol.* 2016;59:651-672.

105. Sisti JS, Collins LC, Beck AH, Tamimi RM, Rosner BA, Eliassen AH. Reproductive risk factors in relation to molecular subtypes of breast cancer: results from the Nurses' Health Studies. *Int. J. Cancer.* 2016;138:2346-2356.

106. Noone AM, Howlander N, Krapcho M, Miller D, Brest A, Yu M, et al. (eds). SEER Cancer Statistics Review, 1975-2015. cancer.gov. https://seer.cancer .gov/csr/1975_2015/. Published April 2018. Accessed June 2018.

107. Eliassen A, Hankinson S. Endogenous hormone levels and risk of breast, endometrial and ovarian cancers: prospective studies. *Adv Exp Med Biol.* 2008;630:148-165.

108. Rice MS, Eliassen AH, Hankinson SE, Lenart EB, Willett WC, Tamimi RM. Breast cancer research in the Nurses' Health Studies: Exposures across the life course. *Am J Public Health.* 2016;106:1592-1598.

109. Gabai-Kapara E, Lahad A, Kaufman B, Friedman E, Segev S, Renbaum P, et al. Population-based screening for breast and ovarian cancer risk due to BRCA1 and BRCA2. *Proc Natl Acad Sci USA.* 2014;111:14205-14210.

110. Turnbull C, Rahman N. Genetic predisposition to breast cancer: past, present, and future. *Annu Rev Genomics Hum Genet.* 2008;9:321-345.

111. Stevens RG. Electric power use and breast cancer: a hypothesis. *Am J Epidemiol.* 1978;125:556-561.

112. Davis DL, Bradlow HL, Wolff M, Woodruff T, Hoel DG, Anton-Culver H. Medical hypothesis: xenoestrogens as preventable causes of breast cancer. *Environ Health Perspect.* 1993;101:372-377.

113. Colborn T, vom Saal FS, Soto AM. Developmental effects of endocrine disrupting chemicals in wildlife and humans. *Environ Health Perspect.* 1993;101:378-384.

114. Kliukiene J, Tynes T, Andersen A. Residential and occupational exposure to 50-Hz magnetic fields and breast cancer in women: a population-based study. *Am J Epidemiol.* 2004;159:852-861.

115. Schoenfeld ER, O'Leary ES, Henderson K, Grimson R, Kabat GC, Ahnn S, et al. Electromagnetic fields and breast cancer on Long Island: a case–control study. *Am J Epidemiol.* 2003;158:47-58.

116. Teitelbaum SL, Gammon MD, Britton JA, Neugut AI, Levin B, Stellman SD. Reported residential pesticide use and breast cancer risk on Long Island, New York. *Am J Epidemiol.* 2007;165:643-651.

117. Xu X, Dailey AB, Talbott EO, Ilacqua VA, Kearney G, Asal NR. Association of serum concentrations of organochlorine pesticides with breast cancer and prostate cancer in U.S. adults. *Environ Health Perspect.* 2010;118:60-66.

118. Macon MB, Fenton SE. Endocrine disruptors and the breast: early life effects and later life disease. *J Mammary Gland Biol Neoplasia.* 2013;18:43-61.

119. Vogel VG, Constantino JP, Wickerham DL, Cronin WM, Cecchini RS, Atkins JN, et al. Effects of tamoxifen vs raloxifene on the risk of developing invasive breast cancer and other diseases: the NSABP Study of Tamoxifen and Raloxifene (STAR) P-2 trial. *JAMA.* 2006;295:2727-2741.

120. Fisher B, Constantino JP, Wickerham DL, Redmond CK, Kavanah M, Cronin WM, et al. Tamoxifen for prevention of breast cancer: report of the National Surgical Adjuvant Breast and Bowel Project P-1 Study. *J Natl Cancer Inst.* 1998;90:1371-1388.

121. Cuzick J, Sestak I, Forbes JF, Dowsett M, Knox J, Cawthorn S, et al. Anastrozole for prevention of breast cancer in high-risk postmenopausal women (IBIS-II): an international, double-blind, randomised placebo-controlled trial. *Lancet.* 2014;383:1041-1048.

122. Goss PE, Ingle JN, Ales-Martinez JE, Cheung AM, Chlebowski RT, Wactawski-Wende J, et al. Exemestane for breast cancer prevention in postmenopausal women. *N Engl J Med.* 2011;364:2381-2391.

123. Siu AL. Screening for breast cancer: U.S. Preventive Services Task Force recommendation statement. *Ann Intern Med.* 2016;164:279.

Chapter Questions

1.　The following data give some of the descriptive epidemiology of gastroschisis in the state of Massachusetts. Gastroschisis is a rare birth defect that is characterized by a herniation of the abdominal wall. Its treatment requires surgical repair.

Number and Prevalence of Gastroschisis by Year of Birth—Massachusetts, 1999–2009	
Year	**Prevalence (per 10,000 live births)**
2000–2001	2.09
2002–2003	2.43
2004–2005	3.09
2006–2007	3.60
2008–2009	3.29

Data from Massachusetts Department of Public Health, *Center for Birth Defects Research and Prevention. Surveillance Reports 1999–2009.* http://www.mass.gov/eohhs/gov/departments/dph/programs/family-health/birth-defect/monitoring/surveillance-reports.html. Accessed October 2017.

Prevalence of Gastroschisis (per 10,000 Live Births) by Maternal Age and Race and Child's Sex—Massachusetts, 2011–2012					
Maternal age (years)		**Maternal race**		**Child's sex**	
< 20	13.31	White	2.75	Male	3.52
20–24	9.99	Black	1.44	Female	2.41
25–29	2.76				

Data from Massachusetts Birth Defects 2011–2012. May 2016. https://www.mass.gov/files/documents/2016/07/sb/report-2011–2012.pdf. Accessed October 2017.

　a.　Based on these data, briefly describe each of the following using words and numbers:
　　i.　The change in prevalence from 2000 to 2009
　　ii.　The trend in prevalence by maternal age
　　iii.　The difference in prevalence between Blacks and Whites
　　iv.　The difference in prevalence by gender

b. Data such as these are used to generate hypotheses about the causes of disease. Using any information in the tables, briefly describe a hypothesis that might explain one of these descriptive features.

c. Data such as these are also used by public health administrators and planners to establish priorities, allocate resources, and plan and evaluate the effectiveness of treatment and prevention programs. Briefly describe how these data might be used to allocate resources for the prevention and treatment of gastroschisis.

2. Define the following terms:
   a. Disease cluster
   b. Outbreak
   c. Epidemic

CHAPTER 6

Overview of Epidemiological Study Designs

LEARNING OBJECTIVES

By the end of this chapter the reader will be able to:
- Distinguish between experimental and observational studies.
- Describe the key characteristics of experimental, cohort, case–control, cross-sectional, and ecological studies regarding subject selection, data collection, and analysis.
- Identify the design of a particular study.
- Discuss the factors that determine when a particular design is indicated.

▶ Introduction

Epidemiology is the study of the distribution and determinants of disease frequency in human populations and the application of this study to control health problems.[1(p1),2(p95)] The term *study* includes both **surveillance**, whose purpose is to monitor aspects of disease occurrence and spread that are pertinent to effective control,[3(p704)] and epidemiological research, whose goal is to harvest valid and precise information about the causes, preventions, and treatments for disease. The term *disease* refers to a broad array of health-related states and events, including diseases, injuries, disabilities, and death.

Epidemiological research encompasses several types of study designs, including experimental studies and observational studies, such as cohort and case–control studies. Each type of epidemiological study design simply represents a different way of harvesting information. The selection of one design over another depends on the particular research question, concerns about validity and efficiency, and practical and ethical considerations. For example, experimental studies, also known as trials, investigate the role of some factor or agent in the prevention or treatment of a disease. In this type of study, the investigator assigns individuals to two or more groups that either receive or do not receive the preventive or therapeutic agent. Because experimental studies closely resemble controlled laboratory investigations, they are thought to produce the most scientifically rigorous data of all the designs.

However, experimental studies are often infeasible because of difficulties enrolling participants, high costs, and thorny ethical issues, most epidemiological research is conducted using an **observational study**, which is considered a "natural" experiment because the investigator lets nature take its course. Observational studies take advantage of the fact that people are exposed to noxious and/or healthy substances through their personal habits, occupation, place of residence, and so on. The studies provide information on exposures that occur in natural settings, and they are not limited to preventions and treatments. Furthermore, they do not suffer from the ethical and feasibility issues of experimental studies. For example, although it is unethical to conduct an experimental study of the effect of drinking alcohol on the developing fetus by assigning newly pregnant women to either a drinking or nondrinking group, it is perfectly ethical to conduct an observational study by comparing women who choose to drink during pregnancy with those who decide not.

The two principal types of observational studies are cohort and case–control studies. A classic cohort study examines one or more health effects of exposure to a single agent. Subjects are defined according to their exposure status and followed over time to determine the incidence of health outcomes. In contrast, a classic case–control study examines a single disease in relation to exposure to one or more agents. Cases that have the disease of interest and controls who are a sample of the population that produced the cases are defined and enrolled. The purpose of the control group is to provide information on the exposure distribution in the population that gave rise to the cases. Investigators obtain and compare exposure histories of cases as well as of controls.

Additional observational study designs include cross-sectional studies and ecological studies. A cross-sectional study examines the relationship between a disease and an exposure among individuals in a defined population at a point in time. Thus, it takes a snapshot of a population and usually measures the exposure prevalence in relation to the disease prevalence. An **ecological study** evaluates an association using the population rather than the individual as the unit of analysis. The rates of disease are examined in relation to factors described on the population level. Both the cross-sectional and ecological designs have important limitations that make them less scientifically rigorous than cohort and case–control studies. These limitations are discussed later in this chapter.

TABLE 6-1 Main Types of Epidemiological Studies	
Type of study	**Characteristics**
Experimental	Studies preventions and treatments for diseases; investigator actively manipulates which groups receive the agent under study.
Observational	Studies causes, preventions, and treatments for diseases; investigator passively observes as nature takes its course.
Cohort	Typically examines multiple health effects of an exposure; subjects are defined according to their exposure levels and followed for disease occurrence.
Case–control	Typically examines multiple exposures in relation to a disease; subjects are defined as cases and controls, and exposure histories are compared.
Cross-sectional	Typically examines the relationship between exposure and disease prevalence in a defined population at a single point in time
Ecological	Examines the relationship between exposure and disease with population-level rather than individual-level data

An overview of these study designs is provided in **TABLE 6-1**. The goal of all these studies is to determine the relationship between an exposure and a disease with validity and precision using minimal resources. **Validity** is defined as the lack of bias and confounding. Bias is an error committed by the investigator in the design or conduct of a study that leads to a false association between the exposure and disease. Confounding, on the other hand, is not the fault of the investigator but rather reflects the fact that epidemiological research is conducted among free-living humans with unevenly distributed characteristics. As a result, epidemiological studies that try to determine the relationship between an exposure and a disease are susceptible to the disturbing influences of extraneous factors known as confounders. Precision is the lack of random error, which leads to a false association between the exposure and disease just by "chance," an uncontrollable force that seems to have no assignable cause.[4(p309)]

Several factors help epidemiologists determine the most appropriate study design for evaluating a particular association, including the hypothesis being tested, state of knowledge, and frequency of the exposure and the disease and expected strength of the association between the two. This chapter provides (1) an overview of epidemiological research designs—experimental, cohort, case–control, case–crossover, ecological, and agent-based modeling—and (2) a description of the settings in which the three main study designs—experimental, cohort, and case–control—are most appropriate.

▶ Overview of Experimental Studies

Definitions and Classification

An experimental study, also known as a trial, investigates the role of some agent in the prevention or treatment of a disease. In this type of study, the investigator assigns individuals to two or more groups that either receive or do not receive the preventive or therapeutic agent. The group that is allocated the agent under study is generally called the **treatment group**, and the group that is not allocated the agent under study is called the **comparison group**. Depending on the purpose of the trial, the comparison group may receive no treatment at all, an inactive treatment such as a placebo, or another active treatment.

The active manipulation of the agent by the investigator is the hallmark that distinguishes experimental from observational studies. In the latter, the investigator acts as a passive observer, merely letting nature take its course. Because experimental studies more closely resemble controlled laboratory investigations, most epidemiologists believe that experimental studies produce more scientifically rigorous results than do observational studies.

Experimental studies are commonly classified by their objective, that is, by whether they investigate a measure that prevents disease occurrence or a measure that treats an existing condition. The former is known as a preventive or prophylactic trial, and the latter is known as a therapeutic or clinical trial. In preventive trials, agents such as vitamins or behavioral modifications such as smoking cessation are studied to determine whether they are effective in preventing or delaying the onset of disease among healthy individuals. In therapeutic trials, treatments such as surgery, radiation, and drugs are tested among individuals who already have a disease. A schematic representation of a typical experimental study is presented in **FIGURE 6-1**.

Selection of Study Population

During the recruitment phase of an experimental study, the study population, which is also called the experimental population, is enrolled on the basis of eligibility criteria that reflect the purpose of the trial as well as scientific, safety, and practical considerations. For example, healthy or high-risk individuals are enrolled in prevention trials, whereas individuals with specific diseases are enrolled in therapeutic trials. Additional inclusion and exclusion criteria may be used to restrict the study population by factors such as gender and age.

The study population must include an adequate number of individuals to determine whether there is a true difference between the treatment and comparison groups. An investigator determines how many subjects to include by using formulas that take into account the anticipated difference between the groups, the background rate of the outcome, and

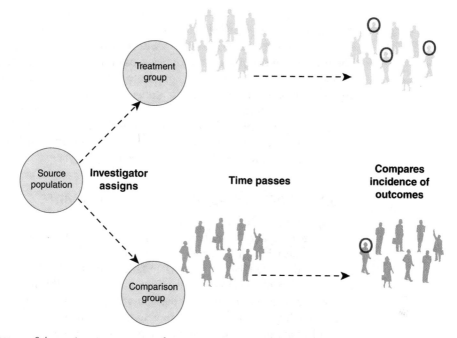

FIGURE 6-1 Schematic representation of experimental study implementation.

the probability of making certain statistical errors.[5(pp142-146)] In general, smaller anticipated differences between the treatment and comparison groups require larger sample sizes.

Consent Process and Treatment Assignment

All eligible and willing individuals must give consent to participate in an experimental study. The process of gaining their agreement is known as informed consent. During this process, the investigator describes the nature and objectives of the study, the tasks required of the participants, and the benefits and risks of participating. The process also includes obtaining the participant's oral or written consent.

Individuals are then assigned to receive one of the two or more treatments being compared. Randomization, "an act of assigning or ordering that is the result of a random process,"[6(p220)] is the preferred method for assigning the treatments because it is less prone to bias than other methods and it produces groups with very similar characteristics if the study size is sufficient. Random assignment methods include flipping a coin or using a random number table (commonly found in statistics textbooks) or a computerized random number generator.

Treatment Administration

In the next phase of a trial, the treatments are administered according to a specific protocol. For example, in a therapeutic trial, participants may be asked to take either an active drug or an inactive drug known as a placebo. The purpose of placebos is to match as closely as possible the experience of the comparison group with that of the treatment group. The principle underlying the use of placebos harkens back to laboratory animal experiments in which, except for the test chemical, all important aspects of the experimental conditions are identical for all groups. Placebos permit study participants and investigators to be masked, or unaware of the participant's treatment assignment. Masking of subjects and investigators helps prevent biased ascertainment of the outcome, particularly when end points involve subjective assessments.

Maintenance and Assessment of Compliance

All experimental studies require the active involvement and cooperation of participants. Although participants are apprised of the study requirements when they enroll, many fail to follow the protocol exactly as required as the trial proceeds. The failure to observe the requirements of the protocol is known as noncompliance, and this may occur in the treatment group, the comparison group, or both. Reasons for not complying include toxic reactions to the treatment, waning interest, and desire to seek other therapies. Noncompliance is problematic because it results in a smaller difference between the treatment and comparison groups than truly exists, thereby diluting the real effect of a treatment.

Because good compliance is an important determinant of the validity of an experimental study, many design features are used to enhance a participant's ability to comply with the protocol requirements.[7] They include designing an experimental regimen that is simple and easy to follow, enrolling motivated and knowledgeable participants, presenting a realistic picture of the required tasks during the consent process, maintaining frequent contact with participants during the study, and conducting a run-in period before enrollment and randomization. The purpose of the run-in period is to ascertain which potential participants are able to comply with the study regimen. During this period, participants are placed on the test or comparison treatment to assess their tolerance and acceptance and to obtain information on compliance.[6(p143)] Following the run-in period, only compliant individuals are enrolled in the trial.

Ascertaining the Outcomes

During the follow-up stage of an experimental study, the treatment and comparison groups are monitored for the outcomes under study. If the study's goal is to prevent the occurrence of disease, the outcomes may include the precursors of disease or the first occurrence of disease (i.e., incidence). If the study is investigating a new treatment among individuals who already have a disease, the outcomes may include disease recurrence, symptom improvement, length of survival, or side effects. The length of follow-up depends on the particular outcome under study. It can range from a few months to a few decades.

Usually, all reported outcomes under study are confirmed to guarantee their accuracy. Confirmation is typically done by masked investigators who gather corroborating information from objective sources, such as medical records and laboratory tests. High and comparable follow-up rates are needed to ensure the quality of the outcome data. Follow-up is adversely affected when participants withdraw from the study (these individuals are called dropouts) or cannot be located or contacted by the investigator (these individuals are termed lost to follow-up). Reasons for dropouts and losses include relocation, waning interest, and adverse reactions to the treatment.

Analysis

The classic analytic approach for an experimental study is known as an intent-to-treat or treatment assignment analysis. In this analysis, all individuals who were randomly allocated to a treatment are analyzed regardless of whether they completed the regimen or received the treatment.[8] An intent-to-treat analysis gives information on the effectiveness of a treatment under everyday practice conditions. The alternative to an intent-to-treat analysis is known as an efficacy analysis, which determines the treatment effects under ideal conditions, such as when participants take the full treatment exactly as directed.

▶ Overview of Cohort Studies

Definitions

A **cohort** is defined as a group of people with a common characteristic or experience. In a cohort study, healthy subjects are defined according to their exposure status and followed over time to determine the incidence of symptoms, disease, or death. The common characteristic for grouping subjects is their exposure level. Usually, two groups are compared: an **exposed** and an **unexposed** group. The unexposed group is called the reference, referent, or comparison group (see **FIGURE 6-2**).

Cohort study is the term that is typically used to describe an epidemiological investigation that follows groups with common characteristics. Other expressions that are used include follow-up, incidence, or longitudinal study. There are several additional terms for describing cohort studies that depend on the characteristics of the population from which the cohort is derived, whether the exposure changes over time and whether there are losses to follow-up. The term **fixed cohort** is used when the cohort is formed on the basis of an irrevocable event, such as undergoing a medical procedure. Thus, an individual's exposure

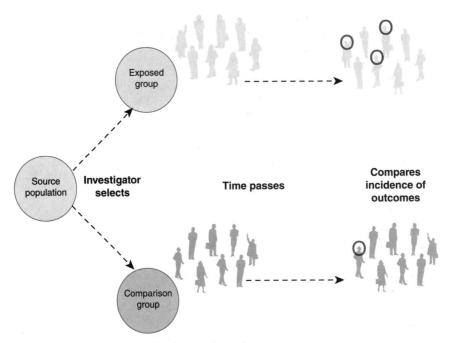

FIGURE 6-2 Schematic representation of cohort study implementation.

in a fixed cohort does not change over time. The term **closed cohort** is used to describe a fixed cohort with no losses to follow-up. In contrast, a cohort study conducted in an **open population**, also known as a **dynamic population**, is defined by exposures that can change over time, such as cigarette smoking. Cohort studies in open populations may also experience losses to follow-up.

Timing of Cohort Studies

Three terms are used to describe the timing of events in a cohort study in relation to the initiation of the study: prospective, retrospective, and ambidirectional. At the initiation of a **prospective cohort study**, participants are grouped on the basis of past or current exposure and are followed into the future to observe the outcomes of interest. When the study commences, the outcomes have not yet developed, and the investigator must wait for them to occur. At the initiation of a **retrospective cohort study**, both the exposures and outcomes have already occurred when the study begins. Thus, this type of investigation studies only prior and not future outcomes. An **ambidirectional cohort study** has both prospective and retrospective components. The decision whether to conduct a retrospective, a prospective, or an ambidirectional study depends on the research question, practical constraints such as time and money, and the availability of suitable study populations and records.

Selection of the Exposed Population

The choice of the exposed group in a cohort study depends on the hypothesis being tested; the exposure frequency; and feasibility considerations, such as the availability of records and ease of follow-up. Special cohorts are used to study the health effects of rare exposures, such as uncommon workplace chemicals, unusual diets, and uncommon lifestyles. Special cohorts are often selected from occupational groups (such as automobile manufacturing workers) or religious groups (such as Mormons) in which the exposures are known to occur. General cohorts are typically assembled for common exposures, such as cigarette smoking and alcohol consumption. These cohorts are often selected from professional groups, such as nurses, or from well-defined geographic areas to facilitate follow-up and accurate ascertainment of the outcomes under study.

Selection of Comparison Group

There are three sources for the comparison group in a cohort study: an internal comparison group, the general population, and a comparison cohort. An internal comparison group consists of unexposed members of the same cohort. An internal comparison group should be used whenever possible because its characteristics will be the most similar to the exposed group. The general population is used for comparison when it is not possible to find a comparable internal comparison group. The general population comparison is based on preexisting population data on disease incidence and mortality. A comparison cohort consists of members of another cohort. It is the least desirable option because the comparison cohort, although not exposed to the exposure under study, is often exposed to other potentially harmful substances and therefore the results can be difficult to interpret.

Sources of Information

Cohort study investigators typically rely on many sources for information on exposures, outcomes, and other key variables. They include medical and employment records, interviews, direct physical examinations, laboratory tests, biological specimens, and environmental monitoring. Some of these sources are preexisting, and others are designed specifically for the study. Because each type of source has advantages and disadvantages, investigators often use several sources to piece together all the necessary information.

Healthcare records are used to describe a participant's exposure history in studies of possible adverse health effects stemming from medical procedures. The advantages of these records include low expense and a high level of accuracy and detail regarding a disease and its treatment. Their main disadvantage is that information on many other key characteristics, apart from basic demographic characteristics, is often missing.

Employment records are used to identify individuals for studies of occupational exposures. Typical employment record data include job title, department of work, years of employment, and basic demographic characteristics. Like medical records, they usually lack details on exposures and other important variables.

Because existing records, such as healthcare and employment records, often have limitations, many studies are based on data collected specifically for the investigation. They include interviews, physical examinations, and laboratory tests. Interviews and self-administered questionnaires are particularly useful for obtaining information on lifestyle characteristics (such as use of cigarettes or alcohol), which are not consistently found in records. Whatever the source of information, it is important to use comparable procedures for obtaining information on the exposed and unexposed groups. Biased results may occur if different sources and procedures are used. Thus, all resources used for one group must be used for the other. In addition, it is a good idea to mask investigators to the exposure status of a subject so they make unbiased decisions when assessing the outcomes. Standard outcome definitions are also recommended to guarantee both accuracy and comparability.

Approaches to Follow-Up

Loss to follow-up occurs either when the participant no longer wishes to take part in the study or he or she cannot be located. Because high rates of follow-up are critical to the success of a cohort study, investigators have developed many methods to maximize retention and trace study participants.[9] For prospective cohort studies, strategies include collection of information (such as full name, Social Security number, and date of birth) that helps locate participants as the study progresses. In addition, regular contact is recommended for participants in prospective studies. These contacts might involve requests for up-to-date outcome information or newsletters describing the study's progress and findings.[9] The best strategy to use when participants do not initially respond is to send additional mailings.

When participants are truly lost to follow-up, investigators employ a number of strategies.[9] They include sending letters to the last known address with "Address Correction requested"; checking telephone directories; directory assistance; Internet resources, such as whitepages.com; vital statistics records; driver's license rosters; and voter registration records and contacting relatives, friends, and physicians identified at baseline.

Analysis

The primary objective of analyzing cohort study data is to compare the occurrence of symptoms, disease, and death in the exposed and unexposed groups. If it is not possible to find a completely unexposed group to serve as the comparison, then the least exposed group is used.

The occurrence of the outcome is usually measured using cumulative incidence or incidence rates, and the relationship between the exposure and outcome is quantified using absolute or relative difference between the risks or rates.

▶ Overview of Case–Control Studies

The case–control study has traditionally been viewed as an inferior alternative to the cohort study. In the traditional view, subjects are selected on the basis of whether they have or do not have the disease. An individual who has the disease is termed a **case**, and someone who does not have the disease is termed a **control**. The exposure histories of cases and controls are then obtained and compared. Thus, the central feature of the traditional view is the comparison of the exposure histories of the cases and controls. This differs from the logic of experimental and cohort study designs in which the key comparison is disease incidence between the exposed and unexposed (or least exposed) groups.

Over the past 3 decades, the traditional view that a case–control study is a backward cohort study has been supplanted by a modern view that asserts that it is merely an efficient way to learn about the relationship between an exposure and a disease.[10] More specifically, a case–control study is a method of sampling a population in which researchers identify and enroll cases of disease and a sample of the source population that gave rise to the cases. The sample of the source population is known as the control group (see **FIGURE 6-3**). Its purpose is to provide information on the exposure distribution in the population that produced the cases so that the rates of disease in exposed and unexposed groups can be compared. Thus, the key comparison in the modern view is the same as that of a cohort study.

Selection of Cases

The first step in the selection of cases for a case–control study is the formulation of a disease or case definition. A case definition is usually based on a combination of signs and symptoms, physical and pathological examinations, and results of diagnostic tests. It is best to use all available evidence to define with as much accuracy as possible the true cases of disease.

Once investigators have created a case definition, they can begin case identification and enrollment. Typical sources for identifying cases are hospital or clinic patient rosters; death certificates; special surveys; and reporting systems, such as cancer or birth defects registries. Investigators consider both accuracy and efficiency in selecting a particular source for case identification. The goal is to identify as many true cases of disease as quickly and cheaply as possible.

Another important issue in selecting cases is whether they should be incident or prevalent. Researchers who study the causes of disease prefer

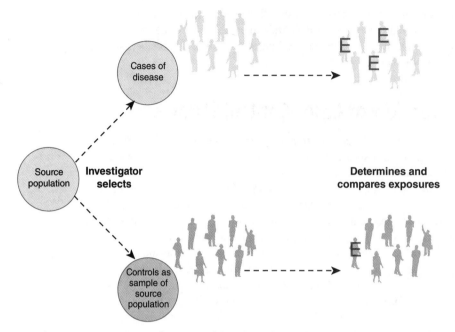

FIGURE 6-3 Schematic representation of case–control study implementation.

incident cases because they are usually interested in the factors that lead to developing a disease rather than factors that affect its duration. However, sometimes epidemiologists have no choice but to rely on prevalent cases (e.g., when studying the causes of insidious diseases whose exact onset is difficult to pinpoint). Studies using prevalent cases must be interpreted cautiously because it is impossible to determine whether the exposure is related to the inception of the disease, its duration, or a combination of the two.

Selection of Controls

Controls are a sample of the population that produced the cases. The guiding principle for the valid selection of controls is that they come from the same base population as the cases. If this condition is met, then a member of the control group who gets the disease under study would end up as a case in the study. This concept is known as "the would criterion," and its fulfillment is crucial to the validity of a case–control study. Another important principle is that controls must be sampled independently of exposure status. In other words, exposed and unexposed controls should have the same probability of selection.

Epidemiologists use several sources for identifying controls in case–control studies. They may sample (1) individuals from the general population, (2) individuals attending a hospital or clinic, (3) friends or relatives identified by the cases, or (4) individuals who have died. Population controls are typically selected when cases are identified from a well-defined population, such as residents of a geographic area. These controls are usually identified using voter registration lists, driver's license rosters, telephone directories, and random digit dialing (a method for identifying telephone subscribers living in a defined geographic area).

Population controls have one principal advantage that makes them preferable to other types of controls. Because of the manner in which population controls are identified, investigators are usually assured that the controls come from the same population as the cases. Thus, investigators are usually confident that population controls are comparable to the cases with respect to demographic and other important variables. However, population controls have several disadvantages. First, they are time consuming and expensive to identify. Second, these individuals do not have the same level of interest in participating as do cases and controls identified from other sources. Third, because they are generally healthy, their recall may be less accurate than that of cases, who are likely reviewing their history in search of a "reason" for their illness.

Epidemiologists usually select hospital and clinic controls when they identify cases from these healthcare facilities. Thus, these controls have diseases or have experienced events (such as a car accident) for which they have sought medical care. The most difficult aspect of using these types of controls is determining which diseases or events are suitable for inclusion. In this regard, investigators should follow two general principles. First, the illnesses in the control group should, on the basis of current knowledge, be unrelated to the exposure under study. For example, a case–control study of cigarette smoking and emphysema should not use lung cancer patients as controls because lung cancer is known to be caused by smoking cigarettes. Second, the control's illness should have the same referral pattern to the healthcare facility as the case's illness. For example, a case–control study of acute appendicitis should use patients with other acute conditions as controls. Following this principle will help ensure that the cases and controls come from the same source population.

There are several advantages to the use of hospital and clinic controls. Because they are easy to identify and have good participation rates, hospital and clinic controls are less expensive to identify than population controls. In addition, because they come from the same source population, they will have characteristics comparable to the cases. Finally, their recall of prior exposures will be similar to the cases' recall because they are also ill. The main disadvantage of this type of control is the difficulty in determining appropriate illnesses for inclusion.

In rare circumstances, deceased and "special" controls are enrolled. Deceased controls are occasionally used when some or all of the cases are deceased by the time data collection begins. Researchers usually identify these controls by reviewing death records of individuals who lived in the same geographic area and died during the same time period as the cases. The main rationale for selecting dead controls is to ensure comparable data collection procedures between the two groups. For example, if researchers collect data via interview, they would conduct proxy interviews with subjects' spouses, children, relatives, or friends for both the dead cases and dead controls.

However, many epidemiologists discourage the use of dead controls because they may not be a representative sample of the source population that produced the cases, which by definition, consists of living people. Furthermore, the investigator must consider the study hypothesis before deciding to use dead controls because they are more likely than living controls to have used tobacco, alcohol, or drugs.[11] Consequently, dead controls may not be appropriate if the study hypothesis involves one of these exposures.

In unusual circumstances, a friend, spouse, or relative (usually a sibling) is nominated by a case to serve as his or her control. These "special" controls are used because, if they are related to the cases, they are likely to share the cases' socioeconomic status, race, age, educational level, and genetic characteristics. However, cases may be unwilling or unable to nominate people to serve as their controls. In addition, biased results are possible if the study hypothesis involves a shared activity among the cases and controls.

Methods for Sampling Controls

Epidemiologists use three main strategies for sampling controls in a case–control study. Investigators can select controls from the "noncases" or "survivors" at the end of the case diagnosis and accrual period. This method of selection, which is known as survivor sampling, is the predominant method for selecting controls in traditional case–control studies. In case–base or case–cohort sampling, investigators select controls from the population at risk at the beginning of the case diagnosis and accrual period. In risk set sampling, controls are selected from the population at risk as the cases are diagnosed.

When case–base and risk set sampling methods are used, the control group may include future cases of disease. Although this may seem incorrect, modern epidemiological theory supports it. Recall that both diseased and nondiseased individuals contribute to the denominators of the risks and rates in cohort studies. Thus, it is reasonable for the control group to include future cases of disease because it is merely an efficient way to obtain the denominator data for the risks and rates.

Sources of Exposure Information

Case–control studies are used to investigate the risk of disease in relation to a wide variety of exposures, including those related to lifestyle, occupation, environment, genes, diet, reproduction, and the use of medications.[12] Most exposures that are studied are complex; therefore, investigators must attempt to obtain sufficiently detailed information on the nature, sources, frequency, and duration of these exposures. Sources available for obtaining exposure data include in-person and telephone interviews; self-administered questionnaires; preexisting medical, pharmacy, registry, employment, insurance, birth, death, and environmental records; and biological specimens.[12] When selecting a particular source, investigators consider its availability and accuracy and the logistics and cost of data collection. Accuracy is a particular concern in case–control studies because exposure data are retrospective. In fact, the relevant exposures may have occurred many years before data collection, making it difficult to gather correct information.

Analysis

As described earlier, controls are a sample of the population that produced the cases. However, in most instances, the sampling fraction is not known; therefore, the investigator cannot fill in the total population in the margin of a two-by-two table or obtain the rates and risks of disease. Instead, the researcher obtains a number called an odds, which functions as a rate or risk. An **odds** is defined as the probability that an event will occur divided by the probability that it will not occur. In a case–control study, epidemiologists typically calculate the odds of being a case among the exposed (a/b) compared to the odds of being a case among the nonexposed (c/d). The ratio of these two odds is expressed as follows:

$$\frac{a/b}{c/d} \text{ or } \frac{ad}{bc}$$

This ratio, known as the disease **odds ratio**, provides an estimate of the relative risk just as the incidence rate ratio and cumulative incidence ratio do. Risk or rate differences are not usually obtainable in a case–control study. However, it is possible to calculate the attributable proportion among the exposed and the attributable proportion in the total population using the odds ratio and the proportion of exposed controls.

Case–Crossover Study

The case–crossover study is a variant of the case–control study that was developed for settings in which the risk of the outcome is increased for only a brief time following the exposure.[13] The period of increased risk following the exposure is termed the **hazard period**.[14] In the case–crossover study, cases serve as their own controls, and the exposure frequency during the hazard period is compared with that from a control period. Because cases serve as their own controls, this design has several advantages, including the elimination of confounding by characteristics such as gender and race and the elimination of a type of bias that results from selecting unrepresentative controls. In addition, because variability is reduced, this design requires fewer subjects than does the traditional case–control study.

▶ When Is It Desirable to Use a Particular Study Design?

The goal of every epidemiological study is to gather correct and sharply defined data on the relationship between an exposure and a health-related state or an event in a population. The three main study designs represent different ways of gathering this information. Given the strengths and weaknesses of each design, there are circumstances for which a particular type of study is clearly indicated. These situations are described in the following paragraphs.

Experimental Studies

Investigators conduct an experimental study when they wish to learn about a prevention or treatment for a disease. In addition, they conduct this type of study when they need data with a high degree of validity that is simply not possible in an observational study. The high degree of validity in an experimental study stems mainly from investigators' ability to randomize subjects to either the treatment group or the comparison group and thereby control for distortions produced by confounding variables. A high level of validity may be needed for studying a prevention or treatment that is expected to have a small effect, usually defined as a difference of 20% or less between groups. A difference of this size is difficult to detect using an observational study because of uncontrolled bias and confounding. When the difference between groups is small, even a small degree of bias or confounding can create or mask an effect.

Although most scientists agree that well-conducted experimental studies produce more scientifically rigorous data than do observational studies, several thorny issues make it difficult to conduct experimental studies. These issues include noncompliance, the need to maintain high follow-up rates, high costs, physician and patient reluctance to participate, and numerous ethical issues. Investigators must address all these issues when considering this design. In particular, it is ethical to conduct experimental studies only when there is a state of equipoise within the expert medical community regarding the treatment. **Equipoise** is a "state of mind characterized by legitimate uncertainty or indecision as to choice or course of action."[6(p88)] In other words, there must be genuine confidence that a treatment may be worthwhile to administer it to some individuals and genuine reservations about the treatment to withhold it from others.

Observational Studies

Observational studies can be used to study the effects of a wider range of exposures than experimental studies, including preventions, treatments, and possible causes of disease. For example, observational studies provide information to explain the causes of disease incidence and the determinants of disease progression to predict the future healthcare needs of a population and to control disease by studying ways to prevent disease and prolong life with disease. The main limitation of observational studies is investigators' inability to have complete control over disturbing influences or extraneous factors. As Susser states, "Observational studies have a place in the epidemiological armament no less necessary and valid than controlled trials; they take second place in the hierarchy of rigor but not in practicability and generalizability. . . . Even when trials are possible, observational studies may yield more of the truth than randomized trials."[15(p156)]

Once an investigator has decided to conduct an observational study, the next decision is usually whether to select a cohort or case–control design. Because a cohort study can provide information on a large number of possible health effects, this type of study is preferable when little is known about the health consequences of an exposure. A cohort study is also efficient for investigating a rare exposure, which is usually defined as a frequency of less than 20%.

Case–control studies are preferable when little is known about the etiology of a disease because they can provide information on a large number of possible risk factors. Case–control studies take less time and cost less money than do cohort studies primarily because the control group is a sample of the source population. Case–control studies are also more efficient than cohort studies for studying rare diseases because fewer subjects are needed and for studying diseases with long induction and latent periods because long-term prospective follow-up is avoided. (A long induction and latent period means that there is a long time between the causal action of an exposure and the eventual diagnosis of disease.[16]) Because of their relatively smaller sample size, case–control studies are preferred when the exposure data are difficult or expensive to obtain. Finally, they are desirable when the population under study is dynamic because it is difficult to keep track of a population that is constantly changing. Tracing is required for a typical cohort study but not for a typical case–control study.

Case–control studies have a few important disadvantages. First, because of the retrospective nature of the data collection, there is a greater chance of bias. Some epidemiologists have argued that case–control studies are not well suited for detecting weak associations (those with odds ratios less than 1.5) because of the likelihood of bias.[17] Second, because data collection is retrospective, it may be difficult to establish the correct temporal relationship between the exposure and disease.

If an investigator has decided to conduct a cohort study, he or she must make one more choice: Should it be a retrospective or prospective cohort study? This decision depends on the particular research question, the practical constraints of time and money, and the availability of suitable study populations and records. For example, a retrospective design must be used to study historical exposures. In making this decision, the investigator must also take into account the complementary advantages and disadvantages of retrospective and prospective cohort studies. For example, retrospective cohort studies are more efficient than prospective studies for studying diseases with long induction and latent periods. However, minimal information is usually available on the exposure, outcome, confounders, and contacts for follow-up because retrospective cohort studies typically rely on existing records that were not designed for research purposes. In addition, the use of retrospective data makes it more difficult to establish the correct temporal relationship between the exposure and disease.

In prospective cohort studies, investigators can usually obtain more detailed information on exposures and confounders because they have more control of the data collection process and can gather information directly from the participants. Follow-up may be easier because the investigator can obtain tracing information from participants and maintain periodic contact with subjects. Prospective cohort studies are considered less vulnerable to bias than retrospective studies because the outcomes have not occurred when the cohort is assembled and the exposures are assessed. In addition, it is easier for investigators to establish a clear temporal relationship between exposure and outcome. A decision tree depicting the choices between the three main study designs is shown in **FIGURE 6-4**.

▶ **Other Types of Studies**

In addition to the three main study designs described in the previous sections, two other types of studies are commonly conducted in epidemiological research: cross-sectional and ecological studies (see **TABLE 6-2**). Although both studies are popular, these designs have important limitations that are not present in the other observational designs. Lastly, agent-based modeling is a new form of research in epidemiology that is gaining popularity.

Cross-Sectional Studies

A **cross-sectional study** "examines the relationship between diseases (or other health-related characteristics) and other variables of interest as they exist in a defined population at one particular time."[2(p64)] Unlike populations studied in cohort and case–control studies, cross-sectional study populations are commonly selected without regard to exposure or disease status. Cross-sectional studies typically take a snapshot of a population at a single point in time and therefore usually measure the disease prevalence in relation to the exposure prevalence. In other words, current disease status is usually examined in relation to current exposure level. However, it is possible for cross-sectional studies to examine disease prevalence in relation to past exposures if the dates of the exposures are ascertained.

Cross-sectional studies are carried out for public health planning and etiologic research. Most governmental surveys conducted by the National

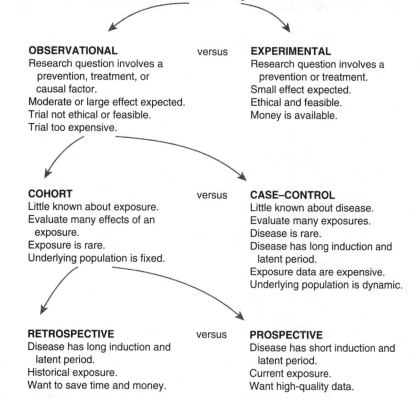

Goal: to harvest valid and precise information on association between exposure and disease using a minimum of resources

OBSERVATIONAL   versus   **EXPERIMENTAL**
Research question involves a   Research question involves a
  prevention, treatment, or   prevention or treatment.
  causal factor.   Small effect expected.
Moderate or large effect expected.   Ethical and feasible.
Trial not ethical or feasible.   Money is available.
Trial too expensive.

COHORT   versus   **CASE–CONTROL**
Little known about exposure.   Little known about disease.
Evaluate many effects of an   Evaluate many exposures.
  exposure.   Disease is rare.
Exposure is rare.   Disease has long induction and
Underlying population is fixed.   latent period.
                                                            Exposure data are expensive.
                                                            Underlying population is dynamic.

RETROSPECTIVE   versus   **PROSPECTIVE**
Disease has long induction and   Disease has short induction and
  latent period.   latent period.
Historical exposure.   Current exposure.
Want to save time and money.   Want high-quality data.

FIGURE 6-4 Decision tree for choosing among study designs.

Center for Health Statistics are cross-sectional in nature. For example, the National Survey of Family Growth is a periodic population-based survey focusing on factors that affect family health and fertility. Its most recent cycle was based on a national probability sample of men and women aged 15 to 49 years. In-person interviews gathered information on marriage and divorce, pregnancy, infertility, and contraception.[18]

Cross-sectional studies are fairly common in occupational settings using data from preemployment physical examinations and company health insurance plans.[19(p144)] For example, investigators conducted a cross-sectional study to determine the relationship between low back pain and sedentary work among crane operators, straddle-carrier drivers, and office workers.[20] All three groups had sedentary jobs that required prolonged sitting. Company records were used to identify approximately 300 currently employed male workers aged 25 through 60 years who had been employed for at least 1 year in their current job. Investigators assessed the "postural load" by observing workers' postures (such as straight upright position and forward or lateral flexion) and movements (such as sitting, standing, and walking). The investigators found that the prevalence of

---

TABLE 6-2 Key Features of Cross-Sectional and Ecological Studies

---

Cross-sectional studies

- Examine association at a single point in time, and therefore measure exposure prevalence in relation to disease prevalence.
- Cannot infer temporal sequence between exposure and disease if exposure is a changeable characteristic.
- Other limitations may include preponderance of prevalent cases of long duration and healthy worker effect.
- Advantages include generalizability and low cost.

Ecological studies

- Examine rates of disease in relation to a population-level factor.
- Population-level factors include summaries of individual population members, environmental measures, and global measures.
- Study groups are usually identified by place, time, or a combination of the two.
- Limitations include the ecological fallacy and lack of information on confounding variables.
- Advantages include low cost, wide range of exposure levels, and the ability to examine contextual effects on health.

current and recent low back pain was more common among crane operators and straddle-carrier drivers than office workers. The crane operators and straddle-carrier drivers had two to three times the risk of low back pain than did the office workers. The authors postulated that these differences resulted from crane operators' and straddle-carrier drivers' more frequent adoption of "non-neutral" trunk positions involving back flexion and rotation while on the job.[20]

Unfortunately, when epidemiologists measure the exposure prevalence in relation to disease prevalence in cross-sectional studies, they are not able to infer the temporal sequence between the exposure and disease. In other words, they cannot tell which came first—the exposure or the disease. This occurs when the exposure under study is a *changeable characteristic*, such as a place of residence or a habit such as cigarette smoking. Consider, for example, a hypothetical cross-sectional study of stress levels and the risk of ovarian infertility conducted among patients seeking treatment at an infertility clinic. The current stress levels of women who have a diagnosis of ovarian infertility is compared with that of fertile women whose husbands are the source of the infertility. If the stress level is three times greater among the infertile women, one could conclude that there is a moderately strong association between stress and ovarian infertility. However, it is difficult to know whether stress caused the infertility because the women may have become stressed after they began having difficulties achieving a pregnancy. This is quite possible given that precise onset of infertility is difficult to determine and that medical treatment for infertility usually does not begin until a couple has been trying to conceive for 6 months to 1 year. This is an important limitation of cross-sectional studies because epidemiologists must establish the correct temporal sequence between an exposure and a disease to support the hypothesis that an exposure causes a disease. Note that the temporal inference problem can be avoided if an unalterable characteristic, such as a genetic trait, is the focus of the investigation. It can also be avoided if the exposure measure reflects not only present but also past exposure. For example, an X-ray fluorescence (XRF) measurement of an individual's bone lead level reflects that person's cumulative exposure over many years.[21] Thus, a cross-sectional study of infertility and bone lead levels using XRF measurements would not suffer from the same temporal inference problem as would the study of infertility and stress just described.

Another disadvantage of cross-sectional studies is that such studies identify a high proportion of prevalent cases of long duration. People who die soon after diagnosis or recover quickly are less likely to be identified as diseased. This can bias the results if the duration of disease is associated with the exposure under study.

Still another bias may occur when cross-sectional studies are conducted in occupational settings. Because these studies include only current and not former workers, the results may be influenced by the selective departure of sick individuals from the workforce. Those who remain employed tend to be healthier than those who leave employment. This phenomenon, known as the **healthy worker effect**, generally attenuates an adverse effect of an exposure. For example, the strength of the association observed in the study of low back pain among sedentary workers may have been biased by the self-selection out of employment of workers with low back pain.

Cross-sectional studies also have several advantages. First, when they are based on a sample of the general population, their results are highly generalizable. This is particularly true of the cross-sectional surveys conducted by the National Center for Health Statistics. Second, they can be carried out in a relatively short period of time, thereby reducing their cost.

Ecological Studies

A classic ecological study examines the rates of disease in relation to a factor described on a population level. Thus, "the units of analysis are populations or groups of people rather than individuals."[2(p89)] The population-level factor may be an aggregate measure that summarizes the individual members of the population (e.g., the proportion of individuals older than 65 years of age), an environmental measure that describes the geographic location where the population resides or works (e.g., the air pollution level), or a global measure that has no analog on the individual level (such as the population density or existence of a specific law or healthcare system).[22(p512)] Thus, the two key features that distinguish a traditional ecological study from other types of epidemiological studies are (1) the population unit of analysis and (2) an exposure status that is the property of the population.

Ecological studies usually identify groups by place, time, or a combination of the two.[22(pp514-517)] In a classic ecological study, researchers examined the association between egg consumption measured on a country level and mortality rates from colon and rectal cancers.[23] The study authors obtained data on cancer mortality rates from the World Health Organization and data on egg consumption from the Food and Agriculture Organization of the United Nations for 34 countries on several continents. The investigators found positive correlations between per capita egg consumption (as a percentage of energy intake) and colon and rectal cancer mortality. That is, countries with high rates of egg consumption (e.g., Israel) tended to have high mortality rates from colon and rectal cancer, whereas those countries with low egg consumption (e.g., Korea) tended to have low mortality rates from these two cancers (see **FIGURE 6-5**).

Ecological studies that identify groups by time often compare disease rates over time in geographically defined populations.[22(pp515-516)] For example, investigators conducted an ecological study to compare human immunodeficiency virus (HIV) seroprevalence changes over time among injecting drug users in cities with and without needle-exchange programs.[24]

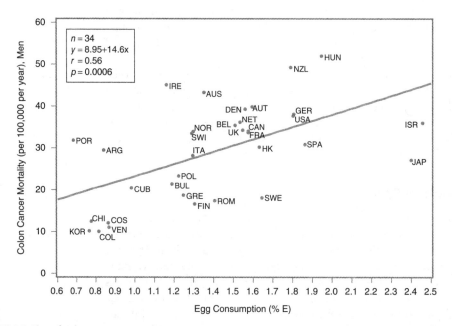

FIGURE 6-5 Plot of colon cancer mortality among men versus egg consumption (as a percentage of energy intake).

Reproduced from Zhang J, Zhao Z, Berkel HJ. Egg consumption and mortality from colon and rectal cancers: an ecological study. *Nutr Cancer*. 2003;46:158-165.

The investigators hypothesized that introduction of needle-exchange programs (programs that allow drug users to obtain clean needles and syringes free of charge) would decrease HIV transmission and lead to lower seroprevalence rates. The authors obtained information on HIV seroprevalence among injecting drug users from published studies and unpublished reports from the Centers for Disease Control and Prevention. They obtained information on the implementation of the needle-exchange programs from published reports and experts. They found that the average HIV seroprevalence increased by 5.9% per year in 52 cities without needle-exchange programs and decreased by 5.8% per year in 29 cities with needle-exchange programs. Thus, the average annual change in seroprevalence was 11.7% lower in cities with needle-exchange programs.

A special type of time-trend ecological study tries to separate the effects of three time-related variables: age, calendar time, and year of birth.[22(p517)] For example, a recent ecological study conducted in India examined the incidence rate of mouth cancer from 1995 through 2009 to better understand these three time-related variables.[25] The authors found that the incidence rate of mouth cancer among men increased annually by 2.7% during this period. Rates were higher among younger men (aged 25–49 years) and among men born in later time periods (1975–1984). The authors concluded that these results likely reflected increased exposure to tobacco and betel quid chewing among Indian men.

Some investigations cannot be classified as traditional ecological studies because they have both ecological and individual-level components. Consider, for example, a partially ecological study that was conducted in Norway to determine whether chlorinated drinking water was associated with the occurrence of birth defects.[26] Chlorinated water contains numerous chemicals called disinfection by-products that may be harmful to developing embryos. Because the study used group-level data on the exposure and individual-level data on the birth defects and confounding variables, it is considered partially ecological. The study population consisted of children born in Norway in the 1990s who lived in an area with information on water chlorination ($n = 141,077$ children). Investigators examined the prevalence of birth defects in relation to the proportion of the population served by chlorinated water. They examined four groups of municipalities: those with 0% chlorinated water, 0.1%–49.9% chlorinated water, 50%–99.9% chlorinated water, and 100% chlorinated water. Individual-level characteristics that were controlled included maternal age and parity and place of birth, as obtained from the children's birth records. The study suggested that there was a 15% increased risk of birth defects overall and a 99% increased risk of urinary tract defects among women whose water was chlorinated. However, the authors acknowledged that the study did not directly measure the concentrations of the disinfection by-products on the individual level.

The lack of individual-level information leads to a limitation of ecological studies known as the "ecological fallacy" or "ecological bias." The **ecological fallacy** means that "an association observed between variables on an aggregate level does not necessarily represent the association that exists at the individual level."[2(p88)] In other words, one cannot necessarily infer the same relationship from the group level to the individual level. In the egg consumption study, we do not know whether the people who had high rates of egg consumption were the same people who died from colon and rectal cancers. Likewise, in the Norway study, we do not know whether the women who drank chlorinated water were the same women who gave birth to babies with defects. This is particularly true for the two middle exposure groups (municipalities with 0.1%–49.9% and 50%–99.9% of the population with chlorinated water) because women with chlorinated and unchlorinated water were grouped together. On a practical level, the ecological bias means that the investigator cannot fill in the cells of a two-by-two table from the data available in a traditional ecological study.

Additional limitations of ecological studies include the investigators' difficulty detecting subtle or complicated relationships (such as a J-shaped or other curvilinear relationship) because of the crude nature of the data and the lack of information on characteristics that might distort the association. For example, although the ecological study of changes in HIV seroprevalence over time suggests that needle-exchange programs reduce HIV transmission, other factors may have accounted for this change, including the simultaneous implementation of other types of HIV prevention strategies.

In spite of these limitations, ecological studies remain a popular study design among epidemiologists for several reasons.[22(pp513-514)] They can be done quickly and inexpensively because they often rely on preexisting data. Their analysis and presentation are generally simple and easy to understand. They have the ability to achieve a wider range of exposure levels than could be expected from a typical individual-level study. Finally, epidemiologists have a genuine interest in ecological effects. For example, ecological studies can be used "to understand how context affects the health of persons and groups through selection, distribution, interaction, adaption, and other responses."[27(p825)] As Susser states, "measures of individual attributes cannot account for these processes; pairings, families, peer groups, schools, communities, cultures, and laws are all contexts that alter outcomes in ways not explicable by studies that focus solely on individuals."[27(p825)] This observation is particularly true for studies of the transmission of infectious disease. For example, investigators conducted an ecological analysis to determine the risk factors for dengue fever (a viral infection transmitted by the *Aedes aegypti* mosquito) in 70 Mexican villages.[28] They measured exposure by the average proportion of *Aedes* larvae among households in each village in relation to the proportion of affected individuals in the village. The study found a strong relationship between dengue antibody levels and the village-level larval concentrations. This association was not seen when an individual-level study was carried out because it did not take into account transmission dynamics at the population level.

Agent-Based Modeling

Agent-based modeling is an increasingly popular form of research in epidemiology. It is not a study design but rather a *method of analysis* that uses computer simulations to study the complex interactions among individuals, their physical and social environments, and time.[29] For example, an agent-based model was recently developed to determine the best strategy for reducing the prevalence of violence-related posttraumatic stress disorder (PTSD). In particular, the model contrasted the effect of hotspot policing (a population-level intervention expected to prevent neighborhood violence) and cognitive behavioral therapy (an individual-level intervention expected to shorten disease duration). The study found that the combination of both interventions produced the greatest reduction in PTSD prevalence.

Summary

Epidemiologists use both experimental and observational study designs to answer research questions. Each type of design represents a different way of harvesting the necessary information. The selection of one design over another depends on the research question and takes into account validity, efficiency, and ethical concerns.

For ethical reasons, experimental studies can be used to investigate only preventions and treatments for diseases. The hallmark of an experimental study is the investigator's active manipulation of the agent under study. Here, the investigator assigns subjects (usually at random) to two or more groups that either receive or do not receive the preventive or therapeutic agent. Investigators select this study design when they need data with a high degree of validity that is simply not possible to obtain in an observational study. However, experimental studies are expensive and often infeasible and unethical, and so most epidemiological research consists of observational studies.

Observational studies can be used to investigate a broader range of exposures, including causes, preventions, and treatments for diseases. The two most important types of observational studies are the cohort study and the case–control study. Epidemiologists use a cohort study when little is known about an exposure because this type of study allows investigators to examine many health effects in relation to an exposure. In a cohort study, subjects are defined according to their exposure levels and followed for disease occurrence. In contrast, investigators use a case–control study when little is known about a disease because this type of study allows researchers to examine many exposures in relation to a disease. In a case–control study, cases with the disease and controls are defined and their exposure histories are collected and compared.

Cross-sectional and ecological studies and agent-based modeling are three other types of observational research. Cross-sectional studies examine exposure prevalence in relation to disease prevalence in a defined population at a single point in time. Ecological studies examine disease rates in relation to a population-level factor. Both types of designs have important limitations absent from the other observational studies. An unclear temporal relationship between exposure and disease arises in cross-sectional studies of changeable exposures. Problems making cross-level inferences from the group to the individual (known as the ecological fallacy) occur in ecological studies. Agent-based modeling is not a study design but rather a method of analysis that uses computer simulations to study complex interactions between individuals, their environment, and time.

References

1. MacMahon B, Trichopoulos D. *Epidemiology Principles and Methods*. 2nd ed. Boston, MA: Little, Brown and Company; 1996.
2. Porta, M. *A Dictionary of Epidemiology*. 6th ed. New York, NY: Oxford University Press; 2014.
3. Heymann, DL. *Control of Communicable Diseases Manual*. 20th ed. Washington, DC: American Public Health Association; 2015.
4. Pickett, JP (exec. ed.). *The American Heritage Dictionary of the English Language*. 4th ed. Boston, MA: Houghton Mifflin; 2000.
5. Colton, T. *Statistics in Medicine*. Boston, MA: Little, Brown and Company; 1974.
6. Meinert, CL. *Clinical Trials Dictionary: Terminology and Usage Recommendations*. Baltimore, MD: The Johns Hopkins Center for Clinical Trials; 1996.
7. Friedman LM, Furberg CD, Demets DL. *Fundamentals of Clinical Trials*. 2nd ed. Littleton, MA: PSG Publishing Co.; 1985.
8. Newell, DJ. Intention-to-treat analysis: implications for quantitative and qualitative research. *Int J Epidemiol*. 1992;21:837-841.
9. Hunt JR, White E. Retaining and tracking cohort study members. *Epidemiol Rev*. 1998;20:57-70.
10. Miettinen OS. The "case-control" study: valid selection of study subjects. *J Chron Dis*. 1985;38:543-548.
11. McLaughlin JK, Blot WJ, Mehl ES, Mandel JS. Problems in the use of dead controls in case–control studies. I. general results. *Am J Epidemiol*. 1985;121:131-139.
12. Correa A, Stewart WF, Yeh HC, Santos-Burgoa C. Exposure measurement in case-control studies: reported methods and recommendations. *Epidemiol Rev*. 1994;16:18-32.
13. Maclure, M. The case-crossover design: a method for studying transient effects on the risk of acute events. *Am J Epidemiol*. 1991;133:144-153.
14. Mittleman MA, Maclure M, Robins JM. Control sampling strategies for case-crossover studies: an assessment of relative efficiency. *Am J Epidemiol*. 1995;142:91-98.
15. Susser M. Editorial: the tribulations of trials—interventions in communities. *Am J Public Health*. 1995;85:156-158.
16. Rothman KJ. Induction and latent periods. *Am J Epidemiol*. 1981;114:253-259.
17. Austin H, Hill HA, Flanders WD, Greenberg RS. Limitations in the application of case-control methodology. *Epidemiol Rev*. 1994;16:65-76.
18. Key statistics from the National Survey of Family Growth. cdc.gov. https://www.cdc.gov/nchs/nsfg/key_statistics.htm. Accessed October 2016.
19. Monson RR. *Occupational Epidemiology*. 2nd ed. Boca Raton, FL: CRC Press; 1990.
20. Burdorf A, Naaktgeboren B, De Groot H. Occupational risk factors for low back pain among sedentary workers. *J Occup Med*. 1993;35:1213-1220.
21. Hu H, Shih R, Rothenberg S, Swartz BS. The epidemiology of lead toxicity in adults: measuring dose and consideration of other methodologic issues. *Environ Health Perspect*. 2007;115:455-462.
22. Morgenstern H. Ecologic studies. In: Rothman KJ, Greenland S, Lash TL (eds.). *Modern Epidemiology*. 3rd ed. Philadelphia, PA: Wolters Kluwer Health/Lippincott Williams and Wilkins; 2008.
23. Zhang J, Zhao Z, Berkel HJ. Egg consumption and mortality from colon and rectal cancers: an ecological study. *Nutr Cancer*. 2003;46:158-165.
24. Hurley SF, Jolley DJ, Kaldor JM. Effectiveness of needle-exchange programmes for prevention of HIV infection. *Lancet*. 1997;349:1797-1800.
25. Shridhar K, Rajaraman P, Koyande S, et al. Trends in mouth cancer incidence in Mumbai, India (1995-2009):

an age-period-cohort analysis. *Cancer Epidemiol.* 2016; 42:66-71.

26. Magnus P, Jaakkola JJK, Skrondal A, et al. Water chlorination and birth defects. *Epidemiology.* 1999;10:513-517.

27. Susser M. The logic in ecological: I. the logic of analysis. *Am J Public Health.* 1994;84:825-829.

28. Koopman JS, Longini IM. The ecological effects of individual exposures and nonlinear disease dynamics in populations. *Am J Public Health.* 1994;84:836-842.

29. Cerda M, Tracy M, Keyes KM, Galea S. To treat or to prevent? Reducing the population burden of violence-related post-traumatic stress disorder. *Epidemiology.* 2015;26:681-689.

Chapter Questions

1. State the main difference between the following study designs:
    a. Observational and experimental studies
    b. Retrospective cohort and prospective cohort studies
    c. Cohort and case–control studies

2. Briefly describe a cross-sectional study and indicate its main limitation.

3. Briefly describe the situations in which the hallmark limitation of a cross-sectional study is avoided.

4. Briefly describe an ecological study and indicate its main limitation.

5. Briefly describe the situations in which an ecological study may be preferred over other observational studies.

6. State which observational study design is best (i.e., most efficient and logical) in each of the following scenarios:
    a. Identifying the causes of a rare disease
    b. Identifying the long-term effects of a rare exposure
    c. Studying the health effects of an exposure for which information is difficult and expensive to obtain
    d. Identifying the causes of a new disease about which little is known
    e. Identifying the short-term health effects of a new exposure about which little is known
    f. Identifying the causes of a disease with a long latent period

7. Which type of study is being described in each of the following scenarios?
    a. A study that examines the death rates from colon cancer in each of the 50 U.S. states in relation to the average percentage of residents in each state undergoing colonoscopy screening
    b. A study that compares the prevalence of back pain among current members of the automobile manufacturing union with that of current members of the bakers and confectionary union
    c. A study that evaluates the relationship between breast cancer and a woman's history of breastfeeding. The investigator selects women with breast cancer and an age-matched sample of women who live in the same neighborhoods as the women with breast cancer. Study subjects are interviewed to determine whether they breastfed any of their children.
    d. A study that evaluates two treatments for breast cancer. Women with stage 1 breast cancer are randomized to receive either cryotherapy (a new treatment involving extreme cold to kill cancer cells) or traditional lumpectomy. Women are followed for 5 years to determine whether there are any differences in breast cancer recurrence and survival.

e. A study that began in 2010 of the relationship between exposure to chest irradiation and subsequent risk of breast cancer. In this study, women who received radiation therapy for postpartum mastitis (an inflammation of the breast that occurs after giving birth) in the 1950s were compared with women who received a nonradiation therapy for postpartum mastitis in the 1950s. The women were followed for 60 years to determine the incidence rates of breast cancer in each group.

8. **Indicate** whether the following statements are true or false:
    a. Observational studies of preventions and treatments are often conducted when experimental studies are unethical or infeasible.
    b. The main limitation of observational studies is the investigator's inability to have complete control of extraneous factors called confounders.
    c. A cross-sectional study of the relationship between blood type and the risk of cataracts will produce misleading results because you cannot tell the correct temporal relationship between the exposure (blood type) and disease (cataracts).
    d. An ecological study was done to determine the relationship between per capita soft drink consumption and mortality rates from diabetes in 10 U.S. states. The investigators found a strong association between soft drink consumption and diabetes mortality. Based on this study, we can conclude that the individuals who consumed the soft drinks were the ones who died from diabetes.
    e. Case–control studies are inherently inferior to cohort studies.
    f. Experimental studies are inherently superior to observational studies.
    g. Prospective cohort studies are inherently superior to retrospective cohort studies.

CHAPTER 7

Experimental Studies

By the end of this chapter the reader will be able to:

- Distinguish between the types of experimental studies, including individual versus community trials, preventive versus therapeutic trials, parallel versus crossover trials, and simple versus factorial trials.
- State the established sequence for conducting trials of new drugs.
- Describe the key features of conducting experimental studies, including the enrollment and consent process, randomization, use of placebos and masking, maintenance and assessment of compliance, follow-up and ascertaining the outcomes, and data analysis.
- Discuss the special ethical issues of experimental studies, including equipoise and use of placebo controls.

▶ Introduction

An **experimental study**, commonly known as a trial, involves the use of designed experiments to investigate the role of some agent in the prevention or treatment of a disease. In this type of study, the investigator assigns individuals to two or more groups that either receive or do not receive a preventive or therapeutic treatment. The active manipulation of the treatment by the investigator is the hallmark that distinguishes experimental from observational studies (see **FIGURE 7-1**).

Because experimental studies more closely resemble controlled laboratory investigations, most epidemiologists believe that, if well conducted, they produce more scientifically rigorous results than do observational studies. In a laboratory experiment, the investigator regulates all important aspects of the experimental conditions, permitting the experimental subjects to differ only for the purpose of testing the hypothesis. For example, a laboratory experiment testing the toxicity of a chemical is conducted on genetically similar animals (such as mice or rats).[1] Animals are assigned (usually by chance) to either the test or control group.

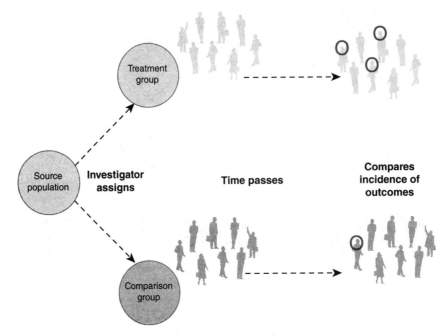

FIGURE 7-1 Schematic representation of experimental study implementation.

Using identical routes of administration (e.g., by mouth or injection), the chemical under investigation is given to the test group, whereas an inert chemical such as a salt solution is dispensed to the control group. All experimental animals are kept in the same physical environment and fed the same diet and follow the same daily schedule. Thus, the only difference between the two groups is the dissimilar chemical (test versus inert) deliberately introduced by the investigator.

Although experimental studies conducted among free-living humans can never achieve the same degree of control as laboratory animal experiments, many aspects of human experimental research emulate the principles of laboratory research. This chapter describes the design, conduct, and analysis of experimental studies among humans. First, an overview of experimental studies is presented, followed by a detailed discussion of each aspect of an experimental study. The chapter concludes with a discussion of the numerous special considerations in experimental studies that make them scientifically rigorous but difficult to perform.

▶ Overview of Experimental Studies

Investigators must formulate a hypothesis before launching an epidemiological study. Hypothesis generation is a creative endeavor in which an investigator proposes a specific idea to explain a set of observations. Next, the epidemiologist must decide which type of study design will efficiently provide valid information to either support or refute the hypothesis. The appropriate study design is determined by considering the state of knowledge, the frequency of the exposure and disease, and the expected strength of the association between the two. In addition, several practical and ethical problems must be solved when experimental studies are conducted.

Once the study has been designed, a research proposal is written and funding is solicited. At this time, the investigators usually request approval for the study from the ethics committee of the participating institutions. The ethics committee, also called the institutional review board, reviews all studies to ensure that the research is ethical and legitimate.[2(p86)] The review is particularly important in experimental studies because a state of equipoise must exist for the study to be ethical. Equipoise is characterized by genuine uncertainty about the risks and benefits of the test treatment. That is, there must be sufficient certainty that the test treatment might be beneficial to administer it to some individuals while sufficient doubt exists about its benefits to withhold it from others. Next, during the recruitment phase, investigators enroll individuals in the study on the basis of specific eligibility criteria. The eligibility criteria consist of inclusion and exclusion criteria that stem from both scientific and practical concerns. For example, the clopidogrel versus aspirin in patients at risk of ischemic events (CAPRIE) experimental study compared the effectiveness of clopidogrel with that of asprin in reducing the risk of heart attacks and strokes among patients with atherosclerotic vascular disease.[3] Inclusion criteria consisted of an established diagnosis of recent stroke, heart attack, or peripheral arterial disease. Exclusion criteria included contraindications to the study drugs because of potential side effects and geographic factors that made participation unrealistic. The eligibility criteria influence the generalizability of the study, which is the larger population to whom the study results are applicable.

Subsequently, eligible individuals must give formal consent to participate, usually by signing a consent form that has been approved by the ethics committee. Investigators then use either random or nonrandom methods to assign individuals to receive one of the two or more treatments being compared. Random assignment, usually termed randomization, is preferred because its unpredictable nature makes it less prone to bias. The group that is allocated to the agent under study is generally called the treatment group, and the other group is called the comparison or control group. The comparison group may receive no treatment at all, an inactive treatment such as a placebo, or another active treatment. Often, the active treatment given to the comparison group is the current standard of care. For example, the CAPRIE study compared a new drug (clopidogrel) with the standard treatment (aspirin). Because the aspirin treatment, while effective, had serious potential side effects, such as gastrointestinal bleeding, there was great interest in finding another effective treatment with fewer adverse effects.[3]

In the next phase of a trial, the treatments are administered according to a specific protocol. For example, the CAPRIE study patients were asked to take tablets of clopidogrel or aspirin every day with their morning meal for at least 1 year.[3]

During the **follow-up** stage, the treatment and comparison groups are monitored for the outcomes under study. If the goal of the study is to prevent the occurrence of disease, the outcome may include the precursors of disease or the first occurrence of disease (i.e., incidence). On the other hand, if the study is testing a new treatment among individuals who already have a disease, outcomes may include disease recurrence, symptom improvement, length of survival, or side effects. In the CAPRIE therapeutic study, outcome measures included the recurrence of stroke and heart attacks, primary brain hemorrhage, and leg amputation.[3]

The length of time that subjects are followed depends on the outcomes being studied. Only a few months may be needed in a short-term study of drug side effects, but a decade may be necessary for examining slowly developing diseases such as cancer. During follow-up, investigators maintain contact with participants through periodic visits, phone calls, or letters. Losses to follow-up and dropouts must be kept to a minimum during this phase to ensure a successful trial. For example, in the CAPRIE study, follow-up visits with physicians took place several times a year for up to 3 years, and therefore the number of losses to follow-up and dropouts was quite low.[3]

All reported outcomes of interest are confirmed to guarantee their accuracy. Confirmation is usually done by masked investigators who gather corroborating information from objective sources such as medical records. **Masking**, which means that the investigator is unaware of the participant's treatment assignment, reduces the chance of making a biased assessment of the outcome and therefore improves the rigor of the study.

During the follow-up stage, investigators assess participants' level of **compliance** with the treatment regimen. That is, they determine whether participants are following exactly the study protocol. In the CAPRIE study, follow-up visits included questions about the use of study medications and any other drugs.[3] Fortunately, less than 1% of the patients were completely noncompliant (i.e., they never took the study drugs as directed). Noncompliance is problematic because it makes it more difficult for investigators to determine whether an experimental treatment is effective.

The classical approach to the analysis of an experimental study is known as an **intent-to-treat analysis**. Here, all individuals allocated to a treatment are analyzed as representing that treatment regardless of whether they completed or even received the treatment. Investigators take this approach to preserve the baseline comparability of the groups and to provide information on the effectiveness of a treatment under real-life conditions.

▶ Types of Experimental Studies

Experimental studies can be classified in several ways depending on their design and purpose. The major types of categorization are described in the following sections and are summarized in **TABLE 7-1**.

Individual Versus Community Trials

Trials are often distinguished according to the unit by which the treatment is assigned. The most commonly conducted trial is an **individual trial**, in which the treatment is allocated to individual persons. For example, an individual trial among adults infected with human immunodeficiency virus (HIV) compared the effectiveness of treatment with three drugs (a protease inhibitor and two nucleoside analogs) versus treatment with two drugs (both nucleoside analogs) in slowing the progression of HIV disease.[4] In this classic study, 1,156 HIV-infected individuals were each randomly assigned to one of two daily regimens, with roughly 580 patients in each group. Each patient was treated and followed for a maximum of 40 weeks. Outcome measures, including disease progression and death, were measured in each patient and later aggregated by treatment group. This was one of the first trials to show the clinical benefits and safety of three drug combinations for treating HIV infection.

TABLE 7-1 Types of Experimental Studies, or Trials	
Type	**Defining characteristics**
Individual	Treatment is allocated to individuals.
Community	Treatment is allocated to entire community.
Preventive	Prophylactic agent is given to healthy or high-risk individuals to prevent disease occurrence.
Therapeutic	Treatment is given to diseased individuals to reduce the risk of recurrence, improve survival, or improve quality of life.
Parallel	Each group receives one treatment. Treatments are administered concurrently.
Crossover	Each group receives all treatments one after another. The treatment order differs for each group. Washout period may intervene between treatments.
Simple	Each group gets one treatment.
Factorial	Each group gets two or more treatments.

In a **community trial**, which is less common, the treatment is allocated to an entire community. A well-known community trial was the Newburgh-Kingston Caries Fluorine Study, which was conducted to determine whether increasing fluoride levels in drinking water would reduce the incidence of dental caries among resident children.[5] Children who lived in the community of Newburgh, New York, served as the treatment group. Beginning in 1944, fluoride was added to the town's drinking water supply to raise its concentration from about 0.1 to 1 part per million (ppm). The children of Kingston, New York, a similarly sized community about 35 miles away, served as the comparison group. The fluoride level (0.1 ppm) of its water supply was left unchanged. Periodic dental examinations were conducted among school-aged children residing in each community for several years. Investigators assessed the efficacy of the fluoride treatment by comparing the prevalence of decayed, missing, or filled teeth among children in Newburgh with that of children in Kingston.

More recently, a community trial was conducted to test the hypothesis that messaging through social media would increase HIV testing among men who have sex with men and transgendered persons.[6] The study assigned two communities to receive social media messages about the importance of HIV testing and the locations of testing services. Two comparison communities, matched on size but geographically distinct from the intervention communities, received no intervention. The investigators collected information on the rates of HIV testing in the intervention and comparison communities before and after the intervention to determine whether there were any changes. At baseline, there were no meaningful differences in HIV testing rates between the two sets of communities. After the intervention was conducted for one year, HIV testing increased by 27.3% in the intervention communities and only 3.5% in the comparison communities, suggesting that social media messages are an effective method for promoting HIV testing among men who have sex with men and transgendered persons.

Preventive Versus Therapeutic Trials

Another way to classify experimental studies is according to their purpose, that is, whether they investigate a measure that prevents disease occurrence, known as a **preventive trial**, or a measure that treats an existing condition, known as a **therapeutic trial**. Trials that prevent or delay the onset of disease among healthy individuals are called primary prevention trials, and trials that prevent or delay progression among diseased individuals are termed secondary prevention trials.[2(pp207,245)]

In some preventive trials, the alleged causal factor is reduced or removed. For example, the Boston Lead Free Kids Study tested the hypothesis that removing lead-contaminated soil from around children's homes would reduce their blood lead levels and their risk of lead poisoning.[7] In this instance, the suspected causal factor—lead-contaminated soil—was removed from yards and replaced with clean soil and ground cover.

In other preventive trials, agents such as vitamins (e.g., folic acid and vitamins A, C, and E), minerals (e.g., selenium and calcium), naturally occurring compounds (e.g., carotenoids and flavonoids), and drugs (e.g., cholesterol-lowering and antihypertensive drugs) are studied to determine whether they are effective in reducing disease occurrence or recurrence.[8] Prevention trials may also involve behavior modifications, such as dietary improvements (e.g., low-cholesterol diet),[9] reducing substance use and antisocial behavior,[10] physical exercise,[11] and preventing sexually transmitted diseases.[12] The well-known Women's Health Initiative, a randomized trial of about 65,000 postmenopausal women, combined several preventive measures as it examined the effects of eating a low-fat diet (with 20% of calories from fat), hormone replacement therapy, and calcium and vitamin D supplementation on the prevention of cancer, cardiovascular disease, and osteoporotic fractures.[13]

Some preventive trials are conducted among the general population. For example, the ANRS 1265 Trial of male circumcision for the reduction of HIV infection risk was conducted in a general population of South Africa, thereby increasing the generalizability of the findings.[14] Other preventive trials are conducted among high-risk individuals. For example, the Women's Health Initiative was conducted among healthy postmenopausal women whose baseline risk of disease was no higher than that of similarly aged women in the general population. On the other hand, the Breast Cancer Prevention Trial (BCPT) determined the ability of tamoxifen to reduce breast cancer incidence and mortality among high-risk healthy women.[15] Here, risk was determined by current age, age at menarche and first live birth, family history of breast cancer, number of benign breast biopsies, and mammographic abnormalities. The BCPT focused on high-risk women rather than women from the general population in part because the benefits of taking tamoxifen presumably outweighed its risks only among high-risk women. Tamoxifen has been associated with an increased risk of endometrial cancer in several experimental and observational studies.[16]

Prevention trials usually take many years to conduct and require tens of thousands of participants because they often focus on reducing the incidence of diseases that typically occur at a yearly cumulative incidence of 1% or less.[17] For example, the BCPT enrolled about 13,000 women and followed them for more than 5 years.[15]

Whereas prevention trials are conducted among individuals without disease, therapeutic trials involve testing treatments such as surgery, radiation, and drugs among individuals who already have a disease. Therapeutic trials are commonly called clinical trials because they are conducted in a clinical setting among diseased patients and often use a clinical outcome measure, such as recurrence or side effects.[2(p34)] In therapeutic trials, a new therapy is usually compared with the standard treatment. The new therapy may consist of a new drug, a novel combination of existing drugs, a new therapy, or a technological improvement of an old therapy. These treatments are meant to reduce the recurrence of disease, improve survival, and improve the quality of life. Because therapeutic trials attempt to reduce the occurrence of relatively common outcomes (such as disease recurrence or death), they usually take only a few years to conduct and generally involve fewer patients than preventive trials.[17]

For example, a therapeutic trial was conducted among women with ovarian cancer to determine whether the standard treatment regimen could be improved with the addition of an angiogenesis inhibitor.[18] Women in the experimental group were treated with the standard two-drug chemotherapy plus bevacizumab, and those in the comparison group were treated with only the standard regimen. The investigators enrolled 1,528 eligible women and followed them for 42 months. The investigators found that the addition of the angiogenesis inhibitor improved the length of progression-free survival. Women who received bevacizumab lived an average of 2.4 more months without the disease worsening than did those who received the standard therapy.

The distinction between preventive and therapeutic trials recently blurred when a study of antiretroviral therapy for HIV infection showed that early initiation of a therapeutic regimen benefited both infected patients and their uninfected partners.[19] This trial of serodiscordant couples found that early therapy reduced both the occurrence of opportunistic infections and deaths among the HIV-infected patients as well as the rate of sexual transmission to the uninfected partner.

New Drug Trials

There is a well-established sequence for carrying out therapeutic trials involving new drugs.[2(pp193-194)] A phase 1 drug trial is conducted to provide preliminary information on drug safety using a relatively small number of normal, healthy volunteers. The exception is for cancer chemotherapeutic agents, which are conducted in patients who usually have advanced disease. This trial provides metabolic and pharmacologic profiles of the drug, including determination of the maximally tolerated dose. Next, a phase 2 trial is conducted on a larger number of diseased individuals to obtain preliminary information on efficacy and additional information on safety, including side effects. Sometimes, the Food and Drug Administration (FDA; the federal agency with the authority to approve drugs and devices for clinical use) approves drugs following phase 2 testing, but usually a phase 3 trial is needed to show an advantage of an experimental therapy over a standard one using an objective outcome, such as improved survival.[20] Phase 3 trials also gather information on a drug's indications of use, recommended doses, and side effects, which are all necessary for administering the drug appropriately in clinical practice.[2(p194)] When a phase 3 trial is complete, the drug manufacturer can request to market the drug for the indication covered by the trial. After approval of the new drug application, a phase 4 trial and post-marketing surveillance may be conducted to determine long-term safety and efficacy of the drug. A phase 4 trial may be needed because rare and slowly developing adverse events may not become evident during the typical 3-year phase 3 trial.

Investigators do not always adhere to this rigid sequence for new drug trials, particularly for life-threatening diseases.[2(p194-195)] For example, two or more phases of a drug trial may be conducted concurrently. In addition, for serious diseases with few treatment options, it has become commonplace for new drugs showing promise in early studies to be made widely available to patients who might benefit from them at the same time as the randomized trials designed to measure any such benefit are undertaken.[21]

Parallel Versus Crossover Trials

Trials can also be described according to the method of treatment administration (see Table 7-1). In the simplest design, known as a **parallel trial**, individuals in each group simultaneously receive one study treatment. For example, in the drug efficacy study among women with ovarian cancer, women in the experimental group received the standard drug regimen plus the angiogenesis inhibitor, and women in the comparison group received the standard drug regimen over the same calendar period.[18] Thus, the treatment and comparison groups consisted of entirely different women, and the treatments were administered during the same general time frame (see **FIGURE 7-2**).

In a **crossover trial**, two or more study treatments are administered one after another to each group. Thus, all trial participants receive all of the treatments and only the order of the treatments differs. In this type of trial, a person may serve as his or her own control. For example, if the drug efficacy trial among ovarian cancer patients were a crossover design, women in the experimental group would first receive the standard treatment and new drug combination and then the standard regimen alone, whereas those in the comparison group would first receive the standard regimen alone and then the standard treatment plus new drug combination. The groups usually switch treatments at the same time, and there is often a washout period between the end of one treatment and the start of another to give the body time to metabolize and excrete the initial treatment.

PARALLEL DESIGN

Group 1 —— Treatment A ——➤ Follow-up and outcome assessment

Group 2 —— Treatment B ——➤ Follow-up and outcome assessment

CROSSOVER DESIGN

Group 1 — Treatment A ➤ Washout ➤ Treatment B ➤ Follow-up and outcome assessment

Group 2 — Treatment B ➤ Washout ➤ Treatment A ➤ Follow-up and outcome assessment

Time ————————————————————————————➤

FIGURE 7-2 Parallel and crossover treatment study designs.

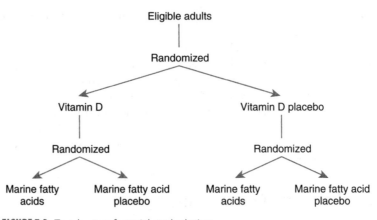

FIGURE 7-3 Two-by-two factorial study design.

Data from Bassuk SS, Manson JE, Lee IM, Cook NR, Christen WG, Bubes VY, et al. Baseline characteristics of participants in the VITamin D and OmegA-3 TriaL (VITAL). *Contemp Clin Trial.* 2016;47:235-243.

Simple Versus Factorial Designs

Trials can also be categorized according to the number of treatments being tested (see Table 7-1). In a **simple trial**, each group receives a treatment consisting of one component (e.g., a single drug). In contrast, two or more treatments are combined in a **factorial trial**. For example, VITamin D and OmegA-3 TriaL (VITAL) investigators used a two-by-two factorial design among nearly 26,000 healthy U.S. adults to test two hypotheses: (1) vitamin D reduces the risk of cancer and cardiovascular disease, and (2) marine omega-3 fatty acids reduce the risk of cancer and cardiovascular disease.[22] As shown in **FIGURE 7-3**, investigators conducted two rounds of randomization (one for each supplement) to assign all possible combinations of the supplements to four groups: (1) active vitamin D and active marine fatty acids, (2) active vitamin D and marine fatty acid placebo, (3) vitamin D placebo and active marine fatty acids, and (4) vitamin D placebo and marine fatty acid placebo. The factorial design allows an investigator to test the separate and combined effects of two or more agents.

▶ Study Population

The study population, also called the experimental population, consists of the people who are considered for enrollment in a trial. Thus, it consists of potential participants. The study population depends on the purpose of the trial and may include healthy, high-risk, or diseased individuals. The study population's characteristics are further defined by specific eligibility criteria. For example, the seminal trial of the efficacy of the antiretroviral drug zidovudine in reducing the risk of maternal–infant HIV transmission enrolled women with the following characteristics: HIV infected; pregnant and between 14 and 34 weeks' gestation; CD4 T lymphocyte counts greater than 200 cells per cubic millimeter;

normal levels of other blood, liver, and urine parameters; and no medical reason for needing antiretroviral therapy.[23] Women were excluded if they had abnormal ultrasound findings, such as fetal anomalies, or if they had received any HIV therapy during the pregnancy. Only women who met all of these criteria were enrolled and randomly assigned to receive either zidovudine or placebo during pregnancy and labor.

Eligibility criteria such as these are based upon scientific, safety, and practical considerations. For example, only HIV-infected, pregnant women were included in the maternal–infant HIV transmission trial because, if the drug were found effective, it was intended to be used by this population.[23] In addition, women were excluded if the fetus had an anomaly that could increase the concentration of zidovudine or its metabolite and endanger its health. Finally, women with a medical reason for needing antiretroviral drugs were excluded because it would be unethical to assign such women to the placebo comparison group.

Although all individuals who meet the eligibility criteria can theoretically participate in a trial, practical constraints usually limit actual enrollment to individuals whom investigators are able to recruit. Thus, participants of therapeutic trials are usually patients at the hospitals and clinics with which the investigators are affiliated. Trials that enroll healthy individuals may also recruit patients at these institutions, or participants may be identified through other sources, such as newspapers and television.

Depending on the number of participants needed for the trial, one or many institutions may take part. A single-center trial is conducted at a single clinical site, whereas a multicenter trial includes two or more sites. Each clinical site enrolls individuals, administers the treatments, and collects data. For example, the maternal–fetal HIV transmission prevention trial was conducted at almost 50 institutions in the United States and France.[23] The large number of institutions was needed to accrue a sufficient number of subjects in a reasonable time frame.

Studies have shown that the characteristics of people who volunteer for trials are different from those who do not. In one study of smoking cessation, participants were more likely than nonparticipants to be White, older, and motivated by financial incentives.[24]

Why do people volunteer for experimental studies? Many enroll because they want the best possible medical care, including new treatments that are otherwise unavailable. Others participate for altruistic reasons, such as a desire to help others with the disease or to leave something for posterity. It is important to keep in mind that the characteristics of trial volunteers may affect the generalizability of the results.

▶ Sample Size

For investigators to determine whether there is a true difference in effectiveness between the treatment and comparison groups, it is crucial that they enroll an adequate number of individuals in the experimental study.

The term *statistical power* refers to "the ability of a study to demonstrate an association if one exists."[25(p221)] Unfortunately, numerous trials have erroneously reported null results (i.e., no difference between the treatment and comparison groups) simply because their sample size was too small and statistical power was too low to detect clinically important differences.[26]

How do investigators decide how many subjects to include in a trial? Usually, they determine the needed sample size using formulas that take into account the following factors: (1) the anticipated difference between the treatment and comparison groups, (2) the background rate of the outcome, and (3) the probability of making statistical errors known as *alpha* and *beta* errors.[27(pp142-146)]

Many therapeutic and most preventive trials require a very large number of participants to have sufficient statistical power to detect a meaningful effect. For most therapeutic trials, the large numbers are necessary primarily because the trial is being conducted to determine whether a test treatment offers a small improvement over an existing treatment. In general, the smaller the anticipated difference between the treatment and comparison groups, the larger the necessary sample size. For the preventive trials, the large sample size is needed because the subjects are healthy at the start and the disease endpoints usually have a low incidence. Some researchers believe that meta-analysis, a statistical procedure that pools data from many small trials, is a viable alternative to conducting large trials.[28]

▶ Consent Process

All eligible individuals must voluntarily agree to participate in a trial. The process of gaining their agreement, known as **informed consent**, must be reviewed and approved by the ethics committee (also called **institutional review board**) of the participating institutions. During the consent process, the investigator must describe, in simple language, the nature and objectives of the study; the treatments being investigated; tasks, procedures, and tests required of participants; method of treatment assignment; data to be collected; and, most important, likely benefits and risks of participating.[2(p51)] Investigators must assure participants that personal information obtained during the course of the study will be kept confidential and that participants may withdraw from the study at any time without jeopardizing their medical care. The consent process includes giving oral or written consent according to a protocol that has been approved by the ethics committee.

▶ Treatment Assignment

After they give their consent, eligible individuals are assigned to either the **treatment group** or the **comparison group**. Nonrandom and random assignments are two general methods for assigning treatments to participants. The nonrandom method most commonly used is **alternation assignment**, which is a systematic assignment method that is based on the order of enrollment. For example, the first enrolled person is assigned to the treatment group, the second is assigned to the comparison group, the third is assigned to the treatment group, and so on.

Although nonrandom assignment methods are simple and easy to follow, they are predictable and thus may lead to situations that allow biased assignment. For example, if two subjects are enrolled at exactly the same time in the alternation assignment scheme, the investigators may have the discretion to assign one individual to the treatment group and the other to the comparison group. If the investigators make this assignment on the basis of a prognostic characteristic, such as severity of illness (e.g., they put the healthier person into the comparison group), and they do this often enough, the study groups would be imbalanced, and the results could be biased.

Random assignment is superior to nonrandom methods because it is less prone to this type of bias. Random treatment assignment, known as **randomization**, is defined as "an act of assigning or ordering that is the result of a random process."[2(p222)] Although the overall probability of being assigned to a particular group is known (e.g., 50% are assigned to each group), there is no way to predict the order of future assignments from that of past ones. The lack of predictability is the key to minimizing bias.

Random methods include flipping a coin or using a random number table (commonly found in statistics textbooks) or a computer random number generator. Large trials often have a central office that handles the randomization so that the investigators who determine eligibility, enroll individuals, and administer the treatments are unaware of the assignment order ahead of time. In smaller trials without a central randomization office, treatment assignments are usually sealed in numbered opaque envelopes to safeguard the process.

Randomization has two main goals. First, as already described, it ensures that treatment assignment occurs in an unbiased fashion. Second, if the sample size is sufficiently large, it will usually control for known and unknown confounding variables by producing treatment and comparison groups with very similar baseline characteristics. (Confounding is a nuisance that can distort results because risk factors are unevenly distributed across compared groups.) For example, in the very large CAPRIE study, approximately 19,000 patients with atherosclerotic vascular disease were randomly assigned to receive clopidogrel ($n = 9,599$) or aspirin ($n = 9,586$).[3] The baseline characteristics of the two groups were quite similar (e.g., exactly the same proportion of males was in each group) (see **TABLE 7-2**). On the other hand, the maternal–infant HIV transmission study randomized a much smaller group of women ($n = 477$) to either the zidovudine or placebo group.[23] Randomization was less successful in achieving baseline comparability (e.g., there was a

TABLE 7-2 Baseline Characteristics of Patients in the Large CAPRIE Study

Characteristic	Clopidogrel group (n = 9,599)	Aspirin group (n = 9,586)
Male (%)	72	72
White (%)	95	95
Current cigarette smoker (%)	29	30
Patients with a history of:		
Hypertension (%)	52	51
Stable angina (%)	22	22
High cholesterol levels (%)	41	41

Data from CAPRIE Steering Committee. A randomized, blinded trial of clopidogrel versus aspirin in patients at risk of ischemic events (CAPRIE). *Lancet.* 1996;348:1329-1339.

10% difference in the proportion of Whites in each group) because the sample size was much smaller (see **TABLE 7-3**).

Investigators often use two additional procedures—blocking and stratification—with randomization to secure balanced groups. **Blocking** is used "to ensure balance in the mix of the treatment groups with regard to time of enrollment" and helps control for "shifts in the nature of persons enrolled over the course of a trial."[2(p24)] When blocking is used, randomization is conducted in groups or blocks of a certain size. For example, in a trial with a projected enrollment of 100 individuals (i.e., 50 participants will ultimately be assigned to each of two groups), blocks of, say, 10 patients may be randomized at a time to ensure that equal numbers of patients are assigned to the two groups throughout the enrollment process.

Stratification accompanies randomization to ensure that key confounding variables are equally distributed between the treatment and comparison groups. In this method, individuals are first stratified or separated according to the confounding characteristic. Then, they are randomly assigned to either the treatment or comparison group within each stratum. For example, women in the maternal–fetal HIV transmission trial were stratified according to the stage of pregnancy at enrollment (one group was from 14 to 26 weeks pregnant, and the other group was greater than 26 weeks pregnant). Then, women in each stratum were randomly assigned to receive either zidovudine or placebo (see **FIGURE 7-4**).[23] This was done because the investigators thought that zidovudine would

TABLE 7-3 Baseline Characteristics of Patients in the Small Maternal–Infant HIV Transmission Trial

Characteristic	Zidovudine group (*n* = 239)	Placebo group (*n* = 238)
Median age at entry (years)	25	25
White (%)	48	38
Gestational age at entry:		
Median (weeks)	26	27
14–26 weeks (%)	52	50
> 26 weeks (%)	48	50
Mean CD4 count at entry	560	538

Data from Connor EM, Sperling RS, Gelber R, Kiselev P, Scott G, O'Sullivan MJ, et al. Reduction of maternal-infant transmission of human immunodeficiency virus type 1 with zidovudine treatment. *N Engl J Med.* 1994;331:1173-1180.

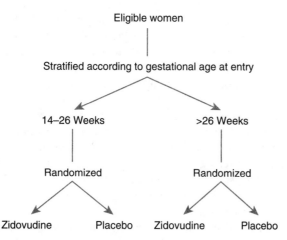

FIGURE 7-4 Depiction of stratified randomization in the maternal–infant HIV transmission study.

Data from Connor EM, Sperling RS, Gelber R, Kiselev P, Scott G, O'Sullivan MJ, et al. Reduction of maternal-infant transmission of human immunodeficiency virus type 1 with zidovudine treatment. *N Engl J Med.* 1994;331:1173-1180.

be more effective if it were started earlier in pregnancy, and therefore they wanted to ensure that the two groups were nearly identical on this important characteristic. As shown in Table 7-3, the median age and the distribution of gestational age at entry were similar in the two groups.

▶ Use of the Placebo and Masking

A **placebo** is defined as a "pharmacologically inactive substance given as a substitute for an active substance, especially when the person taking or receiving it is not informed whether it is an active or inactive substance."[2(p196)] A placebo pill usually consists of a sugar-coated, inert substance. Its purpose is to match as closely as possible the experience of the comparison group with that of the treatment group. The principle underlying the use of placebos harkens back to laboratory animal experiments in which, except for the test chemical, all important aspects of the experimental conditions are identical for the treatment and comparison groups. Thus, when placebo pills are used in drug trials among humans, they are purposely manufactured to be as similar as possible to the active drug in shape, size, texture, color, and taste.

When trials involve procedures rather than pills, "sham" procedures are administered to match as closely as possible the experience of the treatment and comparison groups. A **sham procedure** is defined as "a bogus procedure designed to resemble a legitimate one."[2(p249)] For example, in a study of the effectiveness of acupuncture for the treatment of nausea among cancer patients undergoing radiation therapy, patients in the treatment group were given penetrating acupuncture treatment with sharp needles, and patients in the sham comparison were given a nonpenetrating procedure with blunt needles.[29]

Both placebos and sham procedures permit study participants, healthcare providers, and study investigators to be masked. That is, these parties do not know whether a participant is in the treatment or comparison group. Several terms are commonly used to describe which individuals associated with an experimental study are masked. In a single-masked study, the participants are masked, but the investigators are not. In a double-masked study, both the participants and investigators administering the treatment are masked. In a triple-masked study, the participants, the investigators administering the treatment, and the investigators monitoring the effects of the treatment are masked. The latter investigators are usually members of a treatment effects monitoring committee that is charged with the regular review of collected data for evidence of adverse or beneficial treatment effects while the trial is being conducted and for recommending changes in a study treatment, including ending the trial early.[2(p288)]

Masking of subjects and investigators helps prevent biased ascertainment of the outcome, particularly endpoints that involve subjective assessment. However, in some studies, it is not possible to mask participants or investigators because of the nature of the intervention. For example, both participants and investigators administering the intervention were aware of a participant's group assignment in an HIV prevention trial that investigated the effect of circumcision on HIV incidence in men.[30] However, because the main outcome under study—laboratory-determined HIV seroconversion—was objectively determined, the lack of masking should not have affected the results.

Many researchers have observed that participants who receive the placebos or sham procedures improve over the course of the experimental study. The beneficial effect produced by an inactive control treatment is known as the **placebo effect** and is thought to arise from the power of suggestion. That is, participants assigned to the placebo group improve just because they are told that they will. The related terms **halo effect** and **Hawthorne effect** are also used when the improvement stems from the attention received by participating in a study. This effect is analogous to the Heisenberg uncertainty principle in physics, which states that "the act of observing a phenomenon changes the phenomenon itself."[31(p59)] In epidemiological terms, it means that participants either consciously or unconsciously change their behavior just because they are being studied. For example, cancer patients in the study of acupuncture for the treatment of radiotherapy-induced nausea were asked whether they thought that the treatment was effective.[29] A total of 96% of the sham group and 95% of the treatment group reported that it was very helpful, and similar proportions in each group reported the occurrence of vomiting and use of antiemetic drugs, two objective measures of success.

▶ Maintenance and Assessment of Compliance

All experimental studies require the active involvement and cooperation of participants. In fact, taking part in a trial can be quite intrusive in a person's daily life. For example, required tasks in three therapeutic and preventive trials have included taking pills on a daily basis, exercising three times a week, quitting smoking, and making important dietary changes (see **TABLE 7-4**).[4,9,11]

Although participants are apprised of the study requirements when they enroll, many fail to follow the protocol exactly as required as the trial proceeds. The failure to observe the requirements of the protocol is known as **noncompliance**. There are many reasons for noncompliance, including toxic reactions to the treatment, waning interest, inability to meet the demands of the study, desire to seek other therapies, disease progression, and death.

Noncompliance may occur among members of the treatment group, the comparison group, or both groups. For example, women in the exercising treatment group of a community-based exercise study were noncompliant when they did not participate in the exercise program as directed (see Table 7-4).[11] On the other hand, women in the "usual activity" comparison group were noncompliant when they began exercising during the study period. According to the study investigators, both groups had a moderate level of compliance over the 52-week period.

TABLE 7-4 Required Tasks and Reasons for Noncompliance in Three Experimental Studies

Title/purpose of trial	Tasks required of participants	Reasons for noncompliance

AIDS Clinical Trials Group 320 Study
    Compared effectiveness of three versus two drug regimens for the treatment of HIV among patients with low CD4 counts
	Group 1: Indinavir (every 8 hours), zidovudine (three times a day), and lamivudine (two times a day).
	    Group 2: Indinavir placebo (every 8 hours), zidovudine (three times a day), lamivudine (two times a day).
		Toxic reactions to the treatment, adverse events related to HIV infection, desire to receive other therapies.

Exercise Study for Postmenopausal Women
    Determined the effect of an exercise program on bone mineral density and measures of strength and balance among women with osteopenia
	Exercising group: Participate in 60-minute exercise sessions three times a week for 52 weeks.
	    Comparison group: Maintain usual physical activity level.
		Musculoskeletal pain, other health conditions, lack of interest in the exercising group. Participation in other exercise programs in the comparison group.

Multiple Risk Factor Intervention Trial (MRFIT) Study
    Examined the effect of reducing multiple risk factors on coronary heart disease mortality rates among high-risk men
	Special intervention group: Receive counseling for smoking cessation, dietary advice to lower blood cholesterol levels, and stepped-care treatment for hypertension.
	    Usual care comparison group: Use standard sources of health care.
		Sizable reductions in blood pressure, cigarette smoking, and serum cholesterol occurred in the usual care group because they became more health conscious.

Data from Hammer SM, Squires KE, Hughes MD, Grimes JM, Demeter LM, Currier JS, et al. A controlled trial of two nucleoside analogues plus indinavir in persons with human immunodeficiency virus infection and CD4 cell counts of 200 per cubic millimeter or less. *New Engl J Med.* 1997;337:725-733; Bolton KL, Egerton T, Wark J, Wee E, Matthews B, Kelly A, et al. Effects of exercise on bone density and falls risk factors in post-menopausal women with osteopenia: a randomized controlled trial. *J Sci Med Sport.* 2012;15:102-109; Multiple Risk Factor Intervention Trial: risk factor changes and mortality rates. *JAMA.* 1982;248:1465-1477.

Exercising individuals completed, on average, 78% of their exercise program, and the physical activity level of 75% of the comparison group remained unchanged over the course of the study.[11]

Many studies do not have high levels of compliance. Perhaps the most well-known example of noncompliance in an experimental study was the Multiple Risk Factor Intervention Trial (MRFIT), a randomized primary prevention trial of the effect of smoking, blood cholesterol, and blood pressure reduction on coronary heart disease mortality in 12,866 high-risk men aged 35 to 57 years.[9] MRFIT included two groups of participants: (1) the special intervention group received dietary advice for lowering blood cholesterol levels, smoking cessation counseling, and stepped-care treatment for hypertension, and (2) the usual care group received their typical sources of health care within the community. Noncompliance occurred when men in the usual care group quit smoking and lowered their blood pressure and cholesterol levels. The authors speculated that the comparison group changed their smoking and dietary habits like the rest of the U.S. population during the study period.

Noncompliance is the bane of an investigator's life because it leads to two vexing problems. First, it results in a smaller difference between the treatment and comparison groups than truly exists. For example, the MRFIT study found that the special intervention group had only a 7.1% lower rate of coronary heart disease mortality than the usual care group. Second, noncompliance reduces the statistical power of the study, making it more difficult to detect an effect when it exists. Thus, when a study finds little or no difference between the treatment and comparison groups (null results), noncompliance should be considered as a possible explanation.

Because good compliance is an important determinant of the validity of an experimental study, many study features are designed to enhance a participant's ability to comply with the protocol requirements.[32] First, investigators design experimental regimens that are simple and easy to follow. For example, it is much easier to comply with a regimen that requires taking one pill at the same time each day than one that requires taking numerous pills at different times. When a difficult treatment schedule cannot be avoided, compliance aides, such as blister pill packs resembling monthly calendars and pill boxes with programmed alarms, are used.

Second, investigators enroll motivated and knowledgeable participants who lead fairly organized lives. For example, investigators decided to enroll health professionals in a randomized, double-masked, placebo-controlled primary prevention trial of cardiovascular disease and cancer in part because they believed that the health professionals were more likely to comply with the daily regimen of taking aspirin and/or vitamin E and would be easier to trace.[22]

Third, investigators present a realistic picture of the tasks required by the trial during the informed consent process. In this way, participants know exactly what they are getting themselves into.

Fourth, investigators obtain a detailed medical history from potential subjects so that they can exclude those with conditions that would preclude or make compliance difficult. For example, the CAPRIE trial excluded potential participants who had medical contraindications to the study drugs (e.g., a history of aspirin sensitivity).[3]

Fifth, investigators mask study subjects in placebo-controlled studies because those in the comparison group might be less motivated to comply if they knew that they were receiving the placebo.

Sixth, researchers maintain frequent contact with participants during the study. For example, in the CAPRIE study, follow-up visits involving a physical examination, laboratory tests, and questionnaire administration took place every month for the first 4 months and then every 4 months thereafter.[3]

Finally, investigators conduct a run-in or lead-in period before enrollment and randomization to ascertain which potential participants are able to comply with the study regimen. During this period (which may last several weeks or months), potential participants are placed on the test or control treatment "to assess tolerance or acceptance of a treatment, or to provide information on treatment compliance."[2(p142)] When the run-in is over, investigators enroll only the compliant individuals. For example, in a study of treatment of children with inadequately controlled asthma, 881 children were enrolled in a 4-week run-in period during which all the participants received their study medication.[33] Only 593 children (67%) who were considered good compliers (as evidenced by taking most of their study medication and completing several questionnaires) were randomized and continued in the actual trial.

Even when compliance-enhancement measures are used, investigators must still assess the extent of noncompliance. This can be done in several ways. First, investigators can question participants about the extent of their noncompliance. Second, if the trial requires taking pills, investigators can ask participants to return any unused pills. Investigators in the CAPRIE study used this method and found that only 86 patients (out of more than 19,000) never took any of the study drugs.[3] Recently developed electronic medication monitoring systems that record the date and time when a patient opens a vial of pills has taken these reports to a new level of sophistication.[34] Third, investigators in medication trials can collect biological samples, such as blood or urine, to analyze for the presence of the treatment or its metabolite. For example, in an experimental study of the effectiveness of buspirone, a medication treatment for cannabis dependence, investigators analyzed serum levels of buspirone's main metabolite to assess patient compliance.[35]

▶ Ascertaining the Outcomes

During the follow-up period, investigators monitor the treatment and comparison groups for the outcomes under study. In preventive trials, the outcomes of interest are generally precursors of disease or the first occurrence of disease; in therapeutic trials, the outcomes typically include symptom improvement, length of survival, or disease recurrence. For example, the outcome measure in the HIV-prevention study of early antiretroviral therapy among serodiscordant couples was the incidence of new infections among the HIV-negative partners.[19] Outcome measures in the CAPRIE therapeutic study of patients with atherosclerotic vascular disease included the recurrence of fatal and nonfatal strokes, heart attacks, and brain hemorrhages.[3]

Usually, one of these endpoints is designated as the **primary outcome**, which is the main condition that the trial has been designed to evaluate and the outcome used for the sample size calculations. The remaining endpoints, termed **secondary outcomes**, are considered less important. For example, the primary outcome in the CAPRIE study was the composite outcome cluster of first occurrence of stroke, heart attack, or vascular death.[3] Investigators determined that a sample of at least 18,000 patients was needed based on the expected frequency (14%–25%) of the outcome cluster during the 3-year follow-up period.

In some trials, a surrogate outcome measure, such as a laboratory test result that correlates with a clinical outcome, is used instead of a clinical event.[28] For example, investigators might measure cholesterol levels, which are correlated with the occurrence of heart attacks. The purpose of surrogate measures is to reduce the length of follow-up, sample size, and cost of the study. For example, in experimental studies of AIDS treatments, CD4 T lymphocyte levels and HIV ribonucleic acid (RNA) levels have been used as surrogate measures of a treatment's effectiveness. Although most researchers agree that surrogate markers are useful for identifying promising treatments during the early phases of research, some warn that they may lead to false conclusions because the surrogate markers do not always predict the occurrence of clinical endpoints such as opportunistic infections and survival following HIV infection.[36]

How long must investigators follow subjects to ascertain the outcomes under study? Only a few months may be needed for a short-term study of drug side effects, but a decade may be necessary for examining slowly developing outcomes such as cancer incidence. During the follow-up period, investigators obtain outcome information from participants through periodic medical visits, phone interviews, or mail questionnaires. For example, in the CAPRIE study, follow-up visits with physicians took place for up to 3 years.[3]

Accurate information on the outcomes is crucial to the success of a trial. Investigators work to ensure high-quality outcome data by developing strategies to achieve high follow-up rates and by incorporating a process known as validation in the study design.

Follow-up is adversely affected when participants either withdraw from the study (they are called **dropouts**) or cannot be located or contacted by the investigator (these individuals are termed **losses to follow-up**). Reasons for dropouts and losses include relocation, waning interest, and adverse reactions to the treatment. Dropouts and losses to follow-up pose a problem for researchers because they lead to missing outcome data and ultimately a smaller study.

The problem of missing data is further aggravated if the follow-up rates of the treatment group differ from those of the comparison group and attrition is related to the outcome. This combination of events can lead to incorrect results. For example, if more women in the exercise group than the comparison group dropped out of the exercise study for postmenopausal women and if the bone strength of women who dropped out differed from those who remained, the study results could be biased. Methods for minimizing dropouts and losses include designing a simple protocol, enrolling motivated individuals who lead organized lives, and maintaining frequent contact. In addition, follow-up is often facilitated by obtaining the name of a friend or relative of the study participant at enrollment. Ideally, this person does not live with the participant yet will always know the participant's whereabouts.

The process known as **validation** helps to ensure accurate outcome data. Validation means that investigators verify or corroborate the occurrence of the outcome using several sources. For example, researchers often review medical records to confirm the occurrence of events reported by patients. Whenever possible, corroborating evidence should be objective in nature, such as laboratory test results and physical findings. It is good practice for the investigators who perform the validation to be masked. For example, in the CAPRIE study, masked members of a central validation committee were responsible for determining the accuracy of all nonfatal outcomes and reporting causes of death.[3] The evidence for each reported outcome was reviewed independently by two committee members, and any disagreements were resolved by the entire committee.

▶ Data Analysis

The results of an experimental study may be arranged in a two-by-two table, and the measures of association calculated. For example, let us examine the results of the seminal experimental study of maternal–infant HIV transmission (see **TABLE 7-5**).[23] The cumulative incidence of HIV infection was 13/180 or 7.2% among infants whose mothers received zidovudine and 40/183 or 21.9% among infants whose mothers received placebos. Thus, the relative risk, as estimated by the cumulative

TABLE 7-5 Reduction of Maternal–Infant Transmission of HIV with Zidovudine Treatment

Treatment	Infant HIV infected		
	Yes	No	Total
Yes (Zidovudine)	13	167	180
No (Placebo)	40	143	183

Data from Connor EM, Sperling RS, Gelber R, Kiselev P, Scott G, O'Sullivan MJ, et al. Reduction in maternal–infant transmission of human immunodeficiency virus type 1 with zidovudine treatment. *N Engl J Med.* 1994;331:1173-1180.

incidence ratio, was 0.33. This means that infants whose mothers took zidovudine had one-third the risk of becoming HIV infected than did the infants whose mothers took placebos. Stated differently, there was a 67% reduction in the risk of HIV transmission among the zidovudine group (null relative risk of 1.00 − 0.33 = 0.67 or 67%). The attributable risk or absolute difference in the cumulative incidence of infection was −14.7% (the difference between 7.2% and 21.9%). In other words, nearly 15 HIV infections among every 100 infants whose mothers were given placebos would have been prevented if these mothers had received zidovudine.

Although the mathematical calculations of experimental study data are straightforward, a few conceptual issues regarding the analysis of experimental studies deserve mention. The first relates to composition of the analytic groups. In the classic analytic approach, known as an intent-to-treat or treatment assignment analysis, all individuals who are randomly allocated to a treatment are analyzed regardless of whether they complete or even receive the treatment.[37] An intent-to-treat analysis would compare everyone who was randomly assigned to treatment 1 with everyone who was assigned to treatment 2 (see **FIGURE 7-5**). Thus, this analysis would compare the outcomes of those who completed treatment combined with those who did not complete treatment 1 (groups A and B) with the outcomes of those who completed treatment combined with those who did not complete treatment 2 (groups C and D).

What is the purpose of an intent-to-treat analysis? First, it preserves the benefits of randomization; that is, it preserves baseline comparability of the groups for known and unknown confounders. Second, it maintains the original statistical power if the exposure assumptions remain correct. Third, because good and poor compliers differ from one another on important prognostic factors, it helps ensure that the study results are unbiased.[32] For example, the Coronary Drug Project studied the effect of several lipid-lowering drugs, including clofibrate, among men with a history of myocardial infarction.[38] Investigators found that only 15.0% of the

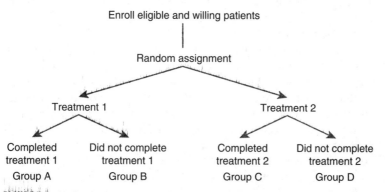

FIGURE 7-5   Analysis groups in a randomized experimental study.

"good" compliers versus 24.6% of the "poor" compliers in the clofibrate group died during the follow-up period. Surprisingly, a similar pattern was seen among the "good" and "poor" compliers who were taking the placebo.

Still another reason for conducting an intent-to-treat analysis is that it gives information on the effectiveness of a treatment under everyday practice conditions. It answers the question "How well does the treatment work among those who are offered it?" If a test treatment is found to be effective, it will be used in clinical settings in which people may not comply exactly with the prescribed regimen because of toxicity, lack of interest, and so forth. Thus, an analysis that excludes noncompliers gives an overly optimistic view of how well the treatment will work in real life.

The alternative to an intent-to-treat analysis is known as an **efficacy analysis**. This type of analysis determines the treatment effects under ideal conditions. It answers the question "How well does the treatment work among those who take the full treatment as directed?"[37] In Figure 7-5, an efficacy analysis would compare the outcomes of those who completed treatment 1 and those who completed treatment 2 (groups A and C) and would ignore the outcomes of participants who failed to complete treatment 1 or treatment 2 (groups B and D). Proponents of this approach argue that it is merely answering a different question than the intent-to-treat analysis. However, others find it problematic because the compared groups (e.g., groups A and C) may not be similar.

Sometimes, investigators conduct both types of analysis in a given study. For example, the CAPRIE study investigators first conducted an intent-to-treat analysis that was based on all randomized patients regardless of their compliance with the study protocol. In addition, they also conducted an "on-treatment" analysis that included only outcomes that occurred while patients were on the study medication or within 28 days of early discontinuation of the medication.[3] In the intent-to-treat analysis, investigators found 939 events during 17,636 person-years at risk in the clopidogrel group and 1,021 events during 17,519 person-years at risk in the aspirin group, resulting in a rate ratio of 0.913. The on-treatment analysis, based on somewhat different numbers, found a similar result of a rate ratio of 0.906.

A second issue that arises in the analysis of experimental studies pertains to determining the effectiveness of the treatment among different subgroups. For example, the maternal–infant HIV transmission study conducted analyses to evaluate the effectiveness of zidovudine in reducing transmission among women of different races, ages, stages of pregnancy, and delivery characteristics.[23] Some investigators pejoratively call such subgroup analyses "data dredging" or "exploratory" because they are usually done on an *ad hoc* basis (i.e., without the benefit of a hypothesis stated at the start of the study).[28] Others believe that it is acceptable to analyze subgroups if they are defined ahead of time and intended. Still others believe that, because data do not magically change on the basis of investigators' prior plans, subgroup analyses provide valuable and valid information regardless of an investigator's original hypothesis. Nevertheless, subgroup analyses are usually based on fewer subjects than analyses using the entire sample. Thus, although results of subgroup analysis may be accurate, they are unlikely to be as precise as those from the whole study population.

▶ Generalizability

Generalizability is a judgment in which the investigator applies "the conclusions of a trial to the broader setting of general medical care and to a more heterogeneous set of patients than those studied."[2(p107)] The group of people to whom the study results may be applied or generalized is termed the **reference population**. The original eligibility criteria that determine the composition of the study population in turn determine the appropriate reference population. Investigators' ability to generalize the results of a study to a broader context is affected by the study participants' physiological, behavioral, and cultural characteristics. For example, the maternal–infant HIV transmission study included only women with mildly symptomatic HIV disease. For this reason, the investigators stated, "It is not clear whether the result of this trial can be extrapolated to . . . women with more advanced disease" because of physiological differences between these groups.[23]

Because the racial and gender compositions of a study population are such important determinants of generalizability, the National Institutes of Health (NIH), a federal agency that provides funding for many experimental studies, has encouraged the inclusion of women and members of minority groups to increase the applicability of trials.[39] Moreover, the NIH requires that every proposed trial include sufficient numbers of women and minorities to enable comparison of treatment responses separately between the gender and racial/ethnic groups.

▶ Special Issues in Experimental Studies

A number of practical issues make it difficult to conduct an experimental study. First, experimental studies are very expensive. Second, many physicians and patients are reluctant to participate in experimental research. Physicians are hesitant to participate because they believe that such trials will hamper their ability to maintain a personalized relationship with their patients.[39] The necessity of standardized approaches to patient workup and monitoring and the additional work and oversight involved in trials also contribute to physician reluctance. In addition, because experimentation still has a negative connotation in our society, patients are often unwilling to serve as "guinea pigs" for the advancement of science.

In addition to these practical issues, epidemiologists must consider numerous ethical issues when designing and conducting experimental studies. Most researchers believe that it is ethical to conduct experimental studies (particularly randomized, placebo-controlled trials) only when there is a state of equipoise or equilibrium regarding the treatment within the expert medical community. **Equipoise** is a "state of mind or belief characterized by a counterbalance of competing values, doubts, or risks."[2(p85)] In other words, there must be genuine confidence that a treatment may be worthwhile to administer it to some individuals and genuine reservations about the treatment to withhold it from others. Furthermore, physicians who already have developed opinions about the effectiveness of a treatment (even though the treatment has not been tested adequately) are reluctant to enroll their patients in a trial if there is a chance that their patients will not get the preferred treatment.

Equipoise is not a static state, and a shift in equipoise sometimes occurs during the course of a trial. The shift often occurs when a clear benefit or adverse effect is observed for the test treatment in an interim data analysis from the ongoing trial. Such an analysis is usually conducted by a treatment-effects monitoring committee, a semi-independent group with varied backgrounds (such as clinicians, medical ethicists, and biostatisticians) who examine the accumulating data for detecting early evidence of harm or benefit that may require early termination. Early terminations have occurred in major trials of both therapeutic and preventive treatments, including the maternal–infant HIV transmission study.[23,40] When the effectiveness of zidovudine in reducing maternal–fetal HIV transmission was observed in the first interim data analysis, study investigators stopped enrolling additional patients, and all women were offered the zidovudine treatment.[23]

Another ethical concern about experimental studies involves the use of placebo controls. Michels and Rothman argue forcefully that randomized clinical trials are unethical when they administer placebos to the comparison group if effective treatments are available.[41] For example, Fabre conducted a trial in 1990 that randomly assigned patients with major depression to either a new medication (buspirone) or a placebo.[42] This study took place at a time when numerous effective treatments were available for severe depression.[43(pp47-76)] When two participants attempted to commit suicide during the course of the study, they were removed from the study and placed on one of the standard medications.[42]

Why do investigators use placebos in these settings? Usually, they offer scientific reasons such as the need to control for the placebo and Hawthorne effects. However, no scientific principle mandates investigators to compare an experimental treatment with a placebo rather than to another effective treatment, and scientific principles should never supersede the well-being of study participants.[41]

Summary

Well-conducted experimental studies are thought to produce more scientifically rigorous results than do observational studies. This is because of several distinctive features of experimental studies, including the random assignment of participants to treatment and comparison groups to eliminate baseline differences between the groups and reduce the likelihood of biased allocation and the use of placebo controls to permit masked ascertainment of the outcomes. On the other hand, several practical issues make it difficult for epidemiologists to conduct experimental studies, including participant noncompliance with the treatment regimen, the need to maintain high follow-up rates over extended periods of time, high cost, and physician and patient reluctance to participate. In addition, experimental studies pose numerous ethical issues. For example, a state of equipoise regarding the treatment must exist within the medical community. That is, there must be genuine confidence that a treatment may be worthwhile to administer it to some individuals and genuine reservations about the treatment to withhold it from others.

References

1. Hodgson E, Guthrie FE (eds.). *Introduction to Biochemical Toxicology.* New York, NY: Elsevier Science Publishing Co.; 1980.

2. Meinert CL. *Clinical Trials Dictionary: Terminology and Usage Recommendations.* 2nd ed. Hoboken, NJ: John Wiley & Sons, Inc.; 2012.

3. CAPRIE Steering Committee. A randomized, blinded, trial of clopidogrel versus aspirin in patients at risk of ischemic events (CAPRIE). *Lancet.* 1996;348:1329-1339.

4. Hammer SM, Squires KE, Hughes MD, Grimes JM, Demeter LM, Currier JS, et al. A controlled trial of two nucleoside analogues plus indinavir in persons with human immunodeficiency virus infection and CD4 cell counts of 200 per cubic millimeter or less. *New Engl J Med.* 1997;337:725-733.

5. Ast DB, Finn SB, McCaffrey I. The Newburgh-Kingston Caries Fluorine Study. *Am J Public Health.* 1950;40:716-724.

6. Rhodes SD, McCoy TP, Tanner AE, Stowers J, Bachmann LH, Nguyen AL, et al. Using social media to increase HIV testing among gay and bisexual men, other men who have sex with men, and transgendered persons: outcomes from a randomized community trial. *Clin Infect Dis.* 2016; 62:1450-1453.

7. Weitzman M, Aschengrau A, Bellinger D, Jones R, Hamlin JS, Beiser A. Lead-contaminated soil abatement and urban children's blood lead levels. *JAMA.* 1993;269:1647-1654.

8. Greenwald P, Kelloff G, Burch-Whitman C, Kramer BS. Chemoprevention. *CA Cancer J Clin.* 1995; 45:31-49.

9. Multiple Risk Factor Intervention Trial: risk factor changes and mortality rates. *JAMA.* 1982;248:1465-1477.

10. Jalling C, Bodin M, Romelsjö A, Källmén H, Durbeej N, Tengström A. Parent programs for reducing adolescent's antisocial behavior and substance use: a randomized controlled trial. *J Child Fam Stud.* 2016;25:811-826.

11. Bolton KL, Egerton T, Wark J, Wee E, Matthews B, Kelly A, et al. Effects of exercise on bone density and falls risk factors in post-menopausal women with osteopenia: a randomised controlled trial. *J Sci Med Sport.* 2012;15:102-109.

12. DiClemente RJ, Wingood GM, Sales JM, Brown JL, Rose ES, Davis TL, et al. Efficacy of a telephone-delivered sexually transmitted infection/human immunodeficiency virus prevention maintenance intervention for adolescents: a randomized clinical trial. *JAMA Pediatr.* 2014;168:938-946.

13. Finnegan LP. The NIH Women's Health Initiative: its evolution and expected contributions to women's health. *Am J Prev Med.* 1996;12:292-293.

14. Auvert B, Taljaard D, Lagarde E, Sobngwi-Tambekou J, Sitta R, Puren A. Randomized, controlled intervention trial of male circumcision for reduction of HIV infection risk: the ANRS 1265 Trial. *PLoS Med.* 2005;2:e298.

15. Fisher B, Constantino JP, Wickerham DL, Redmond CK, Kavanah M, Cronin WM, et al. Tamoxifen for prevention of breast cancer: report of the national Surgical Adjuvant Breast and Bowel Project P-1 Study. *J Natl Cancer Inst.* 1998;90:1371-1388.

16. MacMahon B. Overview of studies on endometrial cancer and other types of cancer in humans: perspectives of an epidemiologist. *Semin Oncol.* 1997;24(1S1):122-139.

17. Prentice RL. On the role, design, and analysis of disease prevention trials. *Control Clin Trials.* 1995;16:249-258.

18. Perren TJ, Swart AM, Pfisterer J, Ledermann JA, Pujade-Lauraine E, Kristensen G, et al. A phase 3 trial of bevacizumab in ovarian cancer. *New Engl J Med.* 2011;365:2484-2496.

19. Cohen MS, Chen YQ, McCauley M, Gamble T, Hosseinipour MC, Kumarasamy N, et al. Prevention of HIV-1 infection with early antiretroviral therapy. *New Engl J Med.* 2011;365:493-505.

20. Kaufman D. Cancer therapy and randomized clinical trial: good medicine? *CA Cancer J Clin.* 1994;44:109-114.

21. Ellenberg SS, Foulkes MA. The utility of large simple trials in the evaluation of AIDS treatment strategies. *Stat Med.* 1994;13:405-415.

22. Bassuk SS, Manson JE, Lee IM, Cook NR, Christen WG, Bubes VY, et al. Baseline characteristics of participants in the VITamin D and OmegA-3 TriaL (VITAL). *Contemp Clin Trials.* 2016;47:235-243.

23. Connor EM, Sperling RS, Gelber R, Kiselev P, Scott G, O'Sullivan MJ, et al. Reduction of maternal-infant transmission of human immunodeficiency virus type 1 with zidovudine treatment. *New Engl J Med.* 1994;331:1173-1180.

24. Dahm JL, Cook E, Baugh K, Wileyto EP, Pinto A, Leone F, et al. Predictors of enrollment in a smoking cessation clinical trial after eligibility screening. *J Natl Med Assoc.* 2009;101:450-455.

25. Porta M. *A Dictionary of Epidemiology.* 6th ed. New York, NY: Oxford University Press; 2014.

26. Moher D, Dulberg CS, Wells GA. Statistical power, sample size, and their reporting in randomized controlled trials. *JAMA.* 1994;272:122-124.

27. Colton T. *Statistics in Medicine.* Boston, MA: Little, Brown and Co.; 1974.

28. Nowak R. Problems in clinical trials go far beyond misconduct. *Science.* 1994;264:1538-1541.

29. Enblom A, Johnsson A, Hammar M, Onelov E, Steineck G, Borjeson S. Acupuncture compared with placebo acupuncture in radiotherapy-induced nausea: a randomized controlled study. *Ann Oncol.* 2012;23(5):1353-1361.

30. Gray RH, Kigozi G, Serwadda D, Makumbi F, Watya S, Nalugoda F, et al. Male circumcision for HIV prevention in men in Rakai, Uganda: a randomized trial. *Lancet.* 2007;369:657-666.

31. Michael M, Boyce WT, Wilcox AJ. *Biomedical Bestiary: An Epidemiologic Guide to Flaws and Fallacies in the Medical Literature.* Boston, MA: Little, Brown and Co.; 1984.

32. Friedman LM, Furberg CD, Demets DL. *Fundamentals of Clinical Trials.* 2nd ed. Littleton, MA: PSG Publishing Co.; 1985.

33. Oliver AJ, Covar RA, Goldfrad CH, Klein RM, Pedersen SE, Sorkness CA, et al. Randomized trial of once-daily fluticasone furoate in children with inadequately controlled asthma. *J Pediatr.* 2016;178:246-253.

34. MEMS® Cap versatile adherence monitoring cap. www.aardexgroup.com/products/mems-cap. Accessed October 2016.

35. McRae-Clark AL, Baker NL, Sonne SC, DeVane CL, Wagner A, Norton J. Concordance of direct and indirect measures of medication adherence in a treatment trial for cannabis dependence. *J Subst Abuse Treat.* 2015;57:70-74.

36. Hullsiek K, Grund B. Considerations for endpoint selection when designing HIV clinical trials. *Curr Infect Dis Rep.* 2012;14:110-118.

37. Newell DJ. Intention-to-treat analysis: implications for quantitative and qualitative research. *Int J Epidemiol.* 1992;21:837-841.

38. Coronary Drug Project Research Group. Influence of adherence to treatment and response of cholesterol on mortality in the Coronary Drug Project. *New Engl J Med.* 1980;303:1038-1041.

39. NIH Policy and Guidelines on the Inclusion of Women and Minorities as Subjects in Clinical Research—Announced October 2001. nih.gov. https://grants.nih.gov/grants/funding/women_min/guidelines.htm. Accessed October 2016.

40. Steering Committee of the Physicians' Health Study Research Group. Final report on the aspirin component of the ongoing Physicians' Health Study. *New Engl J Med.* 1989;321:129-135.

41. Michels KB, Rothman KJ. Update on the unethical use of placebos in randomised trials. *Bioethics.* 2003;17:188-204.

42. Fabre LF. Buspirone in the management of major depression: a placebo controlled comparison. *J Clin Psych.* 1990;51:55-61.

43. *The Internist's Compendium of Drug Therapy.* Lawrenceville, NJ: Core Publishing Division, Excerpta Medica, Inc.; 1990.

Chapter Questions

1. Briefly define each of the following terms that are associated with experimental studies:
    a. Randomization
    b. Reference population
    c. Single-masked study
    d. Double-masked study
    e. Run-in period
    f. Placebo and sham procedure
    g. Equipoise

2. State the main difference between each of the following:
    a. Individual and community trials
    b. Preventive and therapeutic trials
    c. Simple and factorial trial designs

3. Each of the following problems represents a major threat to the validity of an experimental study. Briefly describe one method for avoiding these problems.
    a. Low compliance
    b. Lack of baseline comparability
    c. Biased information on the outcome

4. Describe the essential feature and purpose of an intent-to-treat analysis.
5. What distinctive features of experimental studies enhance their ability to produce scientifically rigorous results?
6. Why are experimental studies difficult to conduct?
7. Indicate whether the following statements are true or false:
    a. A major advantage of a randomized experimental study is that it rules out self-selection of subjects to the treatment and comparison groups.
    b. Randomization controls for confounding equally well in both large and small studies.
    c. Noncompliance in an experimental study makes the compared groups more similar, which reduces the ability of the investigator to detect a difference between the groups.
    d. An important advantage of a placebo-controlled experimental study is that it permits masking of study subjects and study investigators.
    e. Randomization and random selection are alternative terms for the same concept.
    f. Some experimental studies are terminated earlier than planned because of a shift in equipoise.

8. In a double-masked study to evaluate the effectiveness of cranberry juice to reduce the incidence of urinary tract infections (UTIs), participants were randomized to receive cranberry juice or a placebo beverage twice a day for 6 weeks. The intent-to-treat risk difference comparing the incidence of UTIs among those randomized to cranberry juice versus placebo showed an 8% reduction in UTIs among cranberry juice drinkers. Compliance was equally low (about 60%) in both groups. The risk difference from an efficacy analysis would show:
    a. Greater than 8% reduction in UTIs among cranberry juice drinkers
    b. Less than 8% reduction in UTIs among cranberry juice drinkers
    c. An 8% reduction in UTIs among cranberry juice drinkers

9. Suppose that a small, randomized, single-masked experimental study is conducted. Which of the following problems are *surely* avoided in this study?
   a. Noncompliance
   b. Confounding
   c. Biased assessment of the disease outcome
   d. Loss to follow-up

10. Suppose that a randomized intervention study of vitamin D supplementation for the prevention of prostate cancer was conducted among White men aged 50–64 years living in the United States. The results of this study are most generalizable to which of the following groups? Briefly give the reason(s) for your decision.
    a. White men aged 50–64 years living in the United Kingdom
    b. White men aged 65–85 living in the United States.
    c. Black men aged 50–64 years living in the United States.

CHAPTER 8

Cohort Studies

LEARNING OBJECTIVES

By the end of this chapter the reader will be able to:
- Distinguish between the various types of cohort studies, including open, fixed, closed, retrospective, prospective, and ambidirectional designs.
- Describe the key features of conducting cohort studies, including the selection of the exposed and unexposed populations; the sources of information on the exposure, outcomes, and other key variables; approaches to follow-up; calculating person-time; and data analysis.
- Discuss the strengths and limitations of cohort studies.

▶ Introduction

Although experimental studies are scientifically rigorous, they are often infeasible because of difficulties enrolling participants, high costs, and thorny ethical issues. For example, an experimental study of a substance that may increase a person's risk of developing a disease is infeasible because it is unethical to give a potentially harmful substance to a healthy person. Consequently, epidemiological research consists mainly of observational studies. These studies are considered "natural" experiments because the investigator acts as a disinterested observer, merely letting nature take its course. Observational studies take advantage of the fact that people expose themselves to noxious or healthy substances through their personal habits (e.g., drinking alcoholic beverages or taking vitamins), choice of occupation (e.g., asbestos insulation worker), place of residence (e.g., near a lead smelter), and so on. Consequently, many issues that make it infeasible to conduct an experimental study, particularly those related to ethics, are mitigated in an observational study. For example, although it is unethical to conduct an experimental study of the effect of cigarette smoke on the developing fetus by randomly assigning newly pregnant women to either a smoking or a nonsmoking group, it is

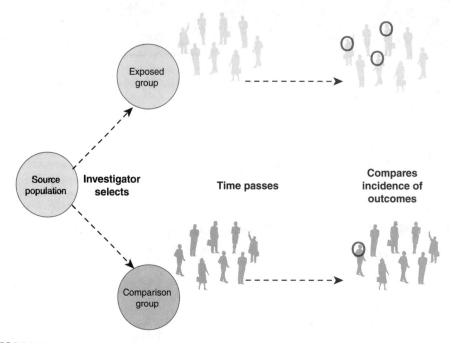

FIGURE 8-1 Schematic representation of cohort study implementation.

perfectly ethical to conduct an observational study by comparing women who choose to smoke during pregnancy with those who choose not to.

The cohort study is one of the two principal types of observational studies. A classic cohort study examines one or more health effects of a single exposure. Subjects are defined according to their exposure status and followed over time to determine the incidence of the health outcomes. A schematic representation of the implementation of a cohort study is presented in **FIGURE 8-1**. This chapter describes the design, conduct, and analysis of cohort studies. First, cohort study terms are defined, and then a detailed discussion of each aspect of these studies is provided. Many design features of cohort studies emulate those of well-done experimental studies because the goal of both types of studies is to obtain high-quality results.

▶ Cohort Study Definitions and Overview

The term *cohort* comes from the Latin word *cohors*, meaning a group of soldiers.[1(p359)] In ancient Rome, a cohort was 1 of 10 divisions of a legion, the major unit of the Roman army. Once a cohort was formed, no new soldiers were added, and therefore soldiers remained in the same cohort for the duration of their service. Attrition occurred mainly through death.

TABLE 8-1 Characteristics of Cohort Studies			
Type of population studied	Defined by	Follow-up	Appropriate measure of disease frequency
Open or dynamic	Changeable characteristic	Members come and go; losses may occur	Incidence rate
Fixed	Irrevocable event	Does not gain members; losses may occur	Incidence rate
Closed	Irrevocable event	Does not gain members; no losses occur	Cumulative incidence

Today, we use the word *cohort* to characterize "any designated group of persons who are followed or traced over a period of time."[2(p49)] The term is also used to describe a group of individuals with a common characteristic or experience. For example, a birth cohort consists of individuals who are born during a particular year or period and therefore share many similar experiences (such as "millennials"). Although *cohort study* is the standard term used to describe an epidemiological investigation that follows groups with common characteristics, some investigators use the terms *follow-up*, *incidence*, and *longitudinal study*.

Several additional terms are used to describe cohort studies. These terms are related to the characteristics of the population from which the cohort is derived and whether the exposure changes over time and there are losses to follow-up (see **TABLE 8-1**).

▶ Types of Populations Studied

The first type of cohort is conducted in an **open population**, also known as a **dynamic population**. Individuals in an open population may enter or leave at any time because its membership is defined by a changeable characteristic, such as smoking cigarettes, drinking alcohol, having a certain occupation, or living in a specific geographic area. For example, a person is a member of the open population of New York City residents only as long as he or she lives in New York City. Cohort studies that are conducted in an open population usually take into account population changes, such as in-and-out migration, and therefore the incidence rate is the most suitable measure of disease frequency for monitoring health outcomes in this setting. For example, consider a hypothetical cohort study of cancer incidence conducted among never-married men who were aged 25 to 44 years and resided in Miami, Florida, from 1985 to

2015. The purpose of these eligibility criteria is to identify a population with a high prevalence of HIV infection. This group is considered an open population because it is defined by the changeable characteristics of marital status, age, and place of residence. If a man got married, aged beyond 44 years, or moved away from Miami, his membership in the population would end, and he would no longer be eligible for the study. The study investigators would have to monitor these eligibility changes among the men enrolled in the study and determine the number of person-years of observation that were accrued during the follow-up period. The person-time data could be used as the denominators for the incidence rates of the diseases under study.

Cohorts may also be formed on the basis of inalterable characteristics (see Table 8-1). A **fixed cohort** is defined by an irrevocable event; for example, undergoing a medical procedure, giving birth to a child, serving in the military, eating contaminated food at a picnic, or being present at a man-made or natural disaster. Thus, exposures in a fixed cohort do not change over time. In addition, the groups are followed from a defined starting point (usually marked by the event) to a defined ending point. The World War II atomic bomb survivors from Hiroshima and Nagasaki, Japan, comprise one of the best-known fixed cohorts to be studied for biological effects of acute radiation exposure.[3] For over half a century, researchers have monitored mortality and cancer incidence rates among approximately 94,000 exposed residents who survived the bombings and 27,000 unexposed residents who were outside the city when the bombs were dropped. The incidence rates of various outcomes have been periodically compared between these two groups during the follow-up period. Incidence rates are the appropriate measure of disease frequency in a fixed cohort when the population experiences losses to follow-up. (**Losses to follow-up** are the participants whom investigators are unable to trace to determine whether they became ill or died.)

The third type of cohort is the **closed cohort**. Like the fixed cohort, a closed cohort is defined by an irrevocable event and has defined starting and ending points for follow-up. The difference between the two is that a closed cohort has no losses to follow-up. For example, a closed cohort study might be conducted among people who attended a party to determine whether eating certain foods increased the risk of gastroenteritis during the week following the party. Thus, everyone who attended the party is a member of the closed population who is eligible for the study. Follow-up would start at the end of the party (assuming that all of the contaminated food was eaten by then and that the illness could occur immediately after ingesting the contaminated food) and would end 7 days later. No members of the population would be lost because the observation period is short. Cumulative incidence or average risk is typically used as the measure of disease frequency in this setting because there are no losses to follow-up.

▶ Characterization of Exposure

Regardless of what type of cohort study is conducted, participants are grouped according to their exposure and followed over time to compare the incidence of symptoms, disease, or death. Usually, two groups are compared, such as an exposed and an unexposed group. The exposed group is called the index group, and the unexposed group is termed the referent or comparison group. It is necessary for the investigator to specify a minimum amount of exposure to qualify for the exposed group. For example, studies of cigarette smoking may use a lifetime history of smoking at least 100 cigarettes to qualify for membership in the exposed smoking group. In addition, when investigators are unable to find truly unexposed people to serve in the comparison group, people with low exposure are usually selected.

It can be difficult to classify the exposure status of subjects, particularly when the exposure changes over time. For example, a woman might begin smoking as a young adult, smoke cigarettes for a few years, stop while she is pregnant, and then return to smoking after giving birth. Thus, depending on the period, this woman could be considered a nonsmoker, a smoker, or an ex-smoker. The investigator might decide to consider a woman exposed if she ever smoked cigarettes at any time in the past. However, such a simplistic exposure definition might miss an association that is confined to certain aspects of the exposure. For example, the association may be present only for high-intensity smoking (e.g., more than two packs per day) or long-duration smoking (e.g., more than 10 years).

Thus, whenever possible, investigators divide the exposed group into levels (e.g., high, medium, and low exposure), enabling investigators to assess the presence of a dose–response relationship. A **dose–response relationship** means that the risk of disease increases as the intensity or duration of exposure increases. This categorization can be complicated because there are many ways to characterize an exposure level. For example, one could use the maximum level ever experienced by the individual, the cumulative level as of a certain date, or the average exposure level over a time period. Exposure to cigarette smoke is often characterized by the number of pack-years that the person has accumulated. This composite measure is calculated by multiplying the average number of packs smoked per day by the number of years smoked at that intensity. Thus, a person who has smoked two packs a day for 20 years has accumulated 40 pack-years of exposure.

▶ Follow-Up and Outcome Assessment

During the follow-up period, the exposed and unexposed groups are monitored for the outcomes under study. As in experimental studies, more than one outcome is typically investigated. The outcomes of interest depend on the research question and may include precursors or first occurrence of disease, disease recurrence, or death. For example, a cohort study of elderly residents of northern Manhattan, New York, examined cardiovascular mortality in relation to leisure-time physical activity.[4] As another example, a cohort study of nurses examined their risk of infertility, that is, the inability to conceive after 12 months of trying to become pregnant.[5]

At the start of follow-up, members of the cohort are at risk for but have not yet experienced the outcome(s) of interest. By the end of the follow-up period, a proportion of the cohort (up to 100%) will have experienced the outcome(s) under study. The length of the follow-up period can range from a few hours for infectious diseases to several decades for diseases such as cancer or cardiovascular disease. The longer the follow-up period, the more difficult it is to trace and maintain contact with study subjects and the more expensive the study. Although follow-up has become even more difficult in recent years because of increased population mobility, newly available resources such as those on the Internet have helped to offset these difficulties. Follow-up rates should be as high as possible to ensure the **validity** of the study. If the health outcomes of those who are lost to follow-up are different from those who are not lost, the study results may be biased. There is no magical follow-up rate that guarantees the validity of a study (other than 100%), but most epidemiologists are satisfied with follow-up rates higher than 90%.

▶ Timing of Cohort Studies

Three terms are used to describe the timing of events at the commencement of a cohort study: (1) prospective, meaning to look forward in time; (2) retrospective, meaning to look back in time; and (3) ambidirectional, meaning to look both ways (see **FIGURE 8-2**). To avoid confusion with other types of studies, the terms *retrospective, prospective,* and *ambidirectional* should always modify the word *cohort* and never be used alone.

At the start of a **prospective cohort study**, participants are grouped on the basis of past or current exposure and followed into the future to observe the outcome(s) of interest. When the study commences, the outcomes have not yet developed, and the investigator must wait for them to occur. The timing of prospective cohort studies is similar to that of experimental studies. For example, a prospective cohort design was used to conduct a major study on the effect of lead exposure on intellectual function in adulthood.[6] Investigators enrolled young children and followed them until they were 38 years old. Investigators obtained the participants' blood lead levels from childhood through adulthood. When the participants reached 38 years of age, investigators conducted tests of cognitive function to determine whether childhood lead exposure was associated with long-term effects on IQ and other measures of cognitive function.

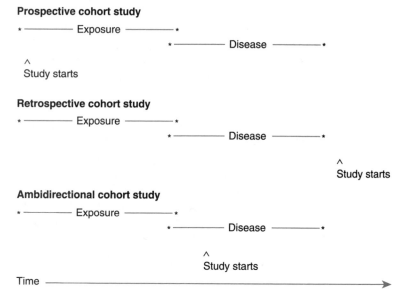

FIGURE 8-2 Timing of cohort studies.

In a **retrospective cohort study**, both the exposures and outcomes have already occurred by the time the study begins. This type of investigation studies only prior outcomes and not future ones. For example, investigators undertook a retrospective cohort study in 2014 to evaluate risk factors for suicide attempts among active-duty members of the U.S. Army during the wars in Afghanistan and Iraq.[7] The study included men and women who served in the Army from 2004 through 2009. Investigators collected data on the occurrence of medically documented suicide attempts as well as information on risk factors, such as mental health diagnoses (such as depression), during this period. Thus, all of the mental health diagnoses and suicide attempts had occurred by the time the investigators conducted the study. The researchers found the occurrence of attempted suicide was 18 times higher among enlisted soldiers with a mental health diagnosis in the month before the suicide attempt as compared to soldiers without a diagnosis.

An **ambidirectional cohort study** has both prospective and retrospective components. For example, the Air Force Health Study is an ambidirectional study of the men who were involved in aerial spraying of herbicides (including the dioxin-contaminated Agent Orange) during the Vietnam War.[8] The purpose of this study is to determine whether these men have an increased risk of adverse health and reproductive outcomes. The retrospective portion of the study conducted analyses of cancer and mortality that occurred from the men's first tour of duty in Vietnam through the 1980s.[9,10] The prospective component will monitor the health of these men for many years to come.[11]

How does an epidemiologist decide whether to conduct a prospective, retrospective, or ambidirectional cohort study? The answer often depends on the research question, the practical constraints of time and money, and the availability of suitable study populations and records. In addition, the decision usually takes into account the complementary advantages and disadvantages of retrospective and prospective cohort studies. For example, retrospective cohort studies are more efficient (they take less time and money) than prospective studies for investigating diseases that take a long time to develop and come to diagnosis. This is because the disease and exposure have already occurred.

Limited information is usually available on the exposure, outcome, and other key variables in retrospective cohort studies because these studies typically rely on existing records that were not designed for research purposes. For example, a retrospective cohort study of agricultural workers who were employed in California vineyards in the 1990s might have to depend on vineyard employment records to identify cohort members. These records may contain only the person's name, date of birth, job title, and dates of employment. A detailed picture of that person's actual job duties and exposures and information on important habits, such as cigarette smoking, may be missing. In addition, follow-up and ascertainment of the outcomes may be hampered because the historical records may not have information to facilitate locating the study subjects many years later.

In contrast, investigators in a prospective cohort study can usually obtain more detailed information on exposures and other key variables because they have more control of the data collection process and can gather information directly from the participants. Follow-up may also be easier because the investigator can obtain tracing information from participants and maintain periodic contact with subjects. In addition, prospective cohort studies are considered less vulnerable to bias because the outcomes have not occurred when the cohort is assembled and the exposures are assessed.

▶ Issues in the Selection of Cohort Study Populations

Emulation of Experimental Studies

The investigator in an experimental study assigns participants to the experimental or comparison group. When the assignment is made randomly and the sample size is sufficiently large, these groups will have nearly identical distributions of baseline characteristics. In contrast, participants in cohort studies enter the exposed and unexposed groups usually on the basis of self-determined behaviors and events. Consequently, the results of cohort studies may be difficult to interpret because of differences between the exposed and unexposed groups that influence the risk of developing the disease. Consider, for example, a cohort study of the effect of maternal cigarette smoking during pregnancy on the risk of birth defects among the offspring. Women who smoke cigarettes during pregnancy are more likely to consume alcoholic beverages than women who do not smoke.[12] Because heavy consumption of alcoholic beverages increases the risk of having a baby with congenital anomalies regardless of whether a woman smokes cigarettes,[13] an association between cigarette smoking and birth defects might really be caused by the alcohol consumption.

Epidemiologists try to minimize these types of problems by translating the key features of experimental studies to cohort studies. First, even though it is not possible to randomly assign exposures in cohort studies, differences between groups can be minimized by carefully selecting the exposed and unexposed groups to be as similar as possible. In fact, the ideal comparison group would consist of exactly the same individuals had they not been exposed. For example, the Air Force Health Study compared an exposed group of 1,300 Air Force servicemen who flew herbicide spraying missions during the Vietnam War with an unexposed group of Air Force servicemen who flew cargo missions in Southeast Asia during the war that did not involve handling or spraying herbicides.[9] The baseline demographic characteristics and health status of the exposed and unexposed groups were quite similar, because all the men underwent the same selection procedures for serving in the Air Force and flying missions during the Vietnam War.

A second key feature of experimental studies that is translated in cohort studies is the use of placebos. Placebos are used in experimental studies to match as closely as possible the experiences of the experimental and comparison groups to permit masking of the study investigators (among others). Although cohort studies cannot use placebos, they can match the experiences of the exposed and unexposed groups by selecting individuals with similar characteristics. Investigators sometimes enhance this process by using special matching criteria when selecting unexposed subjects. For example, if investigators want to ensure that the groups are comparable with respect to age, gender, and race, they would employ a technique known as individual matching. For example, they would select an unexposed 50-year-old Black female for every exposed 50-year-old Black female in the study. Even without placebos, it is relatively easy to mask investigators to the subjects' exposure status during follow-up and outcome ascertainment in a cohort study. One merely keeps this information from the study staff involved in these tasks. Masking guarantees comparable follow-up efforts and outcome ascertainment, which in turn helps ensure valid results.

The third key feature of experimental studies emulated by cohort studies is the method for determining the overall sample size as well as the relative size of the exposed and unexposed groups. Like experimental studies, cohort studies must include an adequate number of individuals to have sufficient statistical power to detect an association if it truly

TABLE 8-2 Similarities and Differences Between Experimental and Cohort Studies

Similarities

- Both make comparisons across two or more exposure groups.
- Both follow participants to monitor outcome rates.
- Both usually monitor more than one outcome.
- Both select groups to achieve comparability and efficiency.
- Relative proportion of subjects in compared groups does not reflect that of the general population.

Differences

- Experimental study investigators allocate exposure to exposure groups. Cohort study participants choose exposures themselves.
- Experimental studies can use randomization to achieve baseline comparability. Cohort study investigators must carefully select groups to achieve comparability.
- Experimental studies can use placebos to match the groups' experiences and permit masking. Cohort study investigators carefully select groups to match as closely as possible. Cohort studies also use masking.
- Experimental studies are prospective. Cohort studies may be prospective, retrospective, or ambidirectional.

exists. Investigators determine the sample size by taking into account the anticipated difference between compared groups, the background rate of the outcome, and the probability of making statistical errors.[14(pp142-146)] The relative sizes of the exposed and unexposed groups are chosen to maximize the power of the study. They are not intended to mimic the frequencies in the general population. For example, an exposure may occur rarely in the general population (e.g., one exposed per 1,000 population), but the frequency in a study population may be 50% (e.g., 1,000 exposed and 1,000 unexposed individuals). The similarities and differences between experimental and cohort studies described so far are summarized in **TABLE 8-2**.

Selection of the Exposed Population

The choice of the exposed group in a cohort study depends on the hypothesis under study; the exposure frequency; and feasibility considerations, such as the availability of records and ease of follow-up. The two main types of cohorts—special cohort and general cohort—are distinguished by the exposure frequency. A **special cohort** is assembled to study the health effects of rare exposures, such as uncommon occupational chemicals, unusual diets or lifestyles, natural or man-made disasters, or medical procedures. A **general cohort** is typically assembled for common exposures, such as use of oral contraceptives, dietary factors such as vitamin use, and habits such as cigarette smoking and alcohol consumption. General cohorts are often selected from professional groups, such as doctors and nurses, volunteers, or residents in well-defined geographic areas to facilitate follow-up and accurate ascertainment of the outcome(s) under study.

When assembling a special cohort, epidemiologists must go to the settings where the exposure has occurred, is occurring, or will occur to identify the exposed population. For example, workplace sites, such as factories, and organizations, such as unions, frequently serve as sources of individuals for occupational cohort studies. Because workers often have more intense and sustained exposures than the general population, cohort studies of occupational groups are an important component of identifying the causes of disease. For example, an occupational cohort study was conducted among 21,863 male and female workers from 12 countries whose jobs involved producing or spraying phenoxy herbicides and chlorophenols to determine whether these workers had an increased risk of cancer deaths.[15] Epidemiologists identified subjects for the cohort study by reviewing employment and other records in businesses involved in manufacturing and spraying these chemicals.

Epidemiologists have conducted special cohort studies among individuals undergoing a medical procedure or treatment involving potentially noxious exposures. For example, important data on the risk of cancer following radiation have come from cohort studies of patients with ankylosing spondylitis (a spinal disorder) who were treated with radiation therapy.[16] Historical records of 87 radiotherapy centers in Great Britain and Northern Ireland were reviewed to identify more than 14,000 patients treated from 1935 to 1954. Investigators found that ankylosing spondylitis patients were more likely than expected to have leukemia and cancers of the lung, bone, and esophagus.

Epidemiologists have conducted cohort studies among groups with unusual diets or lifestyles, such as Seventh Day Adventists and Mormons. For example, Seventh Day Adventists do not consume tobacco, alcohol, or pork, and many of them follow a vegetarian diet. The Adventist Health Study has monitored the morbidity and mortality experience of approximately 96,000 Seventh Day Adventists in the United States and Canada since 2002.[17] The study has found, for example, that participants who followed any one of four vegetarian diets (vegan, lacto-ovo vegetarian, pescovegetarian, and semi-vegetarian) had a lower incidence of colorectal cancer than nonvegetarians. In fact, the lowest risks were seen for pescovegetarians.

As stated previously, epidemiologists assemble a general cohort from professional groups or residents in well-defined geographic areas to study common exposures. One of the best-known cohort studies based on the general population is the Framingham Study, which began in 1948. Its main purpose was to determine the causes of cardiovascular disease.[18(pp14-29)] The risk factors that have been studied include high blood pressure, high blood cholesterol, physical inactivity, obesity, and smoking, which are all fairly common exposures. Investigators initially enrolled about 5,000 healthy adult residents in Framingham, Massachusetts, a town located about 18 miles west of Boston. In 1948, Framingham was a self-contained community of about 28,000 residents who obtained their medical care from local physicians and two hospitals near the center of town. Framingham residents were considered an excellent population for a long-term epidemiological study because (1) the town's population was stable, (2) the investigators could identify a sufficient number of people with and without risk factors for heart disease (e.g., they expected sufficient numbers of smokers and nonsmokers), and (3) local medical doctors were "highly cooperative and well-informed" and wanted to help investigators recruit subjects for the study. All of these factors have contributed to the study's low dropout rate (only 5% after 50 years) and to its numerous important contributions to our understanding of the etiology of heart disease. Today, this important research continues with cohort studies of the offspring and grandchildren of the original cohort study members.[19]

Selection of Comparison Group

In a cohort study, the ideal comparison group would consist of exactly the same individuals in the exposed group had they not been exposed. This theoretical concept is known as the "**counterfactual ideal**."[20(pp54-55)] Because it is impossible for the same person to be exposed and unexposed simultaneously, epidemiologists must select different sets of individuals for the exposed and comparison groups. Even though different people form each group, the investigator chooses groups as similar as possible on characteristics that influence getting the disease. For example, if gender were related to the risk of the disease (i.e., if men had a higher risk than women or vice versa), it would be important for the exposed and unexposed groups to have the same proportion of males and females. The rate of disease in the exposed and comparison groups should be identical if the exposure has no effect on disease occurrence.

The three sources for the comparison group in a cohort study are (1) an internal comparison, (2) the general population, and (3) a comparison cohort (see **TABLE 8-3**). An **internal comparison group** is composed of unexposed members of the same cohort. For example, Boice and Monson conducted a classic retrospective cohort study to determine the risk of breast cancer among female tuberculosis patients who had undergone repeated fluoroscopic X-ray examination of the chest during air collapse therapy.[21] This treatment resulted in considerable radiation exposure to the breast. The comparison group consisted of other female tuberculosis patients who received treatments that did not require fluoroscopic X-ray examinations. Like the exposed group, the women who comprised the internal comparison group were tuberculosis patients at Massachusetts hospitals during the years 1930 to 1954. The study found a 1.8-fold excess of breast cancer cases among the exposed group; however, the risk was higher among women exposed before age 20 years.

TABLE 8-3 Types of Comparison Groups in Cohort Studies

Type of comparison group	Strengths	Weaknesses
Internal	Most comparable to exposed group	May be difficult to identify
General population	Accessible, stable data	Lack of comparability with exposed group; results may suffer from healthy worker effect; data on key variables may be missing
Comparison cohort	Fairly comparable	Results are often difficult to interpret because a comparison cohort often has other exposures

When the general population is the source of the comparison group, preexisting available data on disease occurrence and death in a population are the basis for comparison. In the United States, such data are available from the National Center for Health Statistics. Internationally, excellent mortality statistics are compiled by the World Health Organization. Often, when the comparison group is composed of the general population, the **standardized mortality ratio (SMR)** is used as the measure of association. The SMR is the ratio of the observed number of cases of disease or death to the expected number based on general population rates. SMRs usually "standardize" or control for age, gender, race, and calendar time and are interpreted like risk ratios.

For example, the retrospective cohort study described earlier among workers involved in manufacturing or spraying herbicides compared the cancer mortality experience of 21,863 male and female workers with national mortality data while controlling for gender, age, and calendar time.[15] Because the workers came from 12 countries, mortality data collected by the World Health Organization were used to compute the expected number of deaths. Investigators found 1,083 deaths from cancer among the male workers, whereas 1,012 were expected. These findings resulted in an SMR of 1.07. No increase in cancer mortality rates was seen in female workers.

The general population is used as a comparison group when it is not possible to find a comparable internal comparison. This problem is quite common in occupational studies. For example, it is possible that everyone who works in a factory who manufactures herbicides is exposed to a greater or lesser degree. Although office workers, sales representatives, and company officials may be the least exposed, they usually do not comprise a comparable comparison group for production workers because of differences in gender (office workers are mainly female) and socioeconomic status (sales representatives and company officials have higher incomes).

General population comparison groups are commonly used in occupational studies of mortality because these data are quite accessible to researchers. In addition, the data are stable because they are based on large numbers. The assumption that the general population is unexposed is reasonable because the number of exposed people is generally a small proportion of the total population.

Although there are several advantages to using the general population as a comparison group, there is one main disadvantage. The results are influenced by a form of bias known as the **healthy worker effect**. This means that the rates of death and disease among a working population are usually lower than those of the general population. The lower rates of death and disease occur even when a noxious substance is present that elevates certain disease rates. The healthy worker effect occurs because a relatively healthy working population is being compared with the general population, which consists of ill people as well as healthy people. It is well known that there is selective entry of healthy persons and early removal of unhealthy ones from the workforce. In the study of workers exposed to phenoxy herbicides and chlorophenols, subjects had slightly lower than expected overall mortality rates (SMR = 0.97), which stemmed mainly from fewer deaths from circulatory system diseases (SMR = 0.91) and respiratory diseases (SMR = 0.82).[15]

The third type of comparison group, called the **comparison cohort**, consists of an unexposed cohort from another population. For example, a study compared cardiovascular disease rates among rayon factory workers who were exposed to carbon disulfide with those of paper mill workers who were not exposed to carbon disulfide.[22] Because both groups consisted of blue-collar workers, individual differences in social class and the healthy worker effect were minimized. However, the results of such studies are difficult to interpret because other exposures in the comparison cohort may also influence disease risk. For example, the paper mill workers may be exposed to other chemicals that influence their risk of developing cardiovascular disease.

Epidemiologists have found that the internal comparison group is the best type of comparison group to use in a cohort study. If an internal comparison is not available, the general population is the next best option, and the traditional comparison cohort is the option of last resort.

▶ Sources of Information

Sources of Information on Exposures and Other Key Variables

Depending on the hypothesis being tested, cohort study investigators rely on various sources for information on exposures and other important variables. These sources include medical and employment records, interviews, direct physical examinations, laboratory tests, biological specimens, and environmental monitoring. Some of these sources are preexisting, and others are designed specifically for a study. Each source has advantages and disadvantages; therefore, investigators often use several sources to piece together all the necessary information.

Investigators typically use healthcare records to describe a participant's exposure history in cohort studies of possible adverse health effects stemming from medical procedures. For example, in Boice and Monson's classic study of fluoroscopic X-ray exposure during tuberculosis treatment and the subsequent risk of breast cancer, investigators reviewed medical records to identify female patients who had been treated with air collapse and other therapies from 1930 through 1954.[21] The researchers obtained information from medical records on the stage of the tuberculosis; all treatments received, including the number of fluoroscopic X-ray examinations; and key variables, such as age, race, religion, and other medical conditions.

The advantages of using medical records as an information source include low expense and a high level of accuracy and detail regarding a disease and its treatment. The medical record may be the best source of information about detailed medical events, particularly those that occurred long ago. For example, it is unlikely that a woman in Boice and Monson's study could recall the number of fluoroscopic X-ray exams that she received 30 years ago.[21] Her medical record could provide this important detail to the investigators to allow them to estimate the dose of radiation that the woman received. The main disadvantage of medical records is that information on important variables, apart from basic demographic characteristics, is often missing. For example, Boice and Monson had to send questionnaires to participants to obtain information on breast cancer risk factors, such as family history of the disease and age at first birth, menarche, and menopause.

Employment records are used mainly to identify individuals for studies of occupational exposures. Standard data in employment records include job title; department of work; years of employment; and basic demographic characteristics, such as gender and date of birth. Like medical records, employment records usually lack data on exposure details and key variables, and therefore investigators often have to augment them with other sources. For example, in the study of workers exposed to phenoxy herbicides and other chemicals, investigators identified cohort members not only by reviewing individual job records but also by sending questionnaires to companies about the work environment and types of products manufactured and measuring chemical levels in worker blood and fat tissue.[15] Even with all these sources, the study investigators acknowledged that the exposure assessment was imperfect and that some exposed individuals may have been erroneously classified as unexposed and vice versa. Furthermore, none of the sources had information on variables such as smoking, alcohol use, and other workplace exposures, such as asbestos.

Because existing records have their limitations, many studies are based solely on data collected specifically for the investigation. Data collection sources include questionnaires, physical examinations, laboratory tests, biological specimens, and environmental monitoring. For example, Framingham Heart Study participants underwent interviews, physical exams, laboratory tests, and other tests every 2 years for more than 50 years.[18] The interviews gathered information on each person's medical history, including cigarette smoking, alcohol use, physical activity, dietary intake, and emotional stress. The physical exam and laboratory tests measured, among other things, height and weight; blood pressure; vital signs and symptoms; and cholesterol, hemoglobin, and glucose levels. The biennial exams and interviews allowed investigators to update changes in each person's habits and health.

Study interviews are most often administered by trained personnel either in person or over the telephone. Self-administered questionnaires are also used. Interviews and questionnaires are particularly useful for obtaining information on lifestyle characteristics that are not routinely or consistently recorded in medical and other records (such as alcohol intake, sexual activity, and physical activity). Although these data tend to be better than existing records, questionnaires and interviews must still rely on the ability of participants to know and recall information. Certainly, participants have the ability to recall important characteristics and events (such as history of cigarette smoking or family history of breast cancer), but it may be difficult for them to recall other types of information. For example, many individuals in occupational settings are not aware of the precise chemicals to which they are exposed at their job sites.

Epidemiological studies of environmental pollution typically must conduct environmental monitoring to determine a participant's exposure. For example, investigators in the Six Cities Study, a classic prospective cohort study of the effect of air pollution on mortality, collected data on outdoor air concentrations of total suspended particulate matter, sulfur dioxide, ozone, and suspended sulfates from monitoring stations centrally located in the communities where the participants resided.[23]

When possible and appropriate, epidemiologists also gather exposure data using biological measurements in participants' blood, urine, bone, and toenails. These measurements are known as **biomarkers** of exposure. These markers not only provide measures of the exposure but also provide markers of internal organ dose. For example, a prospective cohort study of the health effects of lead exposure tested children's blood lead levels at age 3 years and several times thereafter.[6] The blood lead data provided an assessment of each child's exposure over the previous 6 weeks. In another cohort study, investigators investigated the risk of hypertension in relation to zinc levels, which were measured in toenail clippings collected from study subjects.[24]

Data collected specifically for a study are of higher quality than those in existing records, but they are more expensive to obtain. For example, a 30-minute telephone interview used in a study to collect information on environmental exposures and confounders costs approximately $100 to $200 per participant.[25] In-person interviews, which were conducted when the subject was too ill to be interviewed by phone, were even more expensive because they involved travel time to the participant's home. Laboratory tests of biological and environmental samples can also be quite expensive. For example, analysis of polychlorinated biphenyls, dioxin, and metabolites of DDT in serum can cost about $1,000 per sample.

Sources of Outcome Information

The sources of outcome information in a cohort study are similar to the sources of exposures information: interviews, self-administered questionnaires, physical examinations, biological specimens, laboratory tests, and medical records. Although accuracy is the primary consideration when selecting a source of outcome data, cost and practical considerations are also important. Investigators often rely on several sources to gather the information because of the advantages and disadvantages described earlier.

For example, the Framingham Heart Study used a combination of interviews, physical examinations, and laboratory tests to gather information on the incidence and precursors of coronary heart disease, stroke, and peripheral artery disease.[18] Medical records and laboratory tests were used to confirm information that was reported in the interview. For example, heart attacks reported by Framingham Study participants were confirmed by electrocardiographic (ECG) changes and enzyme changes diagnostic of the disorder. The presence of Q waves not previously seen was considered definitive evidence that a heart attack had occurred. The ECG evidence was useful in improving the accuracy of the heart attack data; investigators excluded about 20% of heart attacks reported by participants because of equivocal evidence.[18]

Biological specimens supplied by the participant can also provide early evidence of disease. A biological marker is often considered an intermediate outcome because it is on the pathway from exposure to the appearance of clinical disease. For example, CD4 T lymphocyte counts are markers of HIV infection and disease progression. A rapid decline in CD4 counts occurs shortly after infection and continues over time through the onset of clinical disease to death.

Outcome information can be gathered from state and national disease registries (most commonly for cancer occurrence) and departments of vital records (for mortality information). Investigators can collect this type of data without directly involving the participant, which reduces study costs. In fact, mortality data are relatively easy to obtain now that the National Death Index (NDI) is available for medical research. Compiled by the National Center for Health Statistics, the NDI is a computerized central file of death record information beginning with deaths in 1979. Investigators submit identifying information to the NDI personnel, who search their database for a match. The more information submitted, the greater the likelihood that an accurate match will be found. However, although mortality data are readily accessible and complete, the accuracy is often questioned because there are no strict criteria to guide physicians who are completing cause-of-death information on death certificates.

Whatever the source, it is important to follow comparable procedures for determining the outcomes among the exposed and unexposed groups. Investigators' use of differing sources and procedures may lead to inaccurate results. Thus, all resources used for one group must be used for the other. In addition, investigators should be masked to the exposure status of subjects so that they make unbiased decisions when assessing the outcomes. For example, an investigator might have to decide whether an interview report of a "breast tumor" is a malignant or benign tumor. Masking the investigator will ensure that the decision, whatever it is, is unrelated to the participant's exposure status. In addition, investigators should develop standard outcome definitions to guarantee accuracy and comparability. These definitions should be based on information that is readily available from acceptable and accessible procedures. Furthermore, diagnostic criteria should be both sensitive (able to pick up cases of disease) and specific (able to exclude individuals without disease). For example, the diagnosis of angina pectoris might include clinical symptoms such as dull, heavy discomfort in the substernal area, particularly after a meal and with exertion or emotional distress, and evidence of ECG abnormalities at rest and with exercise.

Approaches to Follow-Up

Loss to follow-up occurs when a participant either no longer wishes to take part in a study or cannot be located. Minimizing these losses is crucial for two reasons. First, losses to follow-up effectively decrease the sample size and reduce the ability of the study to detect an association if one is present. Second, those who are lost to follow-up may differ in important ways from those who are successfully traced. Of particular concern is that lost individuals are more likely to have developed the disease under study. If lost individuals are more or less likely to be exposed than those successfully traced, the study results may suffer from a form of bias known as selection bias.

Because high rates of follow-up are critical to the success of a cohort study, investigators have developed a variety of methods to maximize retention and trace study members.[26] For prospective cohort studies, strategies include collection of baseline information that helps to locate participants as the study progresses. This information usually includes the participant's full name; current home address; telephone number; email address; Social Security number; date and place of birth; and the names, addresses, and phone numbers of physicians, friends, and relatives who will always know where the participant is living. Another recommended strategy for prospective studies is regular mail or email contact with participants. These contacts might involve requests for up-to-date outcome information or newsletters describing the study's progress and findings. These communications are used to help participants "bond" with the study and to obtain address corrections from the U.S. Postal Service.[26]

Additional mailings are the best strategy to use when participants do not initially respond. Investigators typically send at least two follow-up letters or postcards by first class or certified mail, emphasizing the importance of the request. If additional mailings are unsuccessful, investigators use telephone calls and even home visits to contact those who have not responded.

When participants are truly lost to follow-up, researchers use a number of additional strategies.[26] Usually, the simplest and least expensive ones are used first, and more difficult and expensive ones are used later. In the early stages of follow-up, letters are sent to the last known address with "Address Correction Requested." In addition, investigators check telephone directories, directory assistance, and Internet resources such as Whitepages.com. An increasingly popular resource is the U.S. Postal Service's National Change of Address (NCOA) system, which has up-to-date change-of-address data for almost the entire country.

If these steps prove unsuccessful, investigators contact relatives, friends, or physicians who were identified at baseline. If this step is unsuccessful, investigators can turn to many local, state, and national resources, including state vital statistics records (for births, marriages, divorces, and deaths); driver's license, voter registration, and public utility records; the NDI; the Social Security Administration; the Centers for Medicare and Medicaid Services; credit bureaus; and commercial companies that specialize in tracing individuals.

Tracing is a laborious and challenging process. It has become even more difficult today because of increased population mobility. However, newly available resources such as those on the Internet offset these difficulties to some degree. The time and monetary investment in follow-up is worthwhile because it helps secure the success of the study.

▶ Analysis of Cohort Studies

The primary objective of the analysis of cohort study data is to compare disease occurrence in the exposed and unexposed groups. Disease occurrence is usually measured using cumulative incidence or incidence rates, and the relationship between exposure and disease occurrence is quantified by the cumulative incidence or incidence rate difference and/or ratio. The calculation of person-time and the concepts of induction and latent periods are discussed here in the context of cohort study analysis.

Calculating Person-Time

Calculating an incidence rate involves determining the amount of person-time accrued by each study subject. It is important to remember

	A	B	C	D	E	F
Year	1930	1950	1960	1995	2010	2015
Age (years)	0	20	30	65	80	–
Milestone	Born	Starts work	Follow-up starts	Retires	Dies	Follow-up ends

FIGURE 8-3 Accrual of person-time.

that **person-time** is, in essence, follow-up time and that follow-up time is calculated only within the context of a study. It is also important to differentiate years of follow-up from years of exposure and years of latency. For example, consider a hypothetical occupational retrospective cohort study in which follow-up starts on January 1, 1960, and ends at the time of death or the closing date of the study (January 1, 2015). Let us consider a hypothetical person who was born on January 1, 1930; started work at age 20 on January 1, 1950; worked for 45 years until 1995; and died at age 80 on January 1, 2010 (see **FIGURE 8-3**).

The maximum number of person-years that any individual can accrue in this study is 55 years (C to F). The number of person-years that our hypothetical individual accrued was 50 years (C to E). The total number of person-years that an individual accrues never changes. However, it is often divided among various exposure categories, such as age and calendar year, when the individual started work, and duration of employment. Note that the number of years that our hypothetical individual worked (B to D) is a measure of exposure duration and is different from the number of person-years that he accrued in the study.

As a real-life example, let us consider Boice and Monson's study of breast cancer after repeated chest fluoroscopies.[21] In this study, years of follow-up were accumulated from the date of the first fluoroscopic examination for exposed women and first sanatorium admission for comparison subjects. Follow-up ended at different points depending on what happened to the women. For women who developed breast cancer, follow-up ended with the diagnosis date. For women who did not develop breast cancer, it ended with the date of death for those who died, the closing date of the study (July 1, 1975) for those who were still alive at the end of the study, and the date last known to be alive for those who were lost to follow-up. Using these start and end dates, the 1,047 women in the exposed group accrued 28,011 person-years of follow-up, and the 717 women in the comparison group accrued 19,025 person-years of follow-up. The maximum possible length of follow-up for any participant was 45 years (from first possible treatment in 1930 to closing date of study in 1975); the average was about 26 years.

Induction and Latent Periods

The analysis of a cohort study typically considers the length of time between the causal action of an exposure and the eventual diagnosis of disease.[27] The causal action of an exposure occurs when sufficient exposure has accrued. The **induction period** that follows is the interval between the action of a cause and disease onset. An example of disease onset might be the transformation of a normal into a cancerous breast cell. The **latent period** is the subsequent interval between disease onset and clinical diagnosis. For example, a clinical diagnosis of breast cancer occurs when the tumor becomes large enough to be detected by either screening mammography or physical examination.

Because the time of disease onset is usually not possible to determine, the induction and latent periods are typically merged into the empirical latent period. For example, in a study of the relationship between tetrachloroethylene-contaminated drinking water and the risk of breast cancer, investigators hypothesized that the water contaminant might act as either a tumor initiator (early in the carcinogenic process) or a promoter (late in the process), and therefore they conducted analyses considering empirical latent periods ranging from 0 to 19 years.[25]

▶ Special Types of Cohort Studies

The comparison group in a cohort study may come from an internal source, another cohort, or the general population. Two special types of cohort studies—**proportional mortality ratio (PMR)** and **standardized mortality ratio (SMR)** studies—are conducted to compare the mortality experience of the exposed group with that of the general population. Both types of studies are common in occupational epidemiology because there is often no truly unexposed group in the workplace.

The difference between PMR and SMR studies is the type of information needed to calculate the measure of association. All the information for the PMR study comes from death certificates (date, age, cause of death). The observed number of deaths from a specific cause in the exposed group is compared with the expected number, which is derived from the proportion of deaths resulting from that cause in the general population. The resulting PMR, which is interpreted like a risk ratio, shows the relative importance of a specific cause of death in relation to all deaths.

For example, investigators compared the mortality patterns of poultry plant workers with those of the U.S. population in a classic PMR study.[28] The study population consisted of members of the Baltimore Meatcutters' Union Local 27 who died from 1954 through 2003 and worked in any of six poultry slaughtering and processing plants during their entire membership in the union. Information on year of birth, gender, race, year of death, and cause of death was abstracted from death certificates. For each cause of death, investigators compared the observed number of deaths with the expected number while controlling for gender, race, age, and calendar year of death. The study found an increased risk of death from diabetes, anterior horn disease, and hypertensive disease and a reduced risk of deaths from intracerebral hemorrhage.

In an SMR study, investigators need additional information to compare the mortality experience of the exposed group with that of the general population. This is because the SMR compares the mortality rates of the two groups, whereas the PMR study compares mortality proportions. Thus, information on person-years of follow-up among the study group is needed to calculate the expected number of deaths.

For example, an industry-wide SMR study of pulp and paper workers in the United States was conducted among 63,025 long-term workers from 51 mills across the country.[29] The workers were required to be employed for at least 10 years to be eligible. Vital status was identified through the mills, Social Security mortality tapes, and the NDI. Investigators calculated SMRs using three comparison populations: the U.S. population, the 20 states in which the mills were located, and the residents of the 330 counties that were within a 50-mile radius of each mill. The latter two comparison populations were used because their demographic characteristics were similar to those of the workers.

A total of 7,171 deaths occurred among cohort members through the end of 1991. Person-time of follow-up was calculated for cohort members starting with 10 years after first employment or when the mill was enrolled in the study (whichever came last) and ending with the termination of the study or death. SMRs were calculated that adjusted for age, calendar time, race, and gender. The investigators found that the overall mortality rate of pulp and paper mill workers was much lower than that of the U.S. population (SMR = 0.74) and that the workers' mortality rate was not elevated for any specific cause of death, including malignancies. However, in a few instances, a higher mortality rate was seen when workers were separated according to the type of pulping process used at their plant.

Because PMR studies take less time and cost less money, they are often done before an SMR study is initiated. However, it is informative to conduct both types of studies in the same population.[30(p131)] Note that SMR studies, and to a lesser extent PMR studies, suffer from the "healthy worker effect."[30(p114)] PMR studies also suffer from the "**seesaw effect**," which means that a higher proportion of deaths from one cause must be counterbalanced by a lower proportion of deaths from another cause. This occurs because the total number of observed deaths in the study population must equal the number of expected deaths derived from the general population.

▶ Strengths and Limitations of Cohort Studies

The goal of every epidemiological study is to harvest valid and precise information about the relationship between an exposure and a disease in a population. The various study designs merely represent different ways of harvesting this information. Each type of design has strengths and

TABLE 8-4 Strengths and Weaknesses of Cohort Studies

Strengths

- Efficient for rare exposures
- Good information on exposures (prospective)
- Can evaluate multiple effects of an exposure
- Efficient for diseases with long induction and latent periods (retrospective)
- Less vulnerable to bias (prospective)
- Can directly measure disease incidence or risk
- Clear temporal relationship between exposure and outcome (prospective)

Weaknesses

- Inefficient for rare outcomes
- Poor information on exposures and other key variables (retrospective)
- Expensive and time consuming (particularly prospective)
- Inefficient for diseases with long induction and latent periods (prospective)
- More vulnerable to bias (retrospective)

weaknesses (see **TABLE 8-4**), which tend to be complementary. For example, the pros and cons of retrospective and prospective cohort studies tend to balance one another. However, under certain circumstances, a cohort study design is clearly indicated. Investigators should use a cohort study when they wish to learn about multiple effects of an exposure or when the exposure is rare, and they should use a retrospective cohort design when the outcome of interest has long induction and latent periods.

Summary

Cohort studies examine the health effects of an exposure by following two or more groups with a common characteristic (exposed and unexposed). Cohort studies may be conducted in populations that are defined by changeable conditions (open or dynamic) or irrevocable events (fixed and closed). The timing of cohort studies can be prospective, retrospective, or ambidirectional. In prospective cohort studies, investigators group participants on the basis of past or current exposure and follow them into the future to observe the outcome(s) of interest. In retrospective cohort studies, investigators group participants on the basis of past exposures and evaluate outcomes that have already occurred. Ambidirectional cohort studies have retrospective and prospective components. Retrospective cohort studies are more efficient than prospective studies for studying diseases with long induction and latent periods. However, prospective studies are less vulnerable to bias than retrospective cohort studies.

Several design features of cohort studies emulate those of experimental studies to produce high-quality results, including the selection of comparable groups and the masking of investigators to subjects' exposure status during follow-up and outcome ascertainment. Regarding the former, the ideal comparison group would consist of the same individuals in the exposed group had they not been exposed. This is known as the "counterfactual ideal." Because it is impossible for the same individuals to be exposed and unexposed simultaneously, the investigator must select different sets of individuals for comparison. The comparison group can come from an internal comparison group, the general population, or a comparison cohort. An internal comparison group consists of unexposed members of the same cohort. A general population comparison group is selected on the basis of preexisting population data, such as mortality rates from the National Center for Health Statistics. A comparison cohort consists of unexposed members of another cohort. The internal comparison group is considered the best of the three because it is most similar to the exposed group.

Depending on the hypothesis being tested, investigators rely on a variety of sources for information on exposures, outcomes, and other key variables. These sources include medical and employment records, interviews, direct physical examinations, laboratory tests, and environmental monitoring. During the follow-up period, the groups are monitored for the outcomes under study. Losses to follow-up occur when participants no longer wish to participate or they can no longer be located. Because follow-up losses are a threat to the validity of the study, epidemiologists use a variety of methods to maximize retention and trace study members, including collection of baseline information to help locate participants as the study progresses.

The main strengths of cohort studies are that they are efficient for studying rare exposures and allow investigators to evaluate multiple health effects of an exposure, and retrospective cohort studies are efficient for studying diseases with long induction and latent periods. The main weaknesses of cohort studies are that they are inefficient for studying rare outcomes, prospective cohort studies are inefficient for studying diseases with long induction and latent periods, and retrospective cohort studies are vulnerable to bias.

References

1. Pickett JP (exec ed.). *The American Heritage Dictionary of the English Language.* 4th ed. Boston, MA: Houghton Mifflin; 2000.
2. Porta M. *A Dictionary of Epidemiology.* 6th ed. New York, NY: Oxford University Press; 2014.
3. Sauvaget C, Lagarde F, Nagano J, Soda M, Koyana K, Kodama K. Lifestyle factors, radiation and gastric cancer in atomic bomb survivors (Japan). *Cancer Cause Control.* 2005;16:773-780.
4. Cheung YK, Moon YP, Kulick ER, et al. Leisure-time physical activitiy and cardiovascular mortality in an elderly population in northern Manhattan: a prospective cohort study. *J Gen Intern Med.* 2017;32:168-174.
5. Mahalingaiah S, Hart JE, Laden F, et al. Adult air pollution exposure and risk of infertility in the Nurses' Health Study II. *Hum Reprod.* 2016; 31:638-647.
6. Reuben A, Caspi A, Belsky DW, et al. Association of childhood blood lead levels with cognitive function and socioeconomic status at age 38 years and with IQ change and socioeconomic mobility

between childhood and adulthood. *JAMA*. 2017;317: 1244-1251.

7. Ursano RJ, Kessler RC, Stein MB, et al. Suicide attempts in the US army during the wars in Afganistan and Iraq, 2004-2009. *JAMA Psychiatry*. 2016; 72:917-926.

8. Lathrop GD, Wolfe WH, Albanese RA, Moynahan PM. *An Epidemiologic Investigation of Health Effects in Air Force Personnel Following Exposure to Herbicides: Baseline Morbidity Results*. Washington, DC: U.S. Air Force; 1984.

9. Wolfe WH, Michalek JE, Miner JC, et al. Health status of Air Force veterans occupationally exposed to herbicides in Vietnam. I. Physical health. *JAMA*. 1990;264:1824-1831.

10. Michalek JE, Wolfe WH, Miner JC. Health status of Air Force veterans occupationally exposed to herbicides in Vietnam. II. Mortality. *JAMA*. 1990;264:1832-1836.

11. Ketchum NS, Michalek JE. Postservice mortality in Air Force veterans occupationally exposed to herbicides during the Vietnam War: 20 year follow-up results. *Mil Med*. 2005;170:406-413.

12. Ethen MK, Ramadhani TA, Scheuerle AE, et al. Alcohol consumption by women before and during pregnancy. *Matern Child Health J*. 2009;13:274-285.

13. Streissguth AP. Fetal alcohol syndrome: an epidemiologic perspective. *Am J Epidemiol*. 1978;107:467-478.

14. Colton T. *Statistics in Medicine*. Boston, MA: Little, Brown and Co.; 1974.

15. Kogevinas M, Becher H, Benn T, et al. Cancer mortality in workers exposed to phenoxy herbicides, chlorophenols, and dioxins: an expanded and updated international cohort study. *Am J Epidemiol*. 1997;145:1061-1075.

16. Darby SC, Doll R, Gill SK, et al. Long term mortality after a single treatment course with x-rays in patients treated for ankylosing spondylitis. *Brit J Cancer*. 1987;55:179-190.

17. Orlich MJ, Singh PN, Sabate J, et al. Vegetarian dietary patterns and the risk of colorectal cancers. *JAMA Intern Med*. 2015;175:767-776.

18. Dawber TR. *The Framingham Study: The Epidemiology of Atherosclerotic Disease*. Cambridge, MA: Harvard University Press; 1980.

19. About the Framingham Heart Study. framinghamheartstudy.org.https://www.framinghamheartstudy.org /fhs-about/. Accessed June 20, 2017.

20. Rothman KJ, Greenland S, Tash TL. *Modern Epidemiology*. 3rd ed. Philadelphia, PA: Wolters Kluwer Health/Lippincott Williams & Wilkins; 2008.

21. Boice JD, Monson RR. Breast cancer in women after repeated fluoroscopic examination of the chest. *J Natl Cancer Inst*. 1977;59:823-832.

22. Hernberg S, Partenen T, Nordman CH, Sumari P. Coronary heart disease among workers exposed to carbon disulfide. *Brit J Ind Med*. 1970;27:313-325.

23. Dockery DW, Pope CA, Xu X, et al. An association between air pollution and mortality in six U.S. cities. *New Engl J Med*. 1993;329:1753-1760.

24. Park JS, Xun P, Li J, et al. Longitudinal association between toenail zinc levels and the incidence of diabetes among American young adults: the CARDIA Trace Element Study. *Sci Rep*. 2016;6:23155. doi: 10.1038/srep23155.

25. Aschengrau A, Rogers S, Ozonoff D. Perchloroethylene-contaminated drinking water and the risk of breast cancer: additional results from Cape Cod, Massachusetts. *Environ Health Perspect*. 2003;111:167-173.

26. Hunt JR, White E. Retaining and tracking cohort study members. *Epidemiol Rev*. 1998;20:57-70.

27. Rothman KJ. Induction and latent periods. *Am J Epidemiol*. 1981;114:253-259.

28. Johnson ES, Yau LC, Zhou Y, Singh KP, Ndetan H. Mortality in the Baltimore union poultry cohort: non-malignant diseases. *Int Arch Occup Environ Health*. 2010;83:543-552.

29. Matanoski G, Kanchanaraksa S, Lees PSJ, et al. Industry-wide study of mortality of pulp and paper mill workers. *Am J Ind Med*. 1998;33:354-365.

30. Monson RR. *Occupational Epidemiology*. Boca Raton, FL: CRC Press; 1990.

Chapter Questions

1. Briefly define each of the following terms that are associated with cohort studies:
    a. Open or dynamic cohort
    b. Fixed cohort
    c. Retrospective cohort study
    d. Prospective cohort study
    e. Ambidirectional cohort study
    f. Standardized mortality ratio (SMR) study

2. State the main similarity and main difference between cohort and experimental studies.
3. What is the ideal but unattainable comparison group in a cohort study?
4. Describe the strengths and weaknesses of the three types of comparison groups used in cohort studies. Which one comes closest to the counterfactual ideal?
5. Among the following studies, which comparison group comes closest to the counterfactual ideal?
   a. A study that compares male breast cancer rates among U.S. Marines who were stationed at Camp Lejeune, North Carolina, and were exposed to solvents in the local drinking water with breast cancer rates among men from the general U.S. population.
   b. A study that compares male breast cancer rates among U.S. Marines who were stationed at Camp Lejeune, North Carolina, and were exposed to solvents in the local drinking water with U.S. Marines who were stationed at Camp Lejeune, North Carolina, but were not exposed to solvents in the local drinking water.
   c. A study that compares male breast cancer rates among U.S. Marines who were stationed at Camp Lejeune, North Carolina, and were exposed to solvents in the local drinking water with U.S. Marines who were stationed at Camp Pendleton, California, and were not exposed to solvents in the local drinking water.
6. State whether or not a cohort study is best suited for each of the following scenarios:
   a. When little is known about a rare exposure
   b. When little is known about a rare disease
   c. When the study population will be difficult to follow
   d. When you want to learn about multiple effects of an exposure
7. Why is it important to minimize losses to follow-up?
8. How is person-time calculated within the context of a cohort study?
9. Indicate whether the following statements are true or false:
   a. A retrospective cohort study is more efficient than a prospective cohort study for studying diseases with long latent and induction periods.
   b. Special cohort studies are the most sensible design for examining many exposures in relation to a single disease.
   c. Losses to follow-up can be a problem in a cohort study but not in an experimental study.
   d. General cohort studies are good for studying common exposures, whereas special cohorts are good for studying rare ones.
10. Which of the following techniques that are commonly used in experimental studies can also be applied in cohort studies?
    a. Masking
    b. Placebo
    c. Randomization
    d. Run-in period
    e. Intent-to-treat analysis

CHAPTER 9

Case–Control Studies

LEARNING OBJECTIVES

By the end of this chapter the reader will be able to:

- Discuss the traditional and modern views of case–control studies.
- List the settings in which case–control studies are desirable.
- Describe the key features of conducting case–control studies, including the selection of cases and controls, the sources of exposure information, and data analysis.
- Describe the key aspects of case–crossover studies.
- Discuss the strengths and limitations of case–control studies.

▶ Introduction

As in other fields in science and public health, ideas about the theoretical framework underlying epidemiological research continue to evolve. This is perhaps most true about epidemiologists' views regarding case–control studies, the second principal type of observational study. The goal of a **case–control study** is identical to that of any other epidemiological study—the valid and precise measurement of the relationship between an exposure and a disease. However, epidemiologists' views about the appropriate way to conceptualize and design this type of study have changed considerably over the past 3 decades. As a consequence of these changes, epidemiologists have come to realize that the quality of a case–control study can be as high as that of a cohort study.

This chapter presents the traditional view of the case–control study and then describes the conceptual shift that has occurred over the past 3 decades. Next, the chapter describes specific features of the design, conduct, and analysis of case–control studies, including the selection of cases and controls, measurement of exposure, and calculation of another measure of association termed the **odds ratio**. Examples are provided to illustrate how case–control studies have been used to answer important public health questions. The chapter concludes with a discussion of the strengths and limitations of case–control studies.

▸ The Changing View of Case–Control Studies

The Traditional View

Traditionally, epidemiologists viewed case–control studies as an alternative to cohort studies. Recall that a cohort study begins with a group of nondiseased people who are categorized according to exposure level and followed to measure the occurrence of disease. In contrast, the subjects in the traditional conceptualization of a case–control study are selected on the basis of whether they have or do not have the disease. Those who have the disease are termed **cases**, and those who do not have the disease are termed **controls**. Investigators obtain and compare the exposure histories of cases and controls.

For example, consider a hypothetical case–control study of pesticide exposure and breast cancer from the traditional standpoint. A series of breast cancer cases are identified and enrolled, and a series of control subjects without breast cancer are also identified and enrolled. Investigators obtain pesticide exposure information by interviewing the women about their prior work and leisure activities (e.g., they might ask participants whether they ever worked on a farm or gardened with pesticides). Next, the investigators compare the exposure histories of the cases and controls. If 75% of breast cancer cases and only 25% of controls have a positive exposure history, the researchers would conclude that there is an association between pesticide exposure and breast cancer.

The central feature of the traditional view is the comparison of the exposure histories of cases and controls. The logic of this approach differs from that of experimental and cohort study designs, in which the key comparison is the disease incidence between the exposed and unexposed (or least exposed) groups. In other words, the traditional view asserts that experimental and cohort studies move from cause to effect and case–control studies move from effect to cause. Thus, many who espouse the traditional view believe that the logic of a case–control study is backward.[1] They also believe that case–control studies are much more prone to bias and are thus inferior to other designs. In fact, the term *TROHOC* study (*cohort* spelled backward) was coined as a disparaging moniker for case–control studies.

The Modern View

Epidemiologists' view of case–control studies began to change in the 1980s with the work of Miettinen, who argued that it is incorrect to consider a case–control study as being merely the reverse of a cohort study.[2] He coined the term *TROHOC fallacy* to describe this erroneous thinking. Miettinen argued that a case–control study is an efficient way to learn about the relationship between an exposure and a disease. More specifically, he stated that the case–control study is a method of sampling a population in which cases of disease are identified and enrolled and a sample of the **source population** that gave rise to the cases is also identified and enrolled. The sample of the source population is known as the **control group**. Its purpose is to provide information on the exposure distribution in the population that produced the cases so that the disease rates in exposed and nonexposed groups can be compared. Thus, Miettinen asserted that the key comparison in a case–control study is the same as that in a cohort study, which is a comparison between the exposed and nonexposed groups.

The following hypothetical example illustrates the modern view of the case–control study. Suppose that investigators undertook a prospective cohort study in 1980 to determine the causes of chronic diseases among middle-aged women in the United States. Investigators decided to conduct a general cohort study, and therefore they assembled a group of 100,000 female teachers aged 45 to 65 years. They planned to examine numerous risk factors (such as use of contraceptives, diet, smoking, alcohol consumption, and environmental exposures), and so they collected data on these characteristics as well as data on health outcomes and other key variables. Investigators used a combination of periodic interviews, physical exams, and laboratory tests to gather this information. In particular, blood was drawn from all participants at baseline, and these samples were processed and frozen for later use.

In 2015, the study investigators became interested in the hypothesis that pesticides, such as dichlorodiphenyltrichloroethane (DDT), increased a woman's risk of breast cancer. Data from other studies suggested that these compounds could increase a woman's risk by mimicking the action of endogenous estrogens.[3] The investigators decided to measure serum levels of dichlorodiphenyldichloroethylene (DDE) (the metabolic by-product of the pesticide DDT) in the frozen blood samples taken from cohort members in 1980. Even though DDT was banned in 1969,[4(pp275-360)] it is quite persistent, and therefore serum levels taken in 1980 should give a fairly accurate estimate of past exposure.

The investigators sent the 100,000 samples to a laboratory for DDE analysis. Upon receipt of the laboratory results, the investigators characterized the cohort according to DDE level (high or low). In addition, they examined the health outcome data collected so far and found that 2,000 study participants had developed breast cancer since the beginning of the study. The investigators arranged the exposure and outcome data into a two-by-two table (see **TABLE 9-1**) and calculated the risk ratio in the usual fashion: by comparing the occurrence of breast cancer (here, cumulative incidence of breast cancer) among women with high DDE levels with that among women with low DDE levels. Thus, the risk ratio, or cumulative incidence ratio, was (500/15,000)/(1,500/85,000), or 1.89.

Unfortunately, there was a major problem in evaluating the hypothesis in this manner: Quantifying DDE serum levels was very expensive at about $100 per sample. Thus, ascertaining DDE exposure levels on all 100,000 study subjects would cost $10 million.

TABLE 9-1 Data from a Hypothetical Cohort Study of Serum DDE Levels and the Risk of Breast Cancer

	Breast cancer		
DDE level	**Yes**	**No**	**Total**
High	500	14,500	15,000
Low	1,500	83,500	85,000
Total	2,000	98,000	100,000

TABLE 9-2 Data from a Hypothetical Case–Control Study of DDE Exposure and Breast Cancer Nested Within a Cohort

	Breast cancer		
DDE level	**Yes**	**No**	**Total**
High	500	600	1,100
Low	1,500	3,400	4,900
Total	2,000	4,000	6,000

Note that the cohort study approach in this setting is prohibitively expensive. What would have happened if the investigators had used a much less costly approach, such as a case–control study nested within the cohort? How would they have gone about conducting such a study? First, they would have analyzed the baseline serum samples of all 2,000 women who were diagnosed with breast cancer (the cases). Next, they would have carefully selected a sample of the cohort to be the control group. Let us assume that they decided to select 4,000 women for the control group. The results of such a study are shown in **TABLE 9-2**.

The investigators could have used these data to estimate the relative risk of breast cancer among women with high versus low DDE levels. The estimate would have been similar to the relative risk calculated for the entire cohort if certain conditions had been met. The most important of these conditions would be the proper selection of controls. (Control selection is discussed in more detail later in this chapter.)

Note that the nested case–control study is much more efficient than the cohort study. The cases are the same as those that would be included in the cohort study, and the controls provide a less expensive and faster way of determining the exposure experience in the population that generated the cases.[5(p123)] Certainly, the cost of determining the DDE exposure levels in the nested case–control study would be much less than that of the cohort study ($600,000 versus $10 million). The analysis of both the case–control and the cohort studies involves comparing the disease frequency among the exposed and nonexposed groups. The cases in both studies form the numerators of the measures of disease frequency. The denominators are slightly different. The total number of persons or person-time forms the denominator in a cohort study, whereas a sample of persons or person-time forms the denominator in a case–control study. This sample is known as the control group.

Thus, the modern view of a case–control study holds that it is a method of sampling a population in which investigators identify and enroll cases of disease and identify and enroll a sample of the population that produced the cases. The purpose of the control group is to determine the relative size of the exposed and unexposed denominators in the source population. The sample is an alternative to obtaining exposure information on the entire study population. As in experimental and cohort studies, the essential comparison is between the exposed and unexposed groups. A schematic representation of the implementation of a case–control study that bridges the traditional and modern viewpoints is presented in **FIGURE 9-1**.

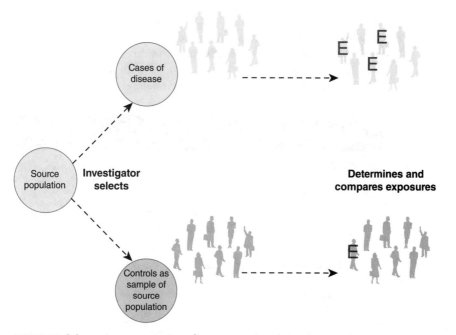

FIGURE 9-1 Schematic representation of case–control study implementation.

▶ When Is It Desirable to Use the Case–Control Method?

Epidemiologists consider many factors to determine which type of study design is most appropriate for investigating a particular hypothesis. These factors include the frequency of the exposure and disease, feasibility, costs, and ethical issues. If an observational study is in order, the choice is typically between a cohort and a case–control study, but how does an investigator decide which type of study is better?

Epidemiologists prefer the case–control study in five types of situations (see **TABLE 9-3**). First, as for the DDE and breast cancer study described earlier, a case–control study is preferable when the exposure data are difficult or expensive to obtain. Collecting exposure data on fewer individuals (typically all of the cases and a sample of the source population) saves both time and money. If control selection is unbiased, the cost savings will not adversely affect the validity of the study.

Second, a case–control study is more efficient than a cohort study when the disease is rare, which is usually defined as a frequency of 20% or less. For example, consider a cohort study of 100,000 subjects examining the relationship between diet and the occurrence of cancer. Although this study would be adequate for examining common types of cancer, such as those occurring in the lung, breast, and colon/rectum, it would not be adequate for examining rare ones, such as cancer of the esophagus. The incidence rate of esophageal cancer is about 4 per 100,000 per year,[6] and therefore only about 40 cases of this cancer would occur in a 100,000-member cohort after 10 years of follow-up. This yield is meager considering the time and expense of following 100,000 individuals for such a long period of time. Furthermore, in a cohort study with only 40 cases, it is unlikely that investigators would be able to detect an association between disease and diet unless it was quite strong.

TABLE 9-3 Situations in Which a Case–Control Study Is Desirable

- Exposure data are difficult or expensive to obtain.
- The disease is rare.
- The disease has a long induction and latent period.
- Little is known about the disease.
- The underlying population is dynamic.

Third, a case–control study is preferable to a cohort study (at least a prospective one) when the disease has long induction and latent periods (i.e., when there is a long time between the causal action of an exposure and the eventual diagnosis of disease).[7] For example, following exposure to ionizing radiation or other workplace exposures, cancers involving solid tumors are thought to have induction and/or latency periods of 10 or more years.[8,9] A prospective cohort study would have to follow participants for a long time to observe these types of outcomes. Follow-up is avoided in a case–control study because it is retrospective (i.e., both the exposure and the outcome have already occurred at the time the subject is enrolled).

Fourth, case–control studies are preferable when little is known about the disease because they allow the investigators to evaluate more than one hypothesis. For example, the earliest etiologic studies of acquired immune deficiency syndrome (AIDS) were case–control studies. Conducted before the human immunodeficiency virus (HIV) was determined to be the cause of AIDS, these studies investigated many possible causes, including illicit drug use, sexual behaviors, and sexually transmitted and viral diseases.[10]

Fifth, case–control studies are desirable when the population under study is dynamic. The membership of a dynamic population is defined by a changeable state or condition, and its membership continually changes with inflow and outflow. The most common type of dynamic population is defined by residence in a particular geographic area. Inflow occurs when someone moves or is born into the geographic area, and outflow occurs when someone moves away or dies. A case–control study is desirable in this setting because it is difficult for researchers to identify and keep track of a population that is constantly changing.

For example, investigators conducted a case–control study on tetrachloroethylene-contaminated drinking water and the risk of breast cancer in the Cape Cod region of Massachusetts, the hook-shaped peninsula in the southeastern part of the state.[11] Tetrachloroethylene (also known as PCE) is a solvent that is commonly used in dry cleaning. From the late 1960s through the early 1980s, the substance leached into the public drinking water supplies in the Cape Cod area from an improperly cured vinyl liner that was placed inside certain water distribution pipes. The Cape Cod population experienced tremendous changes during the period of contamination. In particular, there was a large influx of new residents, mainly elderly retirees.[12] In addition, the region is a popular vacation destination and therefore has a large part-time summer population. The challenge of enumerating and tracking a cohort under these circumstances was one of several reasons the investigators chose to conduct a case–control study to test the hypothesis that exposure to PCE-contaminated drinking water increased the risk of breast cancer.

▶ Selection of Cases

Case Definition

All epidemiological research, including case–control studies, involves composing a disease or **case** definition. This task usually involves dividing subjects into two groups: those who have the disease and those who do not. The criteria that are used to make such decisions are usually based on a combination of signs and symptoms, physical and pathological examinations, and results of diagnostic tests. Which and how many criteria are used to define a case have important implications for determining accurately who has the disease. If nonspecific criteria are used, most but not all people with the disease will be captured, but many people who do not have the disease will be included erroneously. For example, if only chest pain were used to define cases of myocardial infarction, most but not all heart attack cases would be included (people with "silent" heart attacks would be missed), but people with other conditions that produce chest pain (such as indigestion) would be included mistakenly. If restrictive criteria are used, fewer cases will be eligible for inclusion in the study, and therefore the sample size will be smaller. Nonetheless, if given a choice between being inclusive or restrictive, it is better to be restrictive because it leads to fewer classification errors.[13]

In practice, it is best to use all available evidence to define with as much accuracy as possible the true cases of disease. In addition, cases should be defined with the likely causal mechanism in mind, and cases that are likely to result from the same causal mechanism should be grouped together. This approach might seem paradoxical because the purpose of the research is usually to identify the causal mechanism. However, existing knowledge, albeit incomplete, can be used as a guide. For example, we currently know enough about the etiology of uterine cancer to separate cancer of the cervix (the neck of the uterus) from cancer of the uterine corpus (the body of the uterus). In addition, we know enough about the formation of the human heart during gestation to separate infants born with a ventricular septal defect (a hole in the wall separating the two lower chambers of the heart) from infants born with transposition of the great vessels (reversal of the locations of the aorta and pulmonary artery).

Once a case group is formed, it is always possible to divide the cases according to various criteria such as histologic subtype, severity (e.g., mild, moderate, and severe), and the likelihood that the diagnosis is accurate (e.g., definite, probable, or possible). These subdivisions usually improve the accuracy of the case definition by reducing classification errors.

Sometimes, different criteria are used in different studies because epidemiologists disagree about the best way to define the disease. Even when a consensus is reached, disease definitions change over time as more is learned about the condition and its manifestations. For example, the official definition of HIV/AIDS has changed several times as epidemiologists have gained knowledge about its cause and natural history. In either case, it is difficult to compare descriptive statistics and study results when the studies use differing criteria or definitions.

Sources of Case Identification

Once investigators have created a case definition, they can begin identifying and enrolling cases. Typical sources for identifying cases are hospital or clinic patient rosters; death certificates; special surveys, such as the National Health and Nutrition Examination Survey (NHANES); or special reporting systems, including cancer or birth defects registries. Investigators should consider both accuracy and efficiency when selecting a particular source for case identification. The goal is to identify as many true cases of disease as quickly and cheaply as possible. The paragraphs that follow focus on two commonly used sources for case–control studies: hospitals and registries.

Virtually all hospitals in developed countries have computerized databases, including names, addresses, diagnoses, and treatments for all inpatients and outpatients. Investigators can acquire access to these databases to identify subjects for a study after gaining approval from a hospital's ethics committee (which reviews all studies to ensure that the research is ethically and scientifically sound). Investigators can review these databases to find cases. Researchers typically try to identify cases soon after diagnosis, and therefore they review the database frequently. For example, investigators conducted a hospital-based case–control study on the risk of spontaneous abortion following an induced abortion.[14] Women who experienced a pregnancy loss (the cases) were identified each weekday from hospital admissions records so that they could be interviewed before discharge. Women who delivered live infants at the same hospital comprised the control group. They were identified by reviewing delivery logs each weekday, again, so they could be interviewed before discharge. The investigators sought to interview subjects soon after their pregnancy outcomes to obtain accurate information on prior exposures.

Registry systems provide a good source of disease cases. These special reporting systems have been developed mainly for cancer and birth defects. For example, the federally funded Surveillance, Epidemiology, and End Results (SEER) program identifies newly diagnosed cases of cancer in five states and six metropolitan areas across the United States.[15] The portion of the U.S. population covered by SEER includes 26% of African Americans, 38% of Hispanics, and 44% of Native Americans/Alaskan Natives. In addition, the remaining U.S. states, the District of Columbia, Puerto Rico, and the U.S. Pacific Islands also have population-based cancer registries.[16] The Massachusetts Cancer Registry is composed of a network of hospital tumor registrars based in acute-care hospitals, medical practice associations, and certain doctors' offices across the state.[17]

The registrars review medical and laboratory records to identify all newly diagnosed cancers among state residents. When an incident case is found, the registrar reports identifying and demographic information to the central office. This information is confidential, but it can be made available to researchers for epidemiological studies with approval from the registry's ethics committee.

Birth defects and cancer registries have greatly facilitated the conduct of case–control studies because investigators can identify all newly diagnosed cases, say, within a geographic area, using a single source; for example, the case–control study on breast cancer risk in relation to PCE-contaminated drinking water used the Massachusetts Cancer Registry to identify all newly diagnosed breast cancer cases from 1987 through 1993 among residents of eight Cape Cod towns.[11] These cases had been diagnosed and treated in more than 25 hospitals across the state. If they had not had access to the cancer registry, the investigators would have had to gain access to and review discharge records in all 25 hospitals to identify the cases.

Incident or Prevalent Cases

An important issue in the selection of cases is whether they should be incident or prevalent. Recall that prevalence depends on the rate at which new cases develop as well as the duration that the cases have the disease. Duration starts with diagnosis and ends with cure or death. Researchers who study the causes of disease prefer incident cases because they are usually interested in the factors that lead to developing the disease rather than factors that affect the duration of the disease.

Epidemiologists sometimes have no choice but to rely on prevalent cases. For example, many etiologic studies of birth defects have been conducted exclusively on cases identified at birth. Although defects form during the first 3 months of gestation, it is difficult for researchers to identify malformed fetuses that are miscarried or voluntarily aborted; therefore, they rely on the surviving infants who are born 9 months later. Thus, etiologic studies of birth defects must be interpreted cautiously because it is impossible to determine whether the exposure under study is related to the formation of the defect, the survival of the malformed fetus in utero, or a combination of the two.

Complete or Partial Case Ascertainment

There is a common misconception that a case–control study must include all cases of disease occurring within a defined population.[5(pp115,120-121)] This erroneous thinking arises from a desire to make the study results as generalizable as possible. However, validity is the primary goal of an epidemiological study, and validity should never be sacrificed for generalizability. Even when no sacrifice is needed, it is unnecessary to include all cases. It is perfectly legitimate to include only a subset of cases. Thus,

TABLE 9-4 Important Considerations in Case Definition and Selection
■ Criteria for case definition should lead to accurate classification of diseased and nondiseased subjects.
■ Efficient and accurate sources should be used to identify cases.
■ Incident cases are preferable to prevalent cases for causal research.
■ Partial case ascertainment is legitimate as long as the source population can be defined.

it is appropriate to conduct a study using cases identified at only one hospital even when there are many hospitals in the same geographic area. However, regardless of whether ascertainment is complete, one must be able to define the case group's source population so that comparable controls from the same population can be selected. See **TABLE 9-4** for a summary of the important issues in defining and selecting cases for a case–control study.

▶ Selection of Controls

Controls are a sample of the population that produced the cases. Another term for the control group is **referent group** because it "refers to" the exposure distribution in the source population,[2] and another expression for the source population is **study base**. The guiding principle for the valid selection of cases and controls is that they represent the same base population. If this condition is met, then a member of the control group who gets the disease being studied "would" end up as a case in the study. This concept is known as the **would criterion**, and its fulfillment is crucial to the validity of a case–control study.

Another important principle is that controls must be sampled independently of exposure status. In other words, exposed and unexposed controls should have the same probability of selection. This concept is best explained by returning to the hypothetical cohort and case–control studies of serum DDE levels and the risk of breast cancer described earlier in this chapter (see Tables 9-1 and 9-2). Of the 100,000 cohort members, 4,000 were selected as controls; therefore, the overall control sampling fraction was 4,000/100,000, or 4%. The 4% sampling fraction was the same for both the exposed and unexposed groups: $15,000 \times 0.04 = 600$ exposed controls, and $85,000 \times 0.04 = 3,400$ unexposed controls. Thus, this study follows the principle that control selection should be independent of exposure status.

Sources of Control Identification

Investigators can use several sources to identify controls for case–control studies. They can sample individuals from the general population, individuals attending a hospital or clinic, individuals who have died, or friends or relatives identified by the cases. The following section describes each type of control along with its advantages and disadvantages.

Population controls: When cases are identified from a well-defined population (such as residents of a geographic area), population controls are typically selected as the referent group. Population controls can be identified using a variety of sources, including tax lists, voter registration lists, driver's license rosters, telephone directories, and national identity registries. Another method for identifying population controls is through random digit dialing, which is a method for identifying a random sample of telephone subscribers living in a defined geographic area. In the case–control study of PCE-contaminated drinking water and risk of breast cancer, investigators used this method to identify living controls aged 64 years and younger.[11] Although this method has been popular, it is becoming increasingly difficult to use because of the high proportion of the population who use cellular phones and voice mail.

Population controls have one principal advantage that makes them preferable to other types of controls. Because of the manner in which the controls are identified, investigators are usually assured that they come from the same base population as the cases do.

However, population controls have several disadvantages. First, it is time consuming and expensive to identify them, particularly when investigators use random digit dialing. In the study of PCE-contaminated drinking water and breast cancer, investigators had to call 3,402 residential households to interview 157 eligible random digit dial controls. Approximately 68% of households did not have any residents who met the eligibility criteria, 17% never answered the phone after many calls, and about 9% did not respond to the questions that determined eligibility. Ultimately, 190 households were identified with an eligible resident, of which 157 people were interviewed.

Second, it may be difficult to obtain the cooperation of population controls because they usually do not have the same level of interest in participating as do cases and controls identified from other sources. For example, in the study of PCE-contaminated drinking water and breast cancer, 17% of eligible random digit dial controls versus only 8% of contacted and eligible cases refused to participate. Investigators try to improve response rates by sending an introductory letter to potential subjects that describes the general purpose of the study. However, they cannot use this strategy with random digit dial controls because they usually do not know the names and addresses of the individuals.

The third limitation of population controls concerns their recall of past exposures. Because these individuals are generally healthy, their recall may be less accurate than that of the cases who are likely reviewing their history in search of a reason for their illness.

Hospital or clinic controls: When investigators identify cases using hospital and clinic rosters, they typically identify controls from these same records. Thus, hospital and clinic controls have diseases or have experienced events (such as a car accident) for which they must seek medical care. The most difficult aspect of using these types of controls is determining which diseases or events are suitable for the control group. Two general principles should be followed in this regard. First, the illnesses in the control group should, on the basis of current knowledge, be unrelated to the exposure under study. For example, a case–control study of cigarette smoking and myocardial infarction should not use emphysema patients as controls because cigarette smoking is known to be a cause of emphysema. Second, the illness of the controls should have the same referral pattern to the healthcare facility as that of the cases. For example, a case–control study of an acute condition such as a myocardial infarction should identify controls with other acute conditions such as appendicitis or car accident injuries. In theory, following this principle will help ensure that the study base is the same for cases and controls. However, in practice, this strategy may be difficult to implement, particularly given the dramatic changes that are now occurring in healthcare delivery in the United States. Sometimes hospital and clinic controls have a disease that is quite similar to that of cases. For example, birth defect studies often select case infants with one type of defect and control infants with other types of defects that are unrelated to the exposure under study. Because both the cases and controls are ill, parents' recall of past exposures should be comparable. This strategy minimizes recall bias, a type of information bias.

Hospital controls have several advantages, including easy identification and good participation rates, and therefore they are less expensive to identify than population controls. Furthermore, hospital controls are comparable to the cases if they come from the same source population. Finally, their recall of prior exposures is considered comparable to that of cases because they are also ill. Their main disadvantage is the difficulty in determining appropriate illnesses for inclusion. The illness should be unrelated to the exposure under study and have the same referral pattern as cases.

Dead controls: In the past, epidemiologists recommended enrolling deceased controls when a portion or the entire series of cases was deceased when data collection began. These controls were usually identified by reviewing death records of individuals who lived in the same geographic area and died during the same time period as the cases. Investigators' rationale for selecting dead controls was to ensure comparable data collection procedures between the two groups. For example, if investigators collected data by interview, they would conduct proxy interviews for the dead cases and dead controls. These interviews were usually conducted with the subject's spouse, child, relative, or friend because these individuals were knowledgeable and willing to participate on behalf of the subject.

Today, most epidemiologists discourage the use of dead controls because these controls may not be a representative sample of the source population that produced the cases (which, by definition, consists of living people). For example, dead controls are more likely than living controls to have an exposure such as smoking because this activity causes death in a large number of people.[18]

Friend, spouse, and relative controls: In rare circumstances, investigators use a case's friend, spouse, or relative (usually a sibling) as the control. These individuals are usually nominated by cases. They are selected because they are likely to share the cases' socioeconomic status, race, age, and educational level. Furthermore, sibling cases and controls share genetic traits. These individuals are usually willing to participate because they know the cases.

However, several difficulties arise with these controls. First, cases may be unable to nominate people to serve as controls, particularly if they have few appropriate friends, are widowed, or are only or adopted children. Second, cases may be unwilling to nominate anyone because they do not want to reveal their illness or their participation in a study. Third, these controls could possibly share the habits of the cases (such as smoking or drinking), which can lead to biased results if the study hypothesis involves these exposures. For example, in a study of alcohol use and heart disease risk, cases might nominate their drinking partners as controls. This would make the exposure histories of cases and controls similar and bias the results toward the null.

Summary: When selecting a source of controls, epidemiologists must always return to the basic purpose of the control group for guidance: to provide information on the exposure distribution in the population that produced the cases. Thus, controls must represent the source population and be sampled independently of exposure status. To determine whether the source population of cases and controls is the same, investigators must ask the following question: If a member of the control group actually had the disease under study, would he end up as a study case? The answer to this question should always be yes. These and other important considerations for selecting controls are summarized in **TABLE 9-5**.

Ratio of Controls to Cases

When the number of available cases is limited and controls are relatively plentiful, it is possible to increase the power of the study to detect an association by increasing the size of the control group. Control-to-case ratios of up to 4 to 1 help to increase power. Ratios higher than this are not considered worthwhile because of the increased cost of enrolling and gathering data from additional controls.[19] Of course, if the study is based on data that have already been collected, the cost of additional controls is so small that there is no reason to limit the ratio to 4 to 1.

TABLE 9-5 Important Considerations for Selecting Controls

- Controls are a sample of the population that gave rise to the cases.

- The purpose of the control group is to provide information on the exposure distribution in the source population.

- The "would criterion" should be used to determine whether the source population of cases and controls is the same.

- Several sources are available for identifying controls, including the general population; hospital and clinic rosters; death certificates; and cases' friends, spouses, and relatives.

- Each source has advantages and disadvantages. If available, population controls are preferred because investigators are more confident that they come from the source population that produced the cases and population controls avoid problems encountered with other types of controls.

Methods for Sampling Controls

Consider a hypothetical cohort study with 100,000 individuals. Of these, 50,000 are exposed to high arsenic levels in drinking water and 50,000 are exposed to low arsenic levels. Both groups are enrolled in a study in 2005 and are followed for 10 years until 2015. The occurrence of diabetes is the health outcome of interest. Obtaining a biological measure of arsenic exposure is quite expensive, and therefore the investigator decides to conduct a nested case–control study within this cohort. Recall that the controls should be a sample of the source population that produced the cases. Exactly how should the investigator go about selecting controls?

The investigator could use one of three strategies (see **FIGURE 9-2**). In the first strategy, known as **survivor sampling**, the investigator would choose controls from cohort members who are never diagnosed with diabetes during the entire follow-up period. In this scenario, the controls would be selected from the "noncases" or "survivors" at the end of follow-up in 2015. Survivor sampling is the predominant method of selecting controls in traditional case–control studies.

The second approach is to sample controls from the population at risk at the beginning of follow-up in 2005. This approach is called **case–base sampling**, also known as case–cohort sampling.

The third strategy, known as **risk set sampling**, involves longitudinally sampling controls throughout the 10-year follow-up period. In this approach, the investigator selects a control from the population at risk when a case is diagnosed. Thus, when a diabetes case is diagnosed, the investigator selects a control from members of the cohort who are at risk for diabetes at that point in time.

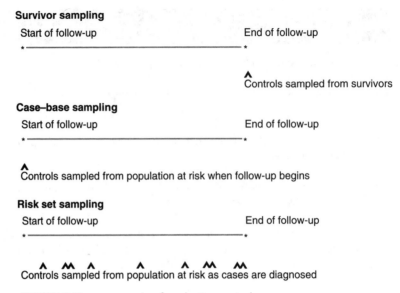

FIGURE 9-2 Three approaches for selecting controls.

Note that when case–base and risk set sampling methods are used, the control group could include future cases of diabetes. Although this may seem incorrect, modern epidemiological theory supports it because both diseased and nondiseased individuals contribute to the denominators of risks and rates in cohort studies. Thus, it is reasonable for the control group to include future cases of disease because it is merely an efficient way to obtain denominator data.

▶ Sources of Exposure Information

Case–control studies have been used to investigate the risk of disease in relation to a wide variety of exposures, particularly those related to lifestyle, occupation, environment, genes, diet, reproduction, and the use of medications.[20] Most exposures are complex; therefore, investigators must attempt to obtain sufficiently detailed information on their nature, sources, frequency, and duration during critical periods in a subject's life. A **critical period** is a time when the subject is susceptible to the action of an exposure. The timing and duration of a critical period depend on the particular exposure; it may be lifelong or limited to a narrow window. An example of the latter is the critical exposure period for teratogens that cause structural birth defects. This interval is limited to the first trimester of pregnancy when the fetal organs are forming.[21(p127)]

Investigators can use a variety of sources to obtain exposure data for case–control studies, including in-person and telephone interviews; self-administered questionnaires; preexisting medical, pharmacy, registry, employment, insurance, birth, death, and environmental records;

TABLE 9-6 Sources of Exposure Information		
Source	**Types**	**Key characteristics**
Questionnaires	Face-to-face, telephone, self-administered	Can obtain information on many exposures with relative ease and flexibility; must be carefully designed and administered to elicit accurate information; expensive
Preexisting records	Administrative, medical, regulatory	May be the only available exposure source; avoids bias; may be incomplete; may lack uniformity and details; inexpensive
Biomarkers	Levels in blood, urine, bone, toenails	Can estimate internal dose; infrequently used because of difficulty identifying valid and reliable markers of exposure to noninfectious agents; expensive

and biological specimens[20] (see **TABLE 9-6**). When selecting a particular source, investigators consider availability, accuracy, logistics, and cost.

Accuracy is a particular concern in case–control studies because exposure data are retrospective. Relevant exposures may have occurred many years before data collection, making it difficult to gather correct information. For example, a case–control study of active and passive cigarette smoking and the occurrence of breast cancer gathered exposure data from participants' childhood through to the present; this approach required most participants to recall their personal exposures over a 50-year span.[22]

In case–control studies, questionnaires serve as the most commonly used source of exposure data.[20] They are usually administered using face-to-face interviews, although telephone interviews (particularly computer-assisted telephone interviews) are becoming increasingly popular. Self-administered questionnaires are used least often mainly because of poor response rates. However, they are inexpensive and good for socially sensitive topics. Whatever the method of administration, the questionnaire respondent is typically the index subject (i.e., the case or control). A surrogate, such as a spouse or other relative, may be interviewed if the index subject cannot participate.

Questionnaires can elicit detailed information on a wide range of exposures with relative ease and flexibility.[20] However, questionnaires depend on the ability of participants to interpret the questions correctly and to remember and report information accurately. Thus, it is important that questions be worded clearly, placed in logical order, and have appropriate response options. In addition, questionnaires should be pretested to identify problems with comprehension, recall, response formulation, and recording. Memory aids, such as a calendar of important life events, are recommended to enhance respondents' recall. Furthermore, investigators must incorporate procedures to minimize interviewer bias, which stems from systematic differences in questioning the cases and controls. One method for reducing this type of bias is to mask interviewers to the outcome status of the study subjects.

Records collected for medical, administrative, and regulatory purposes are another important source of exposure data.[20] Such records may be the only source of information for certain occupational and environmental exposures. For example, most individuals are unaware of the contaminant levels in their drinking water, particularly levels from the past. Thus, investigators rely on routinely collected water-quality data as the source of exposure information for case–control studies of drinking water contaminants and adverse health outcomes.[23,24] Other reasons for using preexisting exposure data include low cost and lack of bias. Because these data are collected before the outcomes occur, investigators are not faced with systematic differences between cases and controls in data availability and collection methods, and therefore the results are not biased. The principal disadvantages of preexisting exposure data include unavailability of records (particularly records from many years earlier) and lack of uniformity and sufficient detail.[20] For example, data on drinking water contaminants are generally not available for private water supplies and for public supplies before 1974, when the federal Safe Drinking Water Act was passed.[25] Furthermore, water samples are usually collected from public taps (often in a town hall or school) and are assumed, rightly or wrongly, to represent the drinking water quality of all households in the area.

Biomarkers are the third main source of exposure data in case–control studies. These cellular, biochemical, and molecular alterations that indicate exposure are usually based on biological measurements of media such as blood, urine, bone, or toenails.[26(p3)] For example, studies have measured urinary cotinine as a measure of exposure to cigarette smoke and urinary alkyl phosphate residues as a measure of organic phosphate pesticide exposure.[26(pp8-9)] Although biomarkers have the potential for estimating the internal dose that a person has absorbed and for improving the accuracy of the exposure assessment, they have been used in only a small portion of case–control studies.[20] This is because it is difficult to identify valid and reliable markers for exposure to noninfectious agents. In addition, if the biomarker is collected after the disease has occurred, the presence of the disease and its treatment could affect its accuracy.

It costs more to collect exposure data specifically for a case–control study than to use existing records. A 30-minute telephone interview in the study of PCE-contaminated drinking water and breast cancer cost approximately $100 to $200 per participant.[11] In-person interviews, which were conducted when the subject was too ill to be interviewed by phone, were even more expensive because they involved travel to the participant's home. Laboratory tests for biomarkers can also be quite expensive. For example, analysis of polychlorinated biphenyls, dioxin, and metabolites of DDT in serum can cost about $1,000 per sample.[27]

▶ Analysis of Case–Control Studies

Calculation of Odds Ratios

Controls are a sample of the population that produced the cases. However, in most instances, investigators do not know the size of the total population that produced the cases. When investigators do not know the sampling fraction, they cannot fill in the total population in the margin of a two-by-two table or obtain rates and risks of disease (see **TABLE 9-7**).

When this situation occurs, investigators calculate a number called an **odds**, which functions as a rate or risk in a case–control study. The odds of an event is the probability that it will occur divided by the probability that it will not occur. For example, the probability of getting heads on one coin toss is 0.50, and the probability of not getting heads on one coin toss is also 0.50. Thus, the odds of getting heads on a coin toss is 0.50/0.50 or 1:1. In a case–control study, we calculate the odds of being a case among the exposed (a/b) and the odds of being a case among the nonexposed (c/d) (see Table 9-7). The ratio of these two odds is known as the **disease odds ratio**. The odds ratio is expressed as follows:

$$\frac{a/b}{c/d} \text{ or } \frac{ad}{bc}$$

The odds ratio can also be conceptualized in another way: the ratio of the odds of being exposed among the cases (a/c) divided by the odds of being exposed among the controls (b/d). This is known as the **exposure odds ratio**, and it is algebraically equivalent to the disease odds ratio. Sometimes, the term **cross-product ratio** is used for both of these odds ratios. In any case, the odds ratio provides an estimate of the relative measure of comparison, just as the incidence rate ratio and cumulative incidence ratio do.

Consider the following example. Investigators conducted a case–control study on the risk of spontaneous abortion among women who had a prior induced abortion.[14] Cases consisted of women who were hospitalized at a Boston hospital for a spontaneous abortion through

TABLE 9-7 Two-by-Two Table in a Case–Control Study

Exposed	Cases	Controls	Total population
Yes	a	b	?
No	c	d	?

TABLE 9-8 Results from a Case–Control Study of the Odds of Spontaneous Abortion Following Induced Abortion

Prior induced abortion	Spontaneous abortion cases	Delivery controls
Yes	42	247
No	107	825

Data from Levin AA, Schoenbaum SC, Monson RR, Stubblefield PG, Ryan KJ. Association of induced abortion with subsequent pregnancy loss. *JAMA*. 1980;243:2495-2499.

27 weeks' gestation. Controls consisted of women who delivered liveborn infants at the same hospital within a few days of the case's pregnancy loss. The exposure—prior induced abortion—could have occurred in the preceding pregnancy, in the more distant past, or not at all. The results for first-trimester pregnancy loss are summarized in **TABLE 9-8**.

Data from this study can be used to calculate the odds of being a case among women with a history of induced abortion (42/247) and the odds of being a case among women without a history of induced abortion (107/825). Thus, the disease odds ratio was $(42/247)/(107/825) = (42 \times 825)/(247 \times 107) = 1.3$. These data can also be used to calculate the exposure odds ratio. For cases, the odds of having a prior induced abortion were 42/107, and the odds of having a prior induced abortion among controls were 247/825. Thus, the exposure odds ratio was $(42/107)/(247/825) = (42 \times 825)/(247 \times 107) = 1.3$. The interpretation of both odds ratios is as follows: Women with a prior induced abortion had a 30% increased odds of experiencing a first-trimester spontaneous abortion as compared with women with no such history.

Interpretation of Odds Ratios

Depending on the method of control selection, the odds ratio from a case–control study estimates different relative measures of comparison.[28] When survivor sampling is conducted, the odds ratio estimates the odds ratio in the base population. When case–base sampling is used, the odds ratio estimates the risk ratio in the base population. When risk set sampling is used, the odds ratio estimates the rate ratio in the base population.

Epidemiologists used to think that the "rare disease assumption" was needed for the odds ratio to estimate the measures just described. However, now we realize that none of these estimates requires this assumption.[28] This assumption is needed only when investigators want one measure to approximate another measure. For example, the odds ratio calculated from a study that has used survivor sampling will be a good estimate of the risk ratio only when the disease is rare.

Calculation of Attributable Proportion

We cannot obtain the actual rate or risk of disease in the exposed and unexposed groups in a case–control study except under special circumstances when the sampling fraction of the controls is known. Thus, it is not usually possible to obtain an absolute measure of comparison such as the risk and rate difference. The odds cannot be used as a substitute because the difference between two odds changes as the size of the control group changes. The ratio of two odds does not.

However, it is possible to obtain a measure of the public health impact of the exposure—the **attributable proportion among the exposed (AP$_e$)**—in case–control studies. This measure estimates the fraction of exposed cases that would be eliminated if the exposure were eliminated or reduced, assuming that the exposure caused the disease. Its formula in case–control studies is as follows:

$$\frac{OR - 1}{OR} \times 100$$

where OR is the odds ratio. Thus, the attributable proportion in the spontaneous abortion study described earlier is $[(1.3 - 1)/1.3] \times 100$, or 23%. This means that 23% of the spontaneous abortions among exposed cases would not have occurred if the cases did not have a history of induced abortion. Of course, this calculation assumes that having an induced abortion causes women to miscarry subsequent pregnancies.

It is also possible to obtain the **attributable proportion in the total population (AP$_t$)** in case–control studies. This measure estimates the proportion of disease among the total study population that would be eliminated if the exposure were eliminated or reduced. Its formula in case–control studies is as follows:

$$\frac{P_e(OR - 1)}{P_e(OR - 1) + 1} \times 100$$

where P_e is the proportion of exposed controls and OR is the odds ratio. Thus, the population attributable proportion in the spontaneous abortion study described earlier is $[(0.23)(1.3 - 1)]/[(0.23)(1.3 - 1) + 1] \times 100$, or 6.5%. This means that 6.5% of the spontaneous abortions among the study population may be attributed to a history of induced abortion and hence would not have occurred if the cases did not have a history of induced abortion. Again, this calculation assumes that having an induced abortion causes women to miscarry subsequent pregnancies.

▶ The Case–Crossover Study: A New Type of Case–Control Study

The **case–crossover study** is a new variant of the case–control study that was developed for situations "when brief exposure causes a transient change in risk of a rare acute-onset disease."[29] Thus, a case–crossover study is suitable for examining the risk of acute myocardial infarction immediately following heavy physical exertion,[30] the risk of motor vehicle collision while using a cellular telephone,[31] the risk of congestive heart failure following short-term increases in particulate air pollution,[32] the risk of unsafe sex following the consumption of alcohol,[33] and the risk of sharps injury in healthcare workers.[34] In each of these settings, the risk of the outcome is increased during or for a brief time after exposure.

The period of increased risk following the exposure is termed the **hazard period**.[30] In the case–crossover study, cases serve as their own controls, and the exposure frequency during the hazard period is compared with that from a control period. The duration of the hazard period depends on the exposure and outcome being studied. For example, the period of increased risk for myocardial infarction following heavy physical activity is less than 1 hour.[35] As its originator states, "The case–crossover design is a scientific way to ask and answer the question clinicians so often ask patients: Were you doing anything unusual just before the episode?"[29]

A somewhat unusual characteristic of the case–crossover study is that cases serve as their own controls. However, this feature is also employed in crossover experimental studies in which the subject receives two treatments in succession and investigators compare outcomes in the same subject.[36] Because each person's response to one treatment is compared with his or her response to the other treatment, the influence of fixed personal characteristics (such as race and gender) is eliminated from the comparison. The notion of cases serving as their own controls also harkens back to the **counterfactual ideal**, meaning that the perfect comparison group for a group of exposed individuals consists of exactly the same individuals had they not been exposed.

The case–crossover method was first used to study the risk of myocardial infarction following heavy physical exertion and other activities.[30] The investigators interviewed 1,228 myocardial infarction patients aged 22 to 92 years within 30 days of their heart attack. The interview obtained detailed data on physical exertion for the 26-hour period before the onset of heart attack symptoms and the usual frequency of physical exertion during the previous year. A person was considered exposed if his or her physical exertion included, for example, jogging, tennis, fast biking, heavy gardening, heavy or deep snow shoveling, or ladder or stair climbing with a 50-pound load. The hazard period was defined as the 1-hour interval immediately before the start of the heart attack.

Control information was based on the case's exposures before the hazard period. In fact, the investigators made several comparisons. First, investigators compared the frequency of heavy exertion during the hazard period with a 1-hour control period at the same time of day on the day before the heart attack. Second, investigators examined the frequency of heavy exertion for several 1-hour control periods during the 25 hours preceding the hazard period. Third, they contrasted the exposure during the hazard period with the individual's usual exposure frequency over the previous year. The investigators obtained similar results regardless of which control period was used. They found that the risk of myocardial infarction was approximately five to seven times higher following heavy exertion than following light or no exertion.

The case–crossover design was also used to investigate the association between cellular telephone calls and motor vehicle accidents.[31] The investigators studied 699 drivers who had cellular phones and were involved in motor vehicle collisions resulting in considerable property damage but no personal injury. Investigators interviewed the subjects and reviewed records of the accident and cellular telephone billing accounts. The hazard period was defined as the 10-minute interval before the time of the accident. Investigators compared the phone activity during the hazard period with a control period at the same time 1 week before the collision. The risk of collision was four times higher when a cellular phone was being used than when it was not in use. Increased relative risks were seen for both men and women, for drivers of all ages, and for drivers with all levels of experience.

Thus, the case–crossover study is a useful design for studying the influence of brief exposures on the risk of onset of acute incidents.[30] Because cases serve as their own controls, these studies have several advantages over traditional case–control studies. First, they are immune to a type of bias (called control selection bias) that arises from the selection of controls that are unrepresentative of the base population that produced the cases. Second, cases and controls have many identical characteristics (such as race and gender). Finally, they are more efficient and require fewer subjects than traditional case–control studies because variability is reduced. The chief features of case–crossover studies are summarized in **TABLE 9-9**.

TABLE 9-9 Key Aspects of Case–Crossover Studies

- The purpose is to study the effect of transient exposures on the risk of acute events.

- Cases serve as their own controls.

- The brief period of increased risk following a transient exposure is termed the hazard period.

- The exposure frequency during the hazard period is compared to a control period.

▶ Applications of Case–Control Studies

Case–control studies are currently being used for determining the causes of disease and for numerous "problem solving activities within the practice of public health and medicine."[37] These problem-solving activities include evaluating the effectiveness of vaccines,[38] evaluating treatment and prevention programs,[39] and investigating outbreaks of disease.[40] Examples of these applications are described in the sections that follow.

Evaluation of Vaccine Effectiveness

Epidemiologists conducted a case–control study in the Ukraine to determine the effectiveness of vaccinating young children against *Haemophilus influenzae* type b (Hib), a leading cause of pneumonia-related death in this age group.[41] Following the introduction of the Hib vaccine to the Ukrainian national childhood immunization program, investigators conducted a case–control study to answer the question, Were children who received the Hib vaccine less likely to be hospitalized for radiologically confirmed pneumonia than children who did not receive the vaccine? They used a case–control design to answer this question because it was less expensive and would take less time than a cohort study.

Cases were identified by reviewing records from 11 public hospitals in Kiev and Dnepropetrovsk. They included children between the ages of 4 and 23 months with radiologically confirmed pneumonia who were eligible to receive the Hib vaccine and had vaccination and medical records available for review. Controls were similarly aged children who were not hospitalized for pneumonia within the past year. Up to four controls were randomly selected for every case from the same medical catchment population that gave rise to the cases. Exposure to the Hib vaccine was determined by reviewing vaccination and medical records.

The investigators found that vaccinated children had a 45% reduced odds of radiologically confirmed pneumonia as compared with nonvaccinated children (the odds ratio was 0.55). The authors concluded that Hib is an important cause of severe pneumonia in young children in Ukraine and that "prevention of pneumonia needs to be incorporated into strategies to communicate the benefits of vaccination against Hib diseases."[41(ps17)]

Evaluation of a Prevention Program

Investigators also used a case–control study to evaluate the role of bicycle helmets in preventing head injuries during bicycle accidents.[42] Cases included 757 individuals treated at one of seven urban emergency departments for bicycle-related injuries or fatalities that involved the head. A head injury was defined as an injury to the part of the head that a helmet would likely protect—the forehead, scalp, ears, skull, brain, and brain stem. Controls were bicyclists treated in the same emergency departments for nonhead injuries. A total of 29% of cases and 57% of controls were wearing helmets when they were injured. After controlling for differences between cases and controls, the investigators found a 69% reduction in the odds of head injuries among those who used bicycle helmets (the odds ratio was 0.31). They concluded that bicycle helmets were very effective in preventing head injuries and recommended a major campaign to increase their use.

Investigation of an Outbreak of Disease

The first case reports of toxic shock syndrome (TSS) were published in the medical literature in 1978.[43] TSS is a "severe, acute disease associated with strains of staphylococci of phage Group 1 that produce[s] a unique epidermal toxin."[43] Little was known about its risk factors, but the case report data suggested that menstruation was associated with its onset. Thus, investigators undertook a case–control study to describe menstrual risk factors for TSS.[44]

The case group consisted of 35 premenopausal, nonpregnant women who were diagnosed with TSS in Wisconsin from 1975 through 1980. The case definition was quite restrictive and included numerous signs, symptoms, and laboratory test results. Controls were selected from a population of premenopausal, nonpregnant women who attended a Wisconsin gynecology clinic for routine care. Three age-matched controls were selected for each case. Cases and controls were interviewed to obtain data on their age, marital status, pattern of tampon and napkin use, preferred brands, birth control methods, vaginal infections, and sexual activities and the intensity and duration of their menstrual flow.

The investigators found that 97% (34/35) of the cases used tampons during the menstrual period near the onset of TSS, and 76% (80/105) of the controls always used tampons during their menstrual periods. Thus, there was almost an 11-fold increased odds of TSS associated with tampon use: $[(34 \times 25)/80 \times 1] = 10.6$. Although they were unsure of the exact role of the tampon in the pathogenesis of the disease, the investigators hypothesized that the highly absorbent tampon fibers might produce mucosal drying and micro-ulcerations that could become infected with *Staphylococcus aureus*, a bacterium commonly isolated from the vagina or cervix of TSS patients.

▶ Strengths and Limitations of Case–Control Studies

The main strength of case–control studies is their efficiency. They take less time and cost less money to conduct than cohort or experimental studies primarily because the control group is a sample of the source population. Case–control studies are particularly efficient for studying

TABLE 9-10 Strengths and Weaknesses of Case–Control Studies

Strengths

- Efficient for rare diseases
- Efficient for diseases with long induction and latent periods
- Can evaluate multiple exposures in relation to a disease, so good for diseases about which little is known

Weaknesses

- Inefficient for rare exposures
- May have poor information on exposures because retrospective
- Vulnerable to bias because retrospective
- Difficult to infer temporal relationship between exposure and disease

rare diseases because fewer subjects are needed than for cohort studies, and for studying diseases with long induction and latent periods because long-term prospective follow-up is avoided. Another strength is their ability to provide information on a large number of possible risk factors, which makes case–control studies particularly useful for studying diseases whose etiology is largely unknown.

The main limitation of case–control studies is the increased possibility of bias because of the retrospective nature of the data collection. In fact, some epidemiologists have argued that case–control studies are not well suited for detecting weak associations (odds ratios less than 1.5) because of the likelihood of bias.[45] Although bias is unlikely to be entirely accountable for a strong association, it may entirely account for a weak association. In addition, because case–control studies rely on retrospective data collection, it is difficult to establish a clear temporal relationship between the exposure and disease. One of the most important guidelines for inferring causation is establishing that the exposure preceded the disease. The strengths and weaknesses of case–control studies are summarized in **TABLE 9-10**.

Summary

Over the past 30 years, epidemiologists' view of the case–control study has changed dramatically. The case–control study is no longer seen as an inferior alternative to a cohort study but rather is regarded as a highly efficient design for learning about exposure–disease relationships. Case–control studies are particularly desirable when (1) the exposure data are difficult or expensive to obtain, (2) the disease is rare or has long latent and induction periods, (3) little is known about the disease, or (4) the underlying population is dynamic. In addition, the case–crossover study, a new variant of the case–control study, was designed to study the acute effects of transient exposures.

Case selection includes composing an accurate disease definition and determining accurate and efficient sources for identifying cases, such as hospital or clinic patient rosters, death certificates, and special reporting systems. Incident cases are preferable over prevalent cases for causal research because investigators are usually interested in factors that lead to developing the disease rather than factors that affect the disease duration.

Controls are a sample of the population that produced the cases, and their purpose is to provide information on the exposure distribution in the source population. The guiding principle for selecting controls is that they must represent the same base population as the cases and thus satisfy the "would criterion." Several sources are available for identifying controls, including the general population; hospital or clinic rosters; death certificates; and friends, spouses, and relatives of cases. One of three sampling frames is used to select controls: noncases at the end of the observation period, the population at risk at the beginning of the observation period, or the population at risk when each case is diagnosed.

Because exposures are complex, sufficiently detailed information must be obtained on their nature, sources, frequency, and duration. Sources of exposure data include in-person and telephone interviews, self-administered questionnaires, preexisting records, and biological specimens. When selecting a particular source, investigators consider availability, accuracy, logistics, and cost. The analysis of case–control studies involves calculating a measure of association termed the odds ratio. This measure is used because disease risks ans rates cannot be calculated in most case–control studies.

The main advantages of case–control studies are efficiency and their ability to inform. Their main disadvantages include an increased possibility of bias and difficulty in establishing a clear temporal relationship between the exposure and disease because of the retrospective nature of the data.

References

1. Feinstein AR. Clinical biostatistics. XX. The epidemiologic TROHOC, the ablative risk ratio, and "retrospective" research. *Clin Pharmacol Ther.* 1973;14:291-307.
2. Miettinen OS. The "case-control" study: valid selection of subjects. *J Chron Dis.* 1985;38:543-548.
3. Davis DL, Bradlow HL, Wolff M, Woodruff T, Hoel DG, Anton-Culver H. Medical hypothesis: xenoestrogens as preventable causes of breast cancer. *Environ Health Perspect.* 1993;101:372-377.
4. Levine R. Recognized and possible effects of pesticides in humans. In: Hays WJ Jr, Laws ER Jr. (eds.). *Handbook of Pesticide Toxicology. Vol 1. General Principles.* San Diego, CA: Academic Press; 1991.
5. Rothman KJ, Greenland S, Lash TL. *Modern Epidemiology.* 3rd ed. Philadelphia, PA: Wolters Kluwer Health/Lippincott Williams & Wilkins; 2008.
6. Howlader N, Noone AM, Krapcho M, Miller D, Bishop K, Kosary CL, et al. (eds.). *SEER Cancer Statistics Review, 1975-2014.* cancer.gov. https://seer.cancer.gov/csr/1975_2014/. Published April 2017. Accessed April 2017.
7. Rothman KJ. Induction and latent periods. *Am J Epidemiol.* 1981;114:253-259.

8. Hall EJ. *Radiobiology for the Radiologist.* 5th ed. Philadelphia, PA: Lippincott Williams & Wilkins; 2000:149.

9. Schottenfeld D, Haas JF. Carcinogens in the workplace. *CA Cancer J Clin.* 1979;29:144-168.

10. Jaffe HW, Choi K, Thomas PA, Haverkos HW, Auerbach DM, Guinan ME, et al. National case-control study of Kaposi's sarcoma and *Pneumocystis carinii* pneumonia in homosexual men: part 1. Epidemiologic results. *Ann Intern Med.* 1983;99:145-151.

11. Aschengrau A, Rogers S, Ozonoff D. Perchloroethylene-contaminated drinking water and the risk of breast cancer: additional results from Cape Cod, Massachusetts, USA. *Environ Health Perspect.* 2003; 111:167-173.

12. STATS Cape Cod. statscapecod.org. http:www.statscapecod.org/benchmarks/balanced/population _trends.php. Accessed October 2016.

13. Lasky T, Stolley PD. Selection of cases and controls. *Epidemiol Rev.* 1994;16:6-17.

14. Levin AA, Schoenbaum SC, Monson RR, Stubblefield PG, Ryan KJ. Association of induced abortion with subsequent pregnancy loss. *JAMA.* 1980;243:2495-2499.

15. Surveillance, Epidemiology, and End Results Program. cancer.gov. https://seer.cancer.gov. Accessed October 2016.

16. National Program of Cancer Registries (NPCR). cdc .gov. www.cdc.gov/cancer/npcr/index.htm. Accessed October 2016.

17. Cancer Incidence Statewide Reports: 2010-2014. August 2017. mass.gov. https://www.mass.gov/lists /cancer-incidence-statewide-reports. Accessed October 2016.

18. McLaughlin JK, Blot WJ, Mehl ES, Mandel JS. Problems in the use of dead controls in case-control studies. I. General results. *Am J Epidemiol.* 1985;121:131-139.

19. Gail M, Williams R, Byar DP, Brown C. How many controls? *J Chronic Dis.* 1976;29:723-731.

20. Correa A, Stewart WF, Yeh H-C, Santos-Burgoa C. Exposure measurement in case-control studies: reported methods and recommendations. *Epidemiol Rev.* 1994;16:18-32.

21. Sadler TW. *Langman's Medical Embryology.* 13th ed. Philadelphia, PA: Wolters Kluwer Health; 2015.

22. Lash TL, Aschengrau A. Active and passive cigarette smoking and the occurrence of breast cancer. *Am J Epidemiol.* 1999;149:5-12.

23. Aschengrau A, Zierler S, Cohen A. Quality of community drinking water and the occurrence of late adverse pregnancy outcomes. *Arch Environ Health.* 1993;48:105-113.

24. Kasim K, Levallois P, Johnson KC, Abdous B, Auger P, Canadian Cancer Registries Epidemiology Research Group. Chlorination disinfection by-products in drinking water and the risk of adult leukemia in Canada. *Am J Epidemiol.* 2006;163:116-126.

25. Understanding the Safe Drinking Water Act. epa .gov. www.epa.gov/sites/production/files/2015-04 /documents/epa816f04030.pdf. Accessed October 2016.

26. Hulka BS, Wilcosky TC, Griffin JD. *Biological Markers in Epidemiology.* New York, NY: Oxford University Press; 1990.

27. Glynn AW, Willett LB. Food frequency questionnaires as a measure of exposure to organochlorines in epidemiological studies. *Ohio State University Bulletin: Special Circular, 1991-1997:163-199.*

28. Pearce N. What does the odds ratio estimate in a case-control study? *Int J Epidemiol.* 1993;22: 1189-1192.

29. Maclure M. The case-crossover design: a method for studying transient effects on the risk of acute events. *Am J Epidemiol.* 1991;133:144-153.

30. Mittleman MA, Maclure M, Robins JM. Control sampling strategies for case-crossover studies: an assessment of relative efficiency. *Am J Epidemiol.* 1995;142:91-98.

31. Redelmeier DA, Tibshirani RJ. Association between cellular-telephone calls and motor vehicle collisions. *New Engl J Med.* 1997;336:453-458.

32. Wellenius GA, Schwartz J, Mittleman MA. Particulate air pollution and hospital admissions for congestive heart failure in seven United States cities. *Am J Cardiol.* 2006;97:404-408.

33. Seage GR, Holte S, Gross M, Koblin B, Marmor M, Mayer KH, et al. Case-crossover study of partner and situational factors for unprotected sex. *J Acquir Immune Defic Syndr.* 2002;31(4):432-439.

34. Kinlin LM, Mittleman MA, Harris AD, Rubin MA, Fisman DN. Use of gloves and reduction of risk of injury caused by needles or sharp medical devices in healthcare workers. *Infect Cont Hosp Ep.* 2010;31(9):908-917.

35. Mittleman MA, Maclure M, Tofler GH, Sherwood JB, Goldberg RJ, Muller JE. Triggering of acute myocardial infarction by heavy exertion: protection against triggering by regular exertion. *New Engl J Med.* 1993;329:1677-1683.

36. Louis TA, Lavori PW, Bailar JC, Polansky M. Crossover and self-controlled designs in clinical research. *New Engl J Med.* 1984;310:24-31.

37. Armenian HK, Lillienfeld DE. Overview and historical perspective. *Epidemiol Rev.* 1994;16:1-5.

38. Comstock GW. Evaluating vaccination effectiveness and vaccine efficacy by means of case-control studies. *Epidemiol Rev.* 1994;16:77-89.

39. Selby JV. Case-control evaluations of treatment and program efficacy. *Epidemiol Rev.* 1994;16:90-101.

40. Dwyer DM, Strickler H, Goodman RA, Armenian HK. Use of case-control studies in outbreak investigations. *Epidemiol Rev.* 1994;16:109-123.

41. Pilishvili T, Chrenyshova L, Bondarenko A, Lapiy F, Sychova I, Cohen A. Evaluation of the effectiveness of *Haemophilus influenzae* type b conjugate vaccine introduction against radiologically-confirmed hospitalized pneumonia in young children in Ukraine. *J Peds.* 2013;163:s12-s18.

42. Thompson DC, Rivara FP, Thompson RS. Effectiveness of bicycle safety helmets in preventing head injuries. *JAMA.* 1996;276(24):1968-1973.

43. Todd J, Fishaut M, Kapral F, Welch T. Toxic-shock syndrome associated with phage-group-I staphylococci. *Lancet.* 1978;2:1116-1118.

44. Davis JP, Chesney PJ, Wand PJ, LaVenture M, Investigation and Laboratory Team. Toxic-shock syndrome: epidemiologic features, recurrence, risk factors, and prevention. *New Engl J Med.* 1980;303: 1429-1435.

45. Austin H, Hill HA, Flanders WD, Greenberg RS. Limitations in the application of case-control methodology. *Epidemiol Rev.* 1994;16:65-76.

Chapter Questions

1. Define each of the following terms:
   a. TROHOC and TROHOC fallacy
   b. Odds ratio
   c. Case–crossover study

2. Describe the situations in which it is desirable to conduct a case–control study.

3. Suppose that a case–control study was conducted in the United States to find out whether a Black woman's exposure to racism during pregnancy influenced her risk of giving birth prematurely. Investigators selected 500 cases who were hospitalized for premature delivery and 1,000 controls. The study found that 90 case mothers and 50 control mothers reported overt incidents of racism during their pregnancy.
   a. Set up the two-by-two table for these data.
   b. Calculate the odds ratio.
   c. State in words your interpretation of this odds ratio.
   d. Suppose that the investigators hire you as an epidemiological consultant to help them design this study. They ask you what type of control group is most appropriate for the study. Briefly describe the control group that you would advise them to select, and justify your choice.
   e. The investigators also ask you to describe the purpose of the control group in a case–control study. What would you tell them?

4. Describe one advantage and one disadvantage of using population controls in a case–control study.

5. Describe the three strategies—survivor sampling, case–base sampling, and risk set sampling—that investigators use to select controls.

6. State the main advantages and disadvantages of case–control studies.

7. Indicate whether the following statements are true or false:
   a. It is possible to obtain a valid estimate of disease prevalence from a typical case–control study.
   b. The purpose of a control group in a case–control study is to provide information on the disease distribution in the source population that produced the cases.
   c. The control group in a case–control study should never include individuals who have the case's disease.

    d.   A case–control study is the most efficient design for studying the health effects of rare exposures, whereas a cohort study is the most efficient design for studying the risk factors for rare diseases.

    e.   Case identification is generally more difficult than control identification in case–control studies.

    f.   The odds of illness are mathematically equivalent to the risk of illness.

    g.   It is preferable to use incident (that is, newly diagnosed) cases in a case–control study.

8.   Why do investigators use the odds ratio used in a case–control study (instead of the risk or rate ratio) to measure the strength of the association between an exposure and a disease?

CHAPTER 10

Bias

LEARNING OBJECTIVES

By the end of this chapter the reader will be able to:

- Describe the key features and provide examples of selection bias, including control selection bias; self-selection bias; loss to follow-up; and differential surveillance, diagnosis, or referral.
- Describe the key features and provide examples of information bias, including recall bias, interviewer bias, and differential and nondifferential misclassification.
- Discuss how the magnitude and direction of bias can affect study results.
- List the ways that selection and information bias can be avoided or minimized.

▶ Introduction

Epidemiological studies generally compare the frequency of disease in two (or more) groups according to a characteristic of interest. The characteristic is usually called the exposure. Those who have it form the exposed group, and those who do not have it form the unexposed group. Epidemiologists compare measures of disease frequency in two ways: (1) absolute measure of comparison, such as **rate or risk difference**, and (2) relative measure of comparison, such as **rate or risk ratio**, **ratio**, and **odds ratio**. These comparisons are commonly called **measures of association** or **measures of effect**. The particular measure that is calculated depends on the study design, the type of data, and the goal of the comparison. Absolute measures typically describe the public health impact of an exposure, and relative measures describe the strength of the causal relationship between an exposure and a disease.

After investigators calculate the measure of association, they must evaluate whether the observed result is true. That is, they must assess the internal **validity** of the study results. A study is considered valid only when the following three alternative explanations have been eliminated:

1. **Bias**: A systematic error in the design or conduct of study that leads to an erroneous association between the exposure and disease.
2. **Confounding**: The mixing of effects between the exposure; the disease; and a third variable, which is termed a confounder. Like bias, confounding distorts the relationship between an exposure and a disease.
3. **Random error**: The probability that the observed result is attributable to **chance**, an uncontrollable force that seems to have no assignable cause.[1(p309)]

If systematic bias, confounding, and random error have been ruled out as alternative explanations, the investigator may conclude that the association is true and the study has internal validity. Only after an observed study result is deemed valid is it appropriate to assess whether the exposure has actually caused the outcome. Making causal inferences is a complicated judgment.

In addition, internal validity must be established before the study results can be generalized to populations beyond the study subjects. The evaluation of **generalizability**, or "external validity," requires review of the study methods; the makeup of the study population; and subject-matter knowledge, such as the biological basis of the association. For example, a valid study of risk factors for coronary artery disease among middle-aged U.S. men might be applicable to middle-aged European men but not to middle-aged U.S. or European women because of biological differences between the genders. On the other hand, an invalid study of coronary artery disease among middle-aged U.S. men is generalizable to no one.

This chapter discusses bias in general terms and then focuses on the two main forms of bias in epidemiological research: selection bias and information bias. Following a definition of each type of bias, the chapter describes the ways in which it arises and methods for avoiding or minimizing it.

▶ Overview of Bias

Epidemiologists define bias as a systematic error that results in an incorrect or invalid estimate of the measure of association. Bias can be introduced at any stage of a study, including during the design, data collection, analysis, or even publication stage. An epidemiologist's definition of bias differs from another common definition of the term: "preference or inclination, especially one that inhibits impartial judgment," or "prejudice."[1(p176)] In epidemiological studies, bias does not usually occur because the investigator is prejudiced but rather because of ignorance or unavoidable decisions made during the course of a study.

Bias can occur in all types of epidemiological studies. However, retrospective studies are more susceptible to bias than prospective studies because of differences in the timing of the study. The two main types of bias are selection bias, which can occur during the selection and follow-up of study participants, and information (or observation) bias, which can occur during data collection.

When evaluating a study for the presence of bias, investigators must (1) identify its source, (2) estimate its magnitude or strength, and (3) assess its direction. Recognizing and carefully dissecting the source of the bias is a prerequisite for assessing the strength and direction of the bias. Regarding its magnitude, a small amount of bias does not usually have a major effect on the study results; however, a large amount of bias can completely alter the study findings. For example, consider a true risk ratio of 2.5. A small amount of bias might alter the estimate of the true risk ratio slightly, say, to 2.3 or 2.8. Even though some bias is present, the conclusion that there is a moderate association is still correct. However, a large amount of bias could alter the estimate of the true risk ratio a great deal, say, to 1.0 or 5.0, and lead to an incorrect conclusion.

The effect of bias also depends on the size of the true measure of association. Bias can account entirely for a weak association, but it is unlikely to account entirely for a strong association. This is one reason epidemiologists have greater confidence that strong associations are valid.

Regarding the direction of the bias, a systematic error can pull the estimate either toward or away from the null. Stated another way, it can either underestimate or overestimate the true measure of association. When the direction of the bias is toward the null, it means that the error causes the true measure of association to be underestimated (see **FIGURE 10-1**). For example, if the true risk ratio is 1.9 (or a 90% increased risk), the observed risk ratio will be lower, say, 1.4 (or a 40% increased risk) if there is a bias toward the null. Similarly, if the true risk ratio is 0.4 (or a 60% reduced risk), the observed risk ratio will be smaller, say, 0.7 (or a 30% reduced risk) if there is a bias toward the null.

On the other hand, bias can pull results away from the null and overestimate the true association (see **FIGURE 10-2**). For example, if the true risk ratio is 2.0, then the observed risk ratio will be greater, say, 2.6, if there is a bias away from the null. Similarly, if the true risk ratio is 0.5, the observed risk ratio will be greater, say, 0.3, if there is a bias away from the null.

Unfortunately, little can be done to fix or remove a bias once it has occurred. Thus, investigators must attempt to avoid bias by carefully designing and conducting the study. For example, epidemiological studies include features such as masking to avoid bias. Key facts about bias are summarized in **TABLE 10-1**.

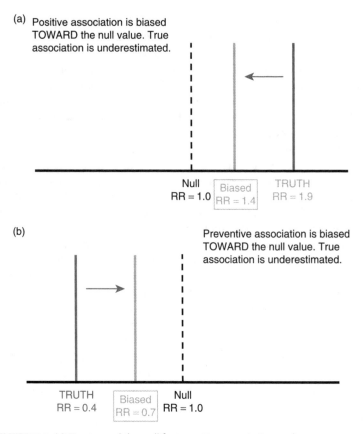

(a) Positive association is biased TOWARD the null value. True association is underestimated.

(b) Preventive association is biased TOWARD the null value. True association is underestimated.

FIGURE 10-1 (a) Bias toward the null for a positive association and (b) a preventive association. RR = risk ratio.

▶ Selection Bias

Selection bias is an error that results "from procedures used to select subjects into the study or the analysis."[2(p258)] Thus, selection bias results from procedures used to choose study subjects that give a result among participants that is different from the result that would occur among all eligible individuals in the source population. See **FIGURE 10-3** for a graphic depiction of this concept. This type of bias is more likely in case–control and retrospective cohort studies because both the exposure and outcome have occurred by the time the subjects are selected. Selection bias can also occur in cohort and experimental studies from differential **losses to follow-up**.

It is often easier to understand selection bias if it is described in the context of a specific study design. Selection bias occurs in a case–control study if selection of cases and controls is based on differing criteria that are related to exposure status. In contrast, selection bias occurs in a retrospective cohort study if selection of exposed and unexposed individuals is related to developing the outcome of interest[3(pp273-274)] or follow-up of

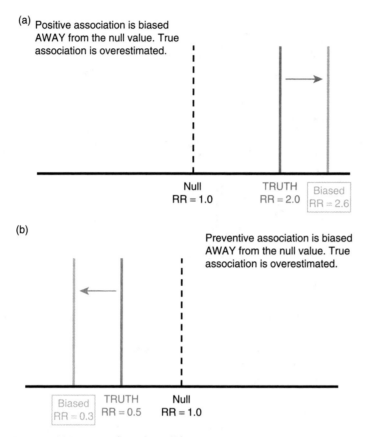

(a) Positive association is biased AWAY from the null value. True association is overestimated.

Null RR = 1.0   TRUTH RR = 2.0   Biased RR = 2.6

(b) Preventive association is biased AWAY from the null value. True association is overestimated.

Biased RR = 0.3   TRUTH RR = 0.5   Null RR = 1.0

FIGURE 10-2 (a) Bias away from the null for a positive association and (b) a preventive association. RR = risk ratio.

TABLE 10-1 Key Facts About Bias

- An alternative explanation for an association

- Usually does not result from a "prejudiced" investigator

- Can pull an association either toward or away from the null

- Amount of bias can be small, moderate, or large

- Is avoided when the study is carefully designed and conducted

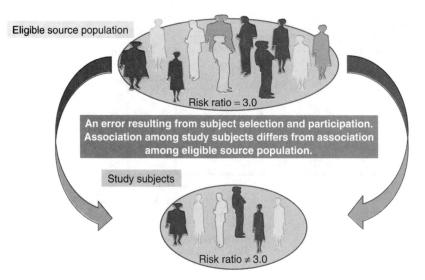

Eligible source population

Risk ratio = 3.0

An error resulting from subject selection and participation. Association among study subjects differs from association among eligible source population.

Study subjects

Risk ratio ≠ 3.0

FIGURE 10-3 Depiction of selection bias.

exposed and unexposed individuals is related to developing the outcome of interest.

Selection bias can occur in several ways, including selection of an inappropriate control group in a case–control study (control selection bias); refusal, nonresponse, or agreement to participate that is related to the exposure and disease (self-selection bias); losses to follow-up that are related to both the exposure and disease; selection of the general population as a comparison group in an occupational cohort study (healthy worker effect); and differential surveillance, diagnosis, or referral of study subjects according to their exposure and disease status.[3(pp273-274)] These problems can bias the results of a study either toward or away from the null. Examples of selection bias in case–control and cohort studies are described in the following sections.

Selection Bias in a Case–Control Study

Control Selection Bias

As an example of **control selection bias**, consider a hypothetical case–control study in which investigators are evaluating the role of Pap smears in the prevention of cervical cancer. Investigators identify newly diagnosed cases of cervical cancer by reviewing medical records from the hospitals where cancer patients are treated. They select population controls from among women who live in the same neighborhoods as cases. Investigators identify controls by canvassing neighborhoods on foot during weekday working hours. Thus, only controls who are at home during canvassing periods are included in the study. The investigators select and enroll 250 cases and 250 controls. Women are considered exposed if they had a Pap smear within 1 year of their diagnosis date (for cases) or an index date (for controls). Comparable index dates are assigned to controls to match the diagnosis dates of the cases. Let us examine the data that are produced by this study (see **TABLE 10-2**).

Exactly 40% of cases and 40% of controls had a Pap smear within the past year. Using the formula for the odds ratio (OR), we find that there is no association between Pap smears and cervical cancer OR = (ad/bc) = $(100 \times 150)/(150 \times 100) = 1.0$.

Unfortunately, this study suffers from control selection bias because the researchers included only controls who were home at the time of recruitment. It turns out that women who are at home during the day are less likely to be employed and therefore are less likely to have regular medical checkups, including Pap smears. Thus, the selected control group has a lower proportion of women with prior Pap smears than does the source population that produced the cases. The data presented in **TABLE 10-3** depict the true relationship between Pap smears and cervical cancer that would have been produced in the absence of selection bias.

Note that 40% of the cases and 60% of the controls had a Pap smear within the past year. Thus, the true odds ratio is $(100 \times 100)/(150 \times 150)$, or 0.44, which means that there is a 56% reduced odds of cervical cancer among women with recent Pap smears. Thus, the results with control selection bias were biased toward the null.

TABLE 10-2 Observed Relationship Between Cervical Cancer and Pap Smears

Pap smear	Cases	Controls
Yes	100	100
No	150	150
Total	250	250

TABLE 10-3 True Relationship Between Cervical Cancer and Pap Smears

Pap smear	Cases	Controls
Yes	100	150
No	150	100
Total	250	250

Returning to the description of selection bias in case–control studies, we can conclude that selection bias occurred in this study because investigators did not use the same criteria to select cases and controls (being home during the day was required for controls but not for cases) and these criteria were related to exposure status (recent Pap smear history). Furthermore, because different criteria were used for selecting cases and controls, the control group did not accurately represent the exposure distribution in the source population that produced the cases. Control selection bias can be avoided by remembering the purpose of the control group: to sample the exposure distribution in the base population that gave rise to the cases. Using identical selection criteria will ensure that cases and controls come from the same source population.

Self-Selection Bias

Case–control studies with low and moderate participation rates are susceptible to **self-selection bias** arising from refusal or nonresponse by participants that is related to both the exposure and disease or agreement to participate that is related to both the exposure and disease. A low or moderate participation rate does not necessarily result in selection bias if the reasons and rates of participation are similar for exposed and unexposed cases and controls. However, if subjects in a particular exposure–disease category (e.g., exposed cases) are more or less likely to participate than subjects in another category, the observed measure of association will be biased. Scenarios with and without self-selection bias are depicted in **TABLE 10-4**.

TABLE 10-4 Scenarios with and Without Self-Selection Bias		
No Self-Selection Bias: Equal Participation Rates		
	Cases*	**Controls***
Exposed	60%	60%
Unexposed	60%	60%
Self-Selection Bias: Unequal Participation Rates That Are Associated with the Exposure and Disease		
	Cases*	**Controls***
Exposed	80%	60%
Unexposed	60%	60%

*The numbers in the cells are participation rates.

The best way to ensure that self-selection bias does not occur is to obtain high participation rates among both cases and controls. Although there is no magical response rate that guarantees the absence of selection bias (other than 100%), most epidemiologists are highly satisfied with participation rates greater than 80%. In addition, investigators can assess the presence of self-selection bias in a study by examining the characteristics of participants and nonparticipants.

Differential Surveillance, Diagnosis, or Referral

Selection bias can occur in a case–control study as a result of differential surveillance, diagnosis, or referral of cases that is related to the exposure.[3(pp273-274)] A well-known example of this type of selection bias occurred in a case–control study on the risk of venous thromboembolism among oral contraceptive users.[4] Cases were women aged 20 to 44 years who were hospitalized for a venous thromboembolism. Controls were similarly aged women who were hospitalized for an acute illness or elective surgery at the same hospitals. Of the cases, 72% reported using oral contraceptives, and only 20% of controls used them. Based on these findings, investigators calculated a 10.2-fold increased odds of thromboembolism among current oral contraceptive users.

The investigators acknowledged that the high odds ratio might be caused by "bias in the criteria for hospital admission."[4] Several reports of the association between oral contraceptives and venous thromboembolism had already been published before this study was conducted. As a result of these previously published studies, healthcare providers were more likely to hospitalize women with symptoms of thromboembolism who were currently taking oral contraceptives than symptomatic women who were not taking oral contraceptives. The tendency to hospitalize patients on the basis of their exposure status led to a stronger observed relationship between oral contraceptives and thromboembolism than truly existed. Another study based on cases that were diagnosed before there was widespread knowledge of this association found only a fourfold increased odds.[5]

How could selection bias have been avoided in this study? First, investigators could have conducted a community-based case–control study that included both hospitalized and nonhospitalized subjects, or the hospital-based study could have been limited to severe cases of thromboembolism for which hospitalization was required. Both of these options would have resulted in an unbiased prevalence of oral contraceptive use in the case group. The former option is preferable to the latter, which restricts the case series by severity and therefore reduces generalizability.

Selection Bias in a Cohort Study

Selection bias occurs in a cohort study when the choice of exposed and unexposed individuals is related to developing the outcome of interest or when losses to follow-up are related to both the exposure and outcome of interest. Retrospective cohort studies are prone to the former type of selection bias because both the exposure and disease have occurred by the time of subject selection. Both retrospective and prospective cohort studies (and experimental studies) can experience the latter form of selection bias.

Losses to Follow-Up

A serious concern in a cohort study, losses to follow-up, arises when subjects can no longer be located or they no longer want to participate in a study. Losses to follow-up are problematic because they can reduce the power of the study to detect associations that are truly present (because of the smaller sample size available for analysis) and can bias the study results.

Nondifferential losses to follow-up refers to losses on one axis (disease or exposure) that are unrelated to the other axis. An example is the loss of diseased individuals that occurs equally among exposed and unexposed individuals. Differential losses to follow-up refers to losses that are related to both exposure and disease. An example is when these losses are more or less likely to occur among exposed individuals who develop the disease than among unexposed individuals who develop the disease.

Whether losses to follow-up bias the results depends on the measure of association being used (i.e., absolute or relative) and whether the losses are nondifferential or differential. For example, nondifferential losses to follow-up that are associated only with disease (e.g., there are equal losses of diseased individuals among exposed and unexposed subjects) result in observed disease incidences that are lower than true incidences. This means that the relative measure of association will not be affected but the absolute measure will be biased toward the null. On the other hand, differential losses to follow-up can bias relative and absolute measures of association either upward or downward. For example, if losses to follow-up occur only among exposed subjects who develop the disease, the observed measure of disease frequency in the exposed group will be lower than the truth, and therefore relative and absolute measures of association will be biased toward the null. On the other hand, if losses to follow-up occur only among unexposed subjects who develop the disease, then the observed measure of disease frequency in the unexposed group will be lower than the truth and both relative and absolute measures of association will be biased upward.

Unfortunately, it is rarely possible to determine whether losses are differential or nondifferential because outcome information is unknown. Thus, it is important to maintain high and similar follow-up rates for compared groups. To achieve this goal, epidemiologists use many methods to maximize retention and trace study subjects, including collecting baseline information to help locate study subjects, maintaining regular mail or personal contact with participants, sending additional mailings to nonrespondents, and checking numerous tracing resources.

Healthy Worker Effect

The **healthy worker effect** is another form of selection bias that occurs in two special types of cohort studies—**proportional mortality ratio (PMR)** and **standardized mortality ratio (SMR)** studies. The healthy worker effect occurs in these studies because the general population, which consists of both healthy and ill people, is selected for comparison to a relatively healthy working population. For example, the radiation-exposed workers in a study of Portsmouth Naval Shipyard workers experienced a 25% lower mortality rate than the general population.[6,7] This was likely because the radiation-exposed workers were required to undergo special physical examination to be eligible for this work, were examined every 3 years, and those with abnormal findings were removed from the program.

In summary, selection bias can be a serious problem in epidemiological studies, which can bias results either toward or away from the null. Because little can be done to correct this bias once it has occurred, epidemiologists must use all available methods to avoid it. The key facts about selection bias are summarized in **TABLE 10-5**.

TABLE 10-5 Key Facts About Selection Bias

- Selection bias is an error that arises from systematic differences in selecting and following the study groups.

- It is more likely to occur in case–control and retrospective cohort studies because both the exposure and disease have occurred by the time of subject selection. It can also occur in prospective cohort and experimental studies when there are differential losses to follow-up.

- Specific types include control selection bias in case–control studies; healthy worker effect in occupational cohort studies; self-selection bias; differential losses to follow-up; and differential surveillance, diagnosis, or referral of subjects according to exposure and disease status.

- Little can be done to fix this bias once it has occurred.

- It can bias an association either toward or away from the null.

- Methods for avoiding it include using the same criteria for selecting cases and controls, obtaining high participation rates, using a variety of methods to successfully trace study subjects, and taking diagnostic and referral practices into account when designing a study.

▶ Information Bias

Information bias is "a flaw in measuring exposure, covariate, or outcome variables that results in different quality (accuracy) of information between comparison groups."[2(p149)] Information bias arises from a systematic difference in the way that the exposure or outcome is measured between compared groups. For example, information bias can occur in a case–control study if different techniques are used for interviewing cases and controls, or it can occur in a cohort study if different procedures are used to obtain outcome information on exposed and unexposed subjects. Information bias can be thought of as a measurement error that distorts the true association between an exposure and a disease. Key features of this bias are that (1) it occurs after the subjects have entered the study, (2) it pertains to how the data are collected, and (3) it often results in incorrect classification of participants as either exposed or unexposed or as diseased or not diseased.

Like selection bias, information bias can create a bias either toward or away from the null. The direction depends on a number of factors, particularly whether the measurement error on one axis (exposure or disease) depends on the other axis (disease or exposure). Information bias can also occur in both prospective and retrospective studies.

The following section describes and provides examples of the different types of information bias, including recall bias, interviewer bias, and differential and nondifferential misclassification. An investigator's decision to use a particular data collection method (such as interviews, preexisting records, or biological specimens) is influenced by its potential for information bias. This bias can be avoided only by carefully designing and conducting the study.

Recall Bias

Recall bias occurs when there is a differential level of accuracy in the information provided by compared groups. Thus, recall bias occurs in a case–control study if cases are more or less likely than controls to recall and report prior exposures, and it occurs in a cohort study if exposed subjects are more or less likely than unexposed subjects to recall and report subsequent diseases. Note that the term *poor recall* is different from recall bias because the former implies a similar level of inaccuracy among groups, that is, equally inaccurate recall for both cases and controls (in a case–control study) and equally inaccurate recall for both exposed and unexposed subjects (in a cohort study).

Differences in reporting accuracy associated with recall bias are thought to result from subjects' failure to report information rather than a tendency to fabricate information. Differential recall can bias the true measure of association either toward or away from the null. The direction depends on which subjects (cases versus controls or exposed versus unexposed subjects) have less accurate recall.

Although recall bias can occur in both case–control and retrospective cohort studies, it is typically described in the context of a traditional case–control study with nondiseased controls. For example, consider a hypothetical case–control study of birth defects that includes malformed infants as cases and healthy infants as controls. Exposure data are collected at postpartum interviews with the infants' mothers. In the classic recall bias scenario, the data gathered from case mothers is more accurate than data from control mothers. This is because mothers of malformed case infants have been carefully reviewing every illness that occurred during the affected pregnancy, every medication taken, every alcoholic beverage consumed, and so forth for a possible reason for their child's defect. In contrast, mothers of healthy control infants have spent less time reviewing their prenatal activities. The results of the hypothetical study are depicted in TABLE 10-6. Note that 100% of the case mothers (20/20) reported their prior exposures and only 75% of healthy control mothers (15/20) did so. Thus, the observed odds ratio is biased upward by 40%. If there had been more underreporting among control mothers, the upward bias would have been even larger.

It is also possible to envision a scenario in which the mothers of the cases underreport their prior exposures. This is likely to occur with socially sensitive exposures, such as drug and alcohol use, that mothers may not wish to admit for fear of being blamed for their child's condition. TABLE 10-7 presents data from a hypothetical study in which all control mothers (20/20) reported their prior exposures and 75% of case mothers (30/40) did so. This differential recall biases the true odds ratio downward by 37% $[(2.7 - 1.7)/(2.7 \times 100\%)] = 37\%$. Here, if more underreporting had occurred among case mothers, the downward bias would have been even larger. The two examples presented in Tables 10-6 and 10-7 demonstrate that the direction of the bias is determined by which group has less accurate recall.

TABLE 10-6 Recall Bias Scenario: Controls Underreport Exposure

| | Truth | | | Observed study data | |
	Case	Control		Case	Control
Exposed	20	20	Exposed	20	15
Unexposed	80	80	Unexposed	80	85
Total	100	100	Total	100	100
	Odds ratio: 1.0			Odds ratio: 1.4	

TABLE 10-7 Recall Bias Scenario: Cases Underreport Exposure

	Truth			Observed study data	
	Case	Control		Case	Control
Exposed	40	20	Exposed	30	20
Unexposed	60	80	Unexposed	70	80
Total	100	100	Total	100	100
	Odds ratio: 2.7			Odds ratio: 1.7	

Now, let us consider a classic example of recall bias that occurred in an actual case–control study of drug exposures among children with congenital heart defects.[8] Cases were infants born with congenital heart disease from 1973 through 1975. Controls were randomly selected infants born in the same time period and geographic area. Information on prenatal drug exposure was obtained by self-administered questionnaires. Data on hormonal drug exposures were obtained from closed-ended questions, and data on nonhormonal drug exposures were obtained from an open-ended question, "Did you take any prescription or nonprescription drugs during your pregnancy?"

The study found an 80% increased risk of cardiac malformations among infants of women who recalled using the antinausea medication Bendectin in early pregnancy. Because information about the use of this medication was derived from the open-ended question, the researchers concluded that it was "likely to be subject to some recall bias." In fact, a later study that was specifically designed to evaluate and remove recall bias found no meaningful increase in the risk of cardiac malformations in association with Bendectin use.[9]

Only a few investigations have been conducted to document the actual occurrence of recall bias. Some of these studies have validated information obtained at postpartum interviews with that found in medical records. For example, Werler and colleagues assessed whether recall bias was present in postpartum interviews with mothers of malformed and nonmalformed infants by comparing interview data with data documented during pregnancy in obstetric records.[10] Mothers of malformed infants were more accurate reporters than mothers of nonmalformed infants for some but not all variables. Mothers of malformed infants were more accurate reporters regarding use of birth control after conception and history of urinary tract infections, but the two groups of mothers showed similar reporting accuracy for history of an elective abortion and over-the-counter drug use. These results suggest that recall bias is not widespread and may be exposure specific.

In other studies, investigators evaluated the presence of recall bias by comparing associations with normal controls to those with malformed controls. These studies have found, for example, that the use of multivitamin supplementation and medications such as decongestants and analgesics during pregnancy was remarkably similar for both types of controls, providing further evidence that concern for recall bias may be overrated.[11]

Although we await more research to determine the true extent of recall bias in epidemiological studies, it is worthwhile to review the steps that epidemiologists take to minimize or avoid its occurrence. The most common method for minimizing recall bias is to select a diseased control group. For example, the study of Bendectin and cardiac malformations compared cases with a specific cardiac malformation to cases with other cardiac malformations.[9] This type of comparison assumes that the exposure is unlikely to cause a general increase in the risk of all types of defects.

Another way to avoid recall bias is to design a structured questionnaire so that exposure ascertainment is complete and accurate. This strategy is important because the opportunity for recall bias increases as exposure ascertainment decreases. For example, a novel study was conducted to examine the effect of questionnaire design on the ascertainment of drug use during pregnancy.[12] Investigators obtained information on drug use in the past year from a sequence of three questions. The first question was open ended: "Were any medications prescribed to you during pregnancy?" The second question asked about drug use for selected indications: "Did you take any medication for the following indications: pain, tension, seizures, or nausea and vomiting?" The third question asked about the use of specifically named drugs: "Did you take any of the following medications? Aspirin, Tylenol, Valium, Compazine, Bendectin." The investigators found that the open-ended question led to vast underreporting of drug use (see **TABLE 10-8**). There was much less underreporting in response to questions about drug use for certain indications and use of specifically named drugs. The investigators concluded that a comprehensive series of questions is necessary to obtain as complete information as possible.

Another way to improve the accuracy of questionnaire data, particularly for socially sensitive topics that the study subject is reluctant to reveal to another individual, is to use either a self-administered questionnaire or audio computer-assisted self-interviewing (ACASI) questionnaire. Self-administered questionnaires are usually scannable to facilitate computer entry. The study subject simply fills out the questionnaire using paper and pencil. A laptop computer with an audio component is used to administer the ACASI questionnaire. The computer reads each question to the subject and waits for the subject to enter a response before moving on to the next question.

Both approaches have been useful for obtaining information on sensitive topics, such as alcohol drinking, illicit drug use, and sexual behaviors. For example, the HIV NET Vaccine Preparedness Study,

TABLE 10-8 Ascertainment of Drug Use According to Type of Question Asked								
	Question asked*							
	Open-ended		**Indication**		**Specific drug name**		**Total users**	
	No.	%	No.	%	No.	%	No.	%
Valium	4	13	18	58	9	29	31	100
Darvon	5	25	8	40	7	35	20	100
Aspirin	2	1	146	77	41	22	189	100
Acetaminophen	0	0	58	61	37	39	95	100

*Asked in sequence.
Data from Mitchell AA, Cottler LB, Shapiro S. Effect of questionnaire design on recall of drug exposure in pregnancy. *Am J Epidemiol*. 1986;123:670-676.

a prospective cohort study of nearly 5,000 individuals at high risk for human immunodeficiency virus, type 1 (HIV-1) infection, compared ACASI with in-person interviews for gathering information on sexual behaviors.[13] Subjects were randomized to receive either personal or computer interviews. The investigators found that men who had sex with men were much more likely to report that they had unprotected receptive anal intercourse using the ACASI format. Although the true prevalence of unprotected receptive anal intercourse was unknown in this population, the higher proportion reported by using ACASI is probably more accurate than that reported in personal interviews.

Either self-administered questionnaires or ACASI can be used in clinical and research settings. For example, the subject can fill out the questionnaire in the clinic waiting room, or a self-administered questionnaire can be mailed to subjects at home to be filled out at their convenience. Of course, self-administered questionnaires require that subjects have an adequate reading and comprehension level; fill out the questionnaire completely; and, if mailed, return the completed questionnaire to the investigator. Although a small token of appreciation is often included with mailed questionnaires (such as cash or movie passes), response rates are typically lower than those from other formats. The ACASI format avoids many of these problems because little or no reading is required and the questionnaire can be taken into the field with laptop computers.

Still another way to avoid recall bias is to forgo questionnaires entirely and rely instead on biological measurements and preexisting records for the necessary study data. For example, medical records are often used to provide detailed information on diseases and their treatment.

These records are also used to validate information provided at interviews and to provide evidence for or against recall bias. For example, exposure data in the case–control study of Bendectin use and congenital heart disease came from two sources: a postdelivery telephone interview and the prenatal obstetric record.[9] Drug use noted in the prenatal record was assumed to be free of recall bias because it was recorded before the pregnancy outcome was known. Investigators analyzed Bendectin exposure according to the interview alone, the obstetric record alone, and both sources combined. They found virtually identical results and therefore provided evidence against differential recall.

Investigators often determine whether recall bias is present by asking subjects about their knowledge of the study hypothesis, usually at the end of the interview. The association between the exposure and outcome is analyzed separately among those with and without knowledge of the hypothesis. Those with knowledge are thought to be more prone to recall bias than those without such knowledge.

For example, women were asked the following questions in a study of periconceptional folic acid exposure and the risk of neural tube defects: "Have you heard there are any vitamins, minerals, or anything else that may cause or reduce the risk of birth defects?" If a participant answered yes, she was asked, "What vitamin or mineral?" and "Is this related to any particular birth defect?"[14] About 17% of case mothers and 3% of control mothers reported that folic acid reduced the risk of neural tube defects. Daily use of folic acid was associated with a 20% decreased risk of neural tube defects among women who were familiar with the study hypothesis and a 60% reduction among women who did not have any knowledge of the hypothesis. These findings led the investigators to conclude that recall bias was present among women who knew the study hypothesis and that they should draw their main conclusions from women without knowledge of the hypothesis.

Interviewer Bias

Interviewer bias is a systematic difference in soliciting, recording, or interpreting information that occurs in studies using in-person or telephone interviews. Interviewer bias can occur in every type of epidemiological study. It can occur in a case–control study when interviewers are aware of the disease status of a subject and question cases and controls differently about their exposures. It can occur in cohort and experimental studies when interviewers are aware of the exposure or treatment status of a subject and query exposed and unexposed subjects differently about their diseases.

Interviewer bias can be avoided by masking interviewers to the subjects' disease (in case–control studies) or exposure status (in cohort and experimental studies). However, masking interviewers is often impossible because of the information they learn while talking with the subjects. For example, a case–control study of the risk of spontaneous abortion among women with a prior induced abortion collected data using personal interviews during the subjects' hospital stay.[15] It was impossible to mask the interviewers to subjects' disease status because cases who had spontaneous abortions were placed on gynecology floors and delivery patient controls were placed on obstetric floors and were frequently interviewed in the presence of their newborn infants.

Another way to avoid interviewer bias is to design standardized questionnaires consisting of closed-ended, easy-to-understand questions with appropriate response options. This decreases the likelihood that the interviewer will interpret the question for the subject or will need to probe the subject for an appropriate response. Understandable questions that are asked in exactly the same manner are key components for reducing interviewer bias.

Writing understandable questions is both an art and a science, which falls under the discipline of psychometrics. Epidemiologists should collaborate with psychometricians when designing questionnaires to avoid several problems.[16(pp309-336)] First, investigators should avoid the use of ambiguous wording that can be interpreted in various ways. For example, the question "Have you ever smoked?" is ambiguous because it is unclear whether cigarettes, cigars, pipes, or a nontobacco product is the intended focus of the question. Second, researchers should avoid using two questions in one, such as "Do you get out of breath when you walk up a hill?" This question is problematic because a negative answer might mean that the respondent does not walk up hills or that he or she does not get out of breath doing so. Third, researchers should avoid the use of words such as medical terms or the names of chemicals that the respondent may not understand. Fourth, they should avoid asking about events and activities that the subjects cannot possibly remember, such as "Tell me the names of all the brands of condoms that you have used since you first started having sex." Fifth, investigators should avoid questions that are not self-explanatory, such as "How is heat delivered to your home?" Although the investigator may be interested in responses such as hot air, steam, gas, or oil, the respondent might reply, "In a truck!" Finally, researchers should avoid questions that have too many ideas, such as "Have you ever used oral contraceptives, condoms, diaphragms, or intrauterine devices?" A positive response will indicate that one or more of these contraceptives has been used but will not indicate which one(s).

Investigators need to write clear questions in the subjects' native language. In addition, given the international nature of epidemiological research and the populations being studied, epidemiologists often need to translate their questionnaires into several languages. Because accurate translation can be tricky, it is standard practice to have one person translate the questionnaire into the foreign language and another person translate it back to English and compare the back translation to the original. Word-for-word translations are often, but not always, the goal, for it is necessary to take into account cultural differences in the conceptualization of health-related events and exposures.

Another way to avoid interviewer bias is to instruct interviewers on appropriate questioning techniques, such as nondirective probing—a neutral way of searching for a suitable answer. These probes are needed when it is clear from a respondent's response that he or she has not understood the question. Nondirective probing techniques include simply repeating the question or asking "What do you mean by . . . ?" It is also important to note that the race, gender, age, and sexual orientation of an interviewer will have an effect on data quality. The demographic characteristics of the interviewer are usually matched to those of the subject to obtain the most accurate responses.

Misclassification

Misclassification, also called measurement error, is probably the most common form of bias in epidemiological research. Misclassification means that there is an error in the classification of the exposure or the disease. For example, misclassification occurs when an exposed individual is classified as unexposed or vice versa. It also occurs when a diseased individual is classified as nondiseased or vice versa. See **FIGURE 10-4** for a graphic depiction of this problem.

Misclassification arises in many ways. In case–control and retrospective cohort studies, the relevant exposures may have occurred many years before data collection, and therefore it is difficult for subjects to recall their exposures accurately. In other words, subjects have poor recall of

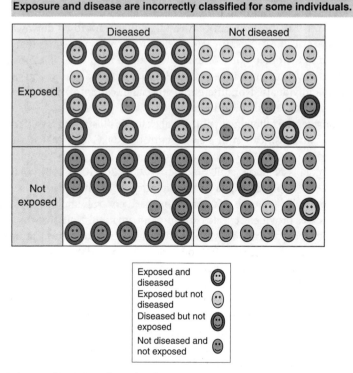

Exposure and disease are incorrectly classified for some individuals.

Exposed and diseased

Exposed but not diseased

Diseased but not exposed

Not diseased and not exposed

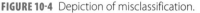

FIGURE 10-4 Depiction of misclassification.

their exposures. For example, a retrospective cohort study of drinking water pollution and pregnancy loss required subjects to recall pregnancy outcomes occurring over a 30-year period.[17] Exposure misclassification also occurs when broad exposure definitions are used. For example, occupational exposure definitions, such as job title (e.g., individuals who ever worked as a plumber), are misclassified because it is unlikely that all individuals with a particular job title actually sustain the exposure(s) of interest. Characteristics of the work environment, such as ventilation, and the use of personal protective equipment also influence whether an individual in a particular job is actually exposed.

Like exposure misclassification, disease misclassification can also occur as a result of an overly broad definition. For example, because birth defects are rare, investigators often group together defects into larger organ group categories, such as cardiovascular defects, central nervous system defects, and so on. This leads to misclassification when the exposure is related to some but not all defects in the group. For example, if all cardiovascular defects are grouped together, misclassification of disease will occur if the exposure increases the risk of one type of cardiovascular defect but not others.

Like losses to follow-up, there are two types of misclassification: nondifferential and differential. **Differential misclassification** refers to errors on one axis (exposure or disease) that are related to the other axis (exposure or disease). For example, if there is an error in exposure classification, it is more or less likely to occur for a diseased individual than a nondiseased individual. Depending on who is misclassified, differential misclassification can bias results either upward or downward. **Nondifferential misclassification** refers to errors on one axis that are unrelated to the other axis. For example, if there is an error in exposure classification, it occurs with equal likelihood among diseased and nondiseased individuals. Nondifferential misclassification of dichotomous variables biases results toward the null.

Consider the following hypothetical example illustrating the effect of exposure misclassification in a case–control study. Completely accurate data are described in **TABLE 10-9**. The odds ratio based on the completely accurate data is as follows: OR $= ad/bc = (200 \times 200/100 \times 100) = 4.0$.

TABLE 10-10 presents data with a high degree of differential misclassification. In this scenario, 50% of the exposed controls and 100% of the exposed cases provide accurate exposure information. Note that the different degree of accuracy between the compared groups is a key feature of differential misclassification. The odds ratio for these data is $(200 \times 250)/(100 \times 50) = 10.0$. In this scenario, differential misclassification biased results away from the null (from 4.0 to 10.0). If there had been less misclassification (say, 75% of the exposed controls gave accurate information), there would have been less bias away from the null.

What happens when the reverse occurs—that is, when exposure information from controls is more accurate than that obtained from cases? A scenario is shown in **TABLE 10-11** in which 50% of the exposed cases and 100% of the controls provided accurate exposure information.

TABLE 10-9 Completely Accurate Exposure Data from a Hypothetical Case–Control Study

	Cases	Controls
Exposed	200	100
Unexposed	100	200
Total	300	300
	Odds ratio: 4.0	

TABLE 10-10 Differential Misclassification of the Exposure in a Hypothetical Case–Control Study: Case Information Is More Accurate Than Control Information

	Cases	Controls
Exposed	200	50
Unexposed	100	250
Total	300	300
	Odds ratio: 10.0	

TABLE 10-11 Differential Misclassification of the Exposure in a Hypothetical Case–Control Study: Control Information Is More Accurate Than Case Information

	Cases	Controls
Exposed	100	100
Unexposed	200	200
Total	300	300
	Odds ratio: 1.0	

Now, the odds ratio is calculated as follows: $(100 \times 200)/(100 \times 200) = 1.0$. In this scenario, differential misclassification biased the results toward the null (from 4.0 to 1.0). Again, if there had been less misclassification, the bias would not have been as strong.

What happens if both cases and controls give similarly inaccurate information on their exposure histories? For example, say that 50% of the exposed cases and 50% of the exposed controls do not remember their exposure and are classified as unexposed (see **TABLE 10-12**). This scenario is an example of nondifferential misclassification because there is the same degree of accuracy between the compared groups.

The odds ratio is now $(100 \times 250)/(50 \times 200) = 2.5$. This is lower than the odds ratio based on the completely accurate data (4.0). Again, there would be less bias toward the null if less nondifferential misclassification had occurred.

This hypothetical example illustrates that differential exposure misclassification can lead to either an upward or a downward bias and that the direction depends on which group has more misclassification. It also illustrates that nondifferential misclassification of a dichotomous exposure biases results toward the null. In fact, it can bias the results beyond the null if misclassification is severe. In the most extreme case, it can lead to a completely inverse association (e.g., a twofold increased risk becomes a 50% decreased risk). The bias is much less predictable when the misclassified exposure variable has three or more categories. Of course, nondifferential exposure misclassification does not affect truly null associations.

A classic example of nondifferential exposure misclassification probably occurred in a well-known study of vaginal spermicides and congenital disorders.[18] This cohort study was conducted among members of the Group Health Cooperative, a Seattle Health Maintenance Organization that provided medical services as well as most prescription drugs. Spermicides were provided either free of charge or at reduced cost to cooperative members. The investigators used the cooperative's computerized health and pharmacy records to compare the prevalence proportions of major

TABLE 10-12 Nondifferential Misclassification of the Exposure in a Hypothetical Case–Control Study

	Cases	Controls
Exposed	100	50
Unexposed	200	250
Total	300	300
	Odds ratio: 2.5	

congenital anomalies among offspring of women who did and did not fill prescriptions for vaginal spermicides. A woman was considered to be a spermicide user if a prescription for any kind of vaginal spermicide was filled within 600 days before the end of a pregnancy and no subsequent prescription for any other contraceptive (except for a diaphragm) was filled after the spermicide prescription and before the conclusion of the pregnancy. The investigators found that the prevalence of major malformations was about twice as high among users than nonusers. In particular, the prevalence of limb reduction defects, congenital neoplasms, chromosomal abnormalities, and hypospadias was increased among spermicide users.

This study had three potential sources of exposure misclassification that stemmed from the operational definition of spermicide use. The first arose from grouping all types of vaginal spermicides into one exposure category. About 80% of spermicide use in the health plan involved products containing the chemical octoxynol, and about 20% involved products containing nonoxynol 9. Grouping these two chemicals into one exposure variable may result in misclassification if only one of the chemicals is related to risk of congenital disorders. The second potential source resulted from investigators' use of pharmacy records to ascertain the exposure. It is quite possible that some women who were considered exposed never used the prescribed spermicides and some women who were considered unexposed used spermicides obtained from other sources (such as the neighborhood drug store). The third source of exposure misclassification resulted from using a wide exposure window—filling a prescription within 600 days before delivery or abortion. The relevant exposure period for the development of most congenital defects in the study is the first 3 months of pregnancy, the period of organogenesis. Although the long exposure window includes this period, it also includes periods during which exposure to spermicides was irrelevant (e.g., after the defect formed). These three potential sources of misclassification were most likely nondifferential. That is, the classification error regarding spermicide use was as likely to occur for a malformed infant as for a normal infant. Thus, the results were likely biased toward the null, and therefore the true relationship between spermicides and congenital disorders is probably stronger than observed.

What can epidemiologists do to reduce misclassification? The main way is to improve the accuracy of the collected data. Investigators can do this by using multiple measurements of exposure and disease. For example, because blood pressure readings are prone to error, investigators typically rely on several readings to determine whether a subject has hypertension. Similarly, because air pollution levels vary widely according to the time of day and location of measurement, investigators sometimes ask study subjects to wear personal air pollution monitors to gather continuous pollutant measurements over the course of their daily activities and environments (e.g. home, work, school, traveling from place to place, etc.).

Another method for improving accuracy is through validation, that is, corroborating the collected data using several sources. For example, investigators often review medical records to confirm the occurrence of self-reported diseases. Whenever possible, the corroborating evidence should be objective in nature, such as laboratory test results.

Still another way to improve data accuracy is to switch to a better information source for the exposure or disease. For example, a retrospective cohort study of Portsmouth Naval Shipyard workers improved upon the exposure assessments used in the earlier PMR study by using employment records and film badges to determine external radiation exposure instead of next-of-kin reports.[6,7] Investigators from the study on vaginal spermicides and congenital disorders could have improved the exposure data accuracy by either augmenting or substituting pharmacy data with participant interviews.[18]

A final way to reduce misclassification is to define the exposure and disease using sensitive and specific criteria. Regarding the exposure, criteria should be able to discern those truly exposed and exclude those who are not. Likewise, criteria for the disease should pick up cases of disease as well as eliminate those without disease. For example, criteria for a myocardial infarction definition should include clinical symptoms, electrocardiogram (ECG) findings, and the results of cardiac enzyme tests. Using only a symptom such as chest pain to define this disease would result in misclassification because people with other conditions that produce chest pain would be erroneously included and people with "silent" heart attacks that occur without chest pain would be missed.

The key facts about information bias are summarized in **TABLE 10-13**. A good epidemiological study incorporates a number of design features to minimize or eliminate this type of bias.

TABLE 10-13 Key Facts About Information Bias

- Information bias is an error that arises from systematic differences in the way information on exposure and disease is obtained from study groups.

- This type of bias results in participants who are incorrectly classified as either exposed or unexposed or as diseased or not diseased.

- It occurs after subjects have entered the study.

- It can occur in both retrospective and prospective studies.

- Specific types include recall bias, interviewer bias, and differential and nondifferential misclassification.

- Methods for avoiding information bias include masking interviewers and subjects to the study hypothesis (interviewer and recall bias); using a control group that is composed of diseased individuals (recall bias); carefully designing the study questionnaire (interviewer and recall bias); relying on noninterview data (interviewer and recall bias); and using multiple measurements, the most accurate information source, and sensitive and specific criteria to define the exposure and disease (misclassification).

Summary

Bias is a systematic error that results in an incorrect estimate of the measure of association. The two main types of bias are selection and information bias. When evaluating a study for the presence of bias, it is necessary to identify its source, assess its strength, and determine its direction. Bias can pull the estimate of association either toward or away from the null. Although a small amount of bias does not usually have a major effect on the results, a large amount of bias can completely alter the study findings. Little can be done to fix or remove a bias once it has occurred; therefore, investigators must avoid it by carefully designing and conducting the study.

Selection bias arises from systematic differences in selecting and following the study groups. The former type of selection bias is more likely in case–control and retrospective cohort studies because the exposure and disease have occurred at the time of subject selection. The latter type can occur in retrospective and prospective cohort studies and in experimental studies. There are several ways that selection bias can occur, including selection of an inappropriate control group in a case–control study (control selection bias); nonresponse or agreement to participate that is related to exposure and disease (self-selection bias); differential loss to follow-up; selection of the general population as a comparison in a cohort study (healthy worker effect); and differential surveillance, diagnosis, or referral of study subjects according to exposure and disease status. Selection bias can be avoided by using the same criteria to select cases and controls, obtaining high participation, using successful methods to retain and trace study subjects, taking diagnostic and referral practices into account when designing the study, and excluding self-referrals from a study.

Information bias is an error that arises from systematic differences in the way that information on exposure and disease is obtained from the study groups. It results in participants whose exposure or disease status is incorrectly classified. There are several ways that information bias may occur, including differential accuracy in the information provided by compared groups (recall bias); systematic differences in the way that interview data are solicited, recorded, or interpreted (interviewer bias); and measurement errors known as differential and nondifferential misclassification. Differential misclassification occurs when misclassification errors on one axis (disease or exposure) are related to the other axis, and nondifferential misclassification occurs when the errors on one axis are unrelated to the other axis. The methods for avoiding information bias include masking interviewers and study subjects to the study hypothesis (interviewer and recall bias), using a control group consisting of diseased individuals (recall bias), carefully designing the study questionnaire (interviewer and recall bias), and obtaining accurate exposure and disease data.

References

1. Pickett JP (exec ed.). *The American Heritage Dictionary of the English Language.* 4th ed. Boston, MA: Houghton Mifflin Co.; 2000.
2. Porta M. *A Dictionary of Epidemiology.* 6th ed. New York, NY: Oxford University Press; 2014.
3. Hennekens CH, Buring JE. *Epidemiology in Medicine.* Boston, MA: Little, Brown and Co.; 1987.
4. Boston Collaborative Drug Surveillance Program. Oral contraceptives and venous thromboembolic disease, surgically confirmed gall bladder disease, and breast tumors. *Lancet.* 1973;1:1399-1404.
5. Sartwell PE, Masi AT, Arthes FG, Greene GR, Smith HE. Thromboembolism and oral contraceptives: an epidemiologic case-control study. *Am J Epidemiol.* 1969;90:365-380.
6. Najarian T, Colton T. Mortality from leukemia and cancer in shipyard workers. *Lancet.* 1978;1:1018.
7. Rinsky RA, Zumwalde RD, Waxweiler RJ, Murray WE Jr, Bierbaum PJ, Landrigan PJ, et al. Cancer mortality at a naval nuclear shipyard. *Lancet.* 1981;1:231-235.
8. Rothman KJ, Fyler DC, Goldblatt A, Kreidberg MB. Exogenous hormones and other drug exposures of children with congenital heart disease. *Am J Epidemiol.* 1979;109:433-439.
9. Zierler S, Rothman KJ. Congenital heart disease in relation to maternal use of Bendectin and other drugs in early pregnancy. *New Engl J Med.* 1985;313:347-352.
10. Werler MM, Pober BR, Nelson K, Holmes LB. Reporting accuracy among mothers of malformed and nonmalformed infants. *Am J Epidemiol.* 1989;129:415-421.
11. Werler MM, Louik C, Mitchell AA. Case-control studies for identifying novel teratogens. *Am J Med Genet Part C Semin Med Genet.* 2011;157:201-208.
12. Mitchell AA, Cottler LB, Shapiro S. Effect of questionnaire design on recall of drug exposure in pregnancy. *Am J Epidemiol.* 1986;123:670-676.
13. Metzger DS, Koblin B, Turner C, Navaline H, Valenti F, Holte S, et al. Randomized controlled trial of audio computer-assisted self-interviewing: utility and acceptability in longitudinal studies. *Am J Epidemiol.* 2000;152:99-107.
14. Werler MM, Shapiro S, Mitchell AA. Periconceptional folic acid exposure and risk of occurrent neural tube defects. *JAMA.* 1993;269:1257-1261.
15. Levin AA, Schoenbaum SC, Monson RR, Stubblefield PG, Ryan PG. The association of induced abortion with subsequent pregnancy loss. *JAMA.* 1980;243:2495-2499.
16. Kelsey JL, Thompson WD, Evans AS. *Methods in Observational Epidemiology.* New York, NY: Oxford University Press; 1986.
17. Aschengrau A, Weinberg J, Gallagher LG, Winter MR, Vieira VM, Webster TF, et al. Exposure to tetrachloroethylene-contaminated drinking water and the risk of pregnancy loss. *Water Qual Expo Health.* 2009;1:23-24.
18. Jick H, Walker AM, Rothman KJ, Holmes LB, Watkins RN, D'Ewart DC, et al. Vaginal spermicides and congenital disorder. *JAMA.* 1981;245:1329-1332.

Chapter Questions

1. Briefly define each of the following terms:
   a. Recall bias
   b. Healthy worker effect
   c. Control selection bias
2. State the main difference between differential and nondifferential misclassification, and state which direction(s) each type of error can bias the study results.
3. A case–control study was conducted to determine whether using antihistamines around the time of conception increased the risk of birth defects in the offspring. No personal interviews were conducted regarding the subjects' antihistamine use. Instead, women were considered exposed if computerized pharmacy records from their health maintenance organization indicated that they had filled at least one prescription for antihistamines within 500 days before the birth of the child.
   a. Which type of information bias is this data collection method most susceptible to? In which direction would this type of error bias the study results?
   b. Which type of information bias is this data collection method least susceptible to?

4. A prospective cohort study was conducted to determine the risk of heart attack among men with varying levels of baldness. Third-year residents in dermatology conducted visual baldness assessments at the start of the study (which was before any heart attacks had occurred). Four levels of baldness were coded: none, minimal, moderate, and severe. The follow-up rate was close to 100%. Which of the following types of bias were surely avoided in this study?
    a. Recall bias of the exposure information
    b. Differential misclassification of the exposure
    c. Nondifferential misclassification of the exposure
    d. Selection bias

5. State the different ways that each of the following biases can be minimized:
    a. Interviewer bias
    b. Recall bias
    c. Selection bias
    d. Misclassification

6. Indicate whether the following statements are true or false:
    a. A study must be valid before its results can be generalized.
    b. Bias is introduced primarily during the analysis stage of a study.
    c. Bias can pull an estimate of association either toward or away from the null.
    d. Using an inaccurate case definition increases the likelihood of nondifferential misclassification of the disease.
    e. Including a large sample size reduces self-selection bias.
    f. Poor recall and recall bias are synonymous terms for the same concept.
    g. Open-ended interview questions are the best way to ascertain exposure information.
    h. It is possible to fix or adjust bias during the analysis phase of a study.
    i. When a positive association is biased toward the null, the true association is underestimated.
    j. When a positive association is biased away from the null, the true association is overestimated.
    k. Using incentives to ensure high rates of participation in a study will decrease selection bias.

7. Selection bias is most likely to occur in:
    a. Case–control studies
    b. Retrospective cohort studies
    c. Experimental studies
    d. Both retrospective cohort and case–control studies
    e. Both retrospective cohort and experimental studies

8. Recall bias is most likely to occur in:
    a. Case–control studies
    b. Prospective cohort studies
    c. Experimental studies
    d. All of the above
    e. None of the above

CHAPTER 11

Confounding

▶ Introduction

Epidemiologists evaluate whether a study result is valid by assessing the presence of random error, bias, and confounding. These three phenomena are considered *alternative explanations* for the observed association between an exposure and a disease. Random error is the probability that the observed result is attributable to chance. Bias is a systematic error committed by the investigator during the course of a study. In contrast, confounding is not the fault of the investigator. It simply reflects the fact that epidemiological research is conducted among free-living humans with unevenly distributed characteristics. As a result, epidemiological studies of the relationship between an exposure and a disease are susceptible to the disturbing influences of extraneous factors called confounders. This chapter provides several definitions of confounding and describes the main methods to control for confounding in the design and analysis of a study.

▶ Definition and Examples of Confounding

Confounding is most simply defined as the *mixing of effects* between an exposure, an outcome, and a third extraneous variable known as a confounder.[1(p129)] In fact, confounding can be considered the "third variable problem." When it is present, the association between the exposure and outcome is distorted because of the relationships between the confounder and the exposure and between the confounder and the disease.

Confounding can also be considered in terms of the **counterfactual ideal**.[1(pp54-55)] The ideal comparison group in a cohort study consists of exactly the same individuals in the exposed group had they not been exposed. Because it is impossible for the same person to be exposed and unexposed simultaneously, epidemiologists select different sets of individuals for the exposed and comparison groups. Even though different people form each group, the investigator chooses groups that are as similar as possible on characteristics that influence getting the disease. Accordingly, the rate of disease in the exposed and comparison groups will be identical if the exposure has no effect on disease occurrence.

Confounding can be thought of as a failure of the **comparison group** to reflect the counterfactual experience of the **exposed group**. Thus, even if the exposure has no effect on disease occurrence, the exposed and comparison groups will have different disease rates because they differ on other risk factors for the disease. In other words, risk factors apart from the exposure are distributed differently between the exposed and unexposed groups when confounding is present.

For example, consider a hypothetical cohort study on the risk of dementia among adults with diabetes. The investigators enrolled a group of newly diagnosed diabetic adults (the exposed group) and a group of adults without diabetes (the unexposed group) and followed them to determine the cumulative incidence of dementia. They found that participants with diabetes were 3.5 times more likely to develop dementia than those without diabetes over a 10-year follow-up period (see **TABLE 11-1**).

Although the results imply that there was a strong association between diabetes and the subsequent occurrence of dementia, the

TABLE 11-1 Hypothetical Data on the Association Between Diabetes and Dementia

Diabetes	Dementia Yes	Dementia No	Total
Yes	380	620	1,000
No	110	890	1,000
Total	490	1,510	2,000
		Risk ratio = 3.5	

findings may be invalid because of the distorting influence of confounding factors. For example, a close inspection of the study population revealed that subjects with diabetes were on average older than subjects without diabetes. Thus, perhaps the reason or part of the reason for the increased incidence of dementia among subjects with diabetes was their older age. This is a plausible explanation because the risk of dementia is influenced by age. When confounding by age was "controlled," the subjects with diabetes were twice as likely to develop dementia as those without diabetes. Thus, the initial results were exaggerated by confounding by age. Confounding occurred because age was associated with diabetes and with dementia. More specifically, the subjects with diabetes were older than those without diabetes, and the risk of dementia increased with age.

A variable must meet several criteria to be a confounder. First, the variable must be associated with the exposure in the population that produced the cases. That is, the confounding variable must be more or less common in the exposed group than in the comparison group. Second, the variable must be an independent cause or predictor of the disease, which means that the association between the confounder and the disease is present among both exposed and unexposed individuals. For example, the association between age and dementia is present for both diabetics and nondiabetics. Third, a confounding variable cannot be an intermediate step in the causal pathway between the exposure and disease. We identify intermediate steps by evaluating the biological mechanism by which the exposure is thought to cause the disease. For example, consider the inverse association between modest alcohol consumption and the risk of heart disease.[2] Modest alcohol consumption is thought to lower the risk of heart disease by increasing the level of high-density lipoproteins (HDLs). In other words, modest alcohol consumption increases a person's HDL level, which in turn decreases his or her risk of heart disease. HDL level is a step in the causal chain between modest alcohol consumption and a lowered risk of heart disease and thus is not a confounder. A variable that is a step in the causal chain (here, HDL level) is called a **mediator**. **FIGURE 11-1** depicts a **directed acyclic graph (DAG)**, which is a visual representation of the relationship between the confounder, the exposure, and the disease, and **FIGURE 11-2** depicts a DAG with a variable that is a step in the causal pathway between an exposure and a disease. DAGs are increasingly common in today's practice of epidemiology to

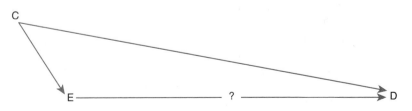

FIGURE 11-1 Directed acyclic graph showing that confounder (C) is associated with both the exposure (E) and the disease (D).

E ─────────────────────────────► S ────────────────────────────► D

FIGURE 11-2 Directed acyclic graph showing that variable (S) is a mediating step in the causal pathway between the exposure (E) and the disease (D) and thus is not a confounder of this relationship.

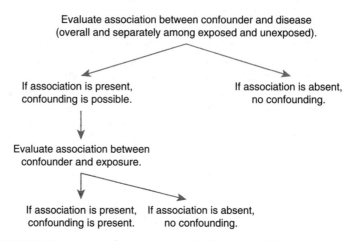

Evaluate association between confounder and disease
(overall and separately among exposed and unexposed).

If association is present,
confounding is possible.

If association is absent,
no confounding.

Evaluate association between
confounder and exposure.

If association is present,
confounding is present.

If association is absent,
no confounding.

FIGURE 11-3 Decision tree for determining whether a variable is a confounder.

help identify confounding and mediating variables and therefore aid in the data collection and analysis of the study.

How do epidemiologists determine whether a variable is a confounder? One way is to evaluate the strength of the associations between the confounder, the exposure, and the disease. First, the strength of the association between the confounder and the disease is evaluated (C and D in Figure 11-1). If there is no association, we can conclude that the variable is not a confounder. If there is an association, we next determine whether this association is present among both exposed and unexposed individuals. If not, we can conclude that the variable is not a confounder. If yes, we determine whether there is an association between the confounder and the exposure (C and E in Figure 11-1). If there is no association, we can conclude that the variable is not a confounder. In summary, epidemiologists conclude that confounding is present if there is an association between the confounder and the disease among the exposed and unexposed groups and between the confounder and the exposure. The decision tree for determining whether a variable is a confounder is depicted in **FIGURE 11-3**.

Consider again the hypothetical cohort study on the risk of dementia among people with diabetes. A visual representation of the relationship between age, diabetes, and the risk of dementia is provided in **FIGURE 11-4**, and numerical data are described in **TABLES 11-2** and **11-3**. Recall that subjects with diabetes had a 3.5-fold increased risk of dementia but that the risk was reduced to a twofold increase after controlling for age. The mixing of effects between age, diabetes, and dementia caused

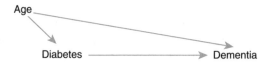

FIGURE 11-4 Directed acyclic graph showing relationship between age, diabetes, and dementia.

TABLE 11-2 Hypothetical Data on the Association Between Age and Dementia Among Diabetics and Nondiabetics

Age	Dementia among participants with diabetes			Dementia among participants without diabetes		
	Yes	No	Total	Yes	No	Total
80–99 years	360	540	900	20	80	100
45–79 years	20	80	100	90	810	900
Total	380	620	1,000	110	890	1,000
			Risk ratio = 2.0			Risk ratio = 2.0

TABLE 11-3 Hypothetical Data on the Association Between Age and Diabetes

Age	Diabetes		
	Yes	No	Total
80–99 years	900	100	1,000
45–79 years	100	900	1,000
Total	1,000	1,000	2,000
		Risk ratio = 9.0	

confounding. Note from the data in Table 11-2 that there was a twofold increased risk of dementia among subjects aged 80 to 99 years as compared with subjects aged 45 to 79 years, which was present for both diabetics and nondiabetics. Thus, there was a positive association between the confounder and the disease among both exposed and unexposed individuals. There was a ninefold increased risk of diabetes with older age (Table 11-3), and therefore there was also an association between the exposure and the confounder. Confounding occurred when these complex associations were ignored in the crude analysis.

Confounding is not an all-or-none condition described merely by its presence or absence. Rather, confounding is a quantitative issue. Thus, it is vital to ask the following questions about the presence of confounding in a particular study. First, what is the magnitude or extent of confounding? Second, what is the direction of confounding? The question regarding the magnitude of confounding can be answered by using the following formula:

$$\text{Magnitude of confounding} = \frac{\text{RR crude} - \text{RR adjusted}}{\text{RR adjusted}}$$

where RR is the risk ratio, rate ratio, odds ratio, or relative risk. Note that the crude **measure of association** (RR crude) has not been adjusted for confounding and the adjusted measure (RR adjusted) has been corrected for confounding. In this example, the crude risk ratio of dementia among participants with diabetes was 3.5, whereas the age-adjusted risk ratio was 2.0. Thus, the magnitude of confounding was $[(3.5 - 2.0)/2.0] \times 100$, or 75%, indicating that a large amount of confounding was present.

Regarding the direction of confounding, confounding pulls the observed association away from the true association. Thus, it can either exaggerate the true association (**positive confounding**) or hide it (**negative confounding**). An example of positive confounding is when the true risk ratio is 1.0 and the confounded risk ratio is 2.0, and an example of negative confounding is when the true risk ratio is 2.0 and the confounded risk ratio is 1.0. In the hypothetical study of the association between diabetes and dementia, age was a positive confounder of the relationship.

Confounding occurs in all types of epidemiological studies. An interesting example of confounding occurred in a study of the relationship between myopia (nearsightedness) and light exposure.[3] In particular, the investigators hypothesized that nighttime ambient light exposure increased the risk of myopia among children. The cross-sectional study included 479 outpatients aged 2 to 16 years from a university pediatric ophthalmology clinic. Children who slept with room lights and night lights before the age of 2 years had an increased risk of myopia as compared with children who slept in darkness during these years. In particular, the investigators observed a 5.5-fold increased risk of myopia associated with full room lights and a 3.4-fold increased risk with night lights. Although the investigators acknowledged that the study was limited by the lack of information on confounders, they concluded, "It seems prudent that infants and young children sleep at night without artificial lighting in the bedroom."[3]

In retrospect, this conclusion was incorrect given the lack of information on crucial confounding factors. That is, no data were collected on independent risk factors for myopia that were also associated with the use of lighting. A subsequent study of this relationship found that family history of myopia was an important confounder.[4] In particular, the study found that families with two myopic parents were much more likely to employ nighttime lighting aids for their children and to have myopic children. The investigators hypothesized that the parents' own poor visual acuity necessitated the lighting.

▶ Confounding by Indication and Severity

Two special types of confounding occur in observational studies of the intended effects of treatments: confounding by indication and confounding by severity. Confounding by indication reflects the fact that treatments are given to individuals with a particular disease, and therefore there is a mixing of effects between the treatment, the disease for which the treatment is given, and the outcome under study.[5] For example, studies of the association between antidepressant drug use and cognitive deficits need to consider depression (the indication for the drug treatment) as a confounder. This is because antidepressant drug use is associated with depression (patients are not given the drug unless they have the condition) and depression itself is a known risk factor for memory deficits.[6] Confounding by indication occurs when individuals who are treated for their condition are compared with individuals who have neither the condition nor the treatment. Thus, a common way to control for this type of confounding is to compare different treatments for the same condition. For example, investigators could compare one antidepressant drug with another drug among individuals who have a diagnosis of depression.

Confounding by severity is a type of confounding "in which not only the disease that forms the indication but also its severity is the potential confounder. . . . Here, the stage of the disease and its corresponding severity and complications are important."[7(p982)] For example, a study found that the initiation of combination therapy with protease inhibitors for human immunodeficiency virus (HIV) infection during pregnancy was associated with a more severe disease.[8] In particular, pregnant women who initiated this type of antiretroviral therapy had more compromised immune systems and higher viral loads than did pregnant women who did not initiate such therapy. Confounding by severity in observational studies usually makes the therapy appear less effective than it appeared in experimental studies. For example, because antiretroviral therapy is more likely to be given to patients with a more severe disease and hence worse prognoses, this treatment is associated with higher crude mortality rates than other treatments. Experimental studies do not suffer from this problem mainly because randomization balances the severity distribution of the compared groups.

▶ Controlling for Confounding: General Considerations

Epidemiologists control or adjust for confounding variables because they consider confounders nuisance variables that distort the true association between an exposure and a disease. Confounding can be controlled in either the design phase, the analysis phase, or a combination of the two. To control for confounding, the investigator must have information on all variables that are potential confounders. Except for randomization, it is impossible to control for a confounder without data.

Epidemiologists typically determine which variables are potential confounders by conducting a literature review to ascertain all currently known risk factors for the disease under study. At this point, it is also helpful to draw a DAG to depict the interrelationships among the risk factors, the exposure, and the disease. Note that risk factors include variables that either increase or decrease a person's risk of disease. For example, potential confounders in a study of the relationship between chemical exposure and the risk of breast cancer included age at diagnosis of breast cancer, race, religion, age at first livebirth or stillbirth, prior history of breast cancer, family history of breast cancer, body mass index (BMI), and prior history of medical treatment with radiation. In particular, the risk of breast cancer is increased among older women, women with a positive family history, and women whose first birth occurs at a later age (older than 29 years).[9]

After determining which variables are potential confounders and collecting data on them, epidemiologists determine whether the variable is an actual confounder. This is typically accomplished by comparing the crude and adjusted estimates of the measure of association. If the crude and adjusted measures differ appreciably, then the variable that has been controlled is considered an actual confounder. The definition of an "appreciable" difference is arbitrary. Epidemiologists commonly use a 10% to 20% difference. Age clearly met this criterion in the diabetes–dementia relationship.

▶ Controlling for Confounding in the Design

There are three main ways to control for confounding in the design stage of a study: randomization, restriction, and matching (see **TABLE 11-4**). **Randomization** is the "act of assigning or ordering that results from

TABLE 11-4 Methods to Control for Confounding in the Design and Analysis Stages

Design stage

- Randomization
- Restriction
- Matching

Analysis stage

- Standardization
- Stratified analysis
- Matched analysis (needed for case–control studies but not for cohort or experimental studies)
- Multivariable analysis

a random process."[10(p220)] Random methods include flipping a coin or using a random number table or a computerized random number generator. Randomization ensures that the treatment assignment occurs in an unbiased fashion and will on average result in a balanced distribution of both known and unknown confounders if the sample size is large enough. Consider, for example, the clopidogrel versus aspirin in patients at risk of ischemic events (CAPRIE) study, which enrolled about 19,000 patients with atherosclerotic vascular disease and randomly assigned them to receive either clopidogrel or aspirin.[11] Randomization achieved baseline comparability of the patients in the two arms of the CAPRIE study because the size of the study was so large.

A unique advantage of randomization is that it will control for variables that study investigators are unable to measure. Although there is no absolute guarantee that randomization will control for unknown confounders (it may not work just by chance), known and unknown confounding is considered unlikely if the sample size is sufficient. Randomization is one of the few aspects of epidemiological research for which there are numerous advantages and no disadvantages. Unfortunately, it can be used only in experimental studies.

Restriction, another method investigators use to control for confounding in the design phase, means that admissibility criteria for study subjects are limited. In other words, entrance into the study is confined to individuals who fall within a specified category of the confounder. For example, confounding by age can be reduced by restricting a study to individuals within a narrow age range, say, from 25 to 35 years. Other examples of restriction include limiting the study population to one gender or only one race. The goal of restriction (and all other methods to control for confounding) is to eliminate or reduce the variability of the confounder. It is important to remember that a variable is a confounder only if its distribution differs between compared groups. Thus, when a study is restricted to one confounder category, the compared groups are identical on that variable. For example, a study restricted to men cannot be confounded by gender.

The advantages of restriction include its simplicity, convenience, low expense, and effectiveness. Confounding can be completely eliminated if a categorical variable such as gender is restricted. In addition, confounding can be greatly reduced if a continuous variable such as age is restricted. How much confounding is reduced depends on the narrowness of the range. For example, for most exposure–disease relationships, restricting to ages 25 to 30 years will control for confounding by age better than restricting to ages 25 to 45 years.

Restriction also has a few drawbacks. First, it makes it difficult to find enough study subjects, and therefore it is usually applied to only a few variables. Second, it limits the generalizability of the study. For example, when investigators restrict a study to men, its results may not be generalizable to women because of biological, social, and other differences between the genders.

Another way to control for confounding in the design stage is to match on one or more confounders. **Matching** is defined as "the process of making the distribution of the matching factors to be identical across study groups."[12(p177)] Matching means that investigators select the study subjects so that potential confounders are distributed in an identical manner. Thus, there will be identical confounder distributions among exposed and unexposed groups in a cohort study and among cases and controls in a case–control study.

The most common forms of matching are individual matching and frequency matching. Both types of matching are used more often in case–control studies than in cohort studies. Individual matching involves "identifying individual subjects for comparison, each resembling a study subject on the matched variable(s)."[12(p177)] For example, consider a cohort study on the relationship between exercise and the risk of colon cancer. A literature review reveals that potential confounders of this association include age, gender, and obesity. Thus, when an exposed subject (an exerciser) is enrolled who is a 55-year-old male with a normal BMI, an unexposed subject (a nonexerciser) would be enrolled who is a 55-year-old male with a normal BMI. (BMI is a measure of obesity.) If it is difficult to find an exact match on a continuous variable such as age, a looser match may be acceptable, say, 55 years plus or minus a few years.

Frequency matching is a type of category matching that balances the proportion of people with a confounding factor in the compared groups. For example, consider a cohort study in which exposed subjects had the following age distribution: 20% were aged 40 to 49 years, 40% were 50 to 59 years, 20% were 60 to 69 years, and 20% were 70 years and older. Frequency matching would ensure that 20% of the unexposed subjects were aged 40 to 49 years, 40% were aged 50 to 59 years, and so on. Once investigators filled a particular age category, they would select no more unexposed individuals in that category. Frequency matching is less exact than individual matching, which makes it easier to find matches.

When matching is conducted in a cohort study, exposed and unexposed groups have the same distribution of the matched confounder, and therefore the crude measure of association is not confounded by the matched variable(s). However, matching in the design of a case–control study does not control confounding by itself. The investigator must perform a special matched analysis. The reason for matching in the design phase of a case–control study is to ensure sufficient numbers of subjects in each category of the matched variable to conduct the matched analysis efficiently. In fact, the crude odds ratio from a matched case–control study will be biased toward the null because matching makes the exposure histories of the cases and controls more similar because the matching variable is associated with the exposure.

Matching has several disadvantages. First, it is not possible for investigators to study the relationship between the matching factor and outcome in a case–control study. Second, it is difficult and expensive to find subjects who are appropriate matches. Third, it is possible to "overmatch" on a confounder in a case–control study. This can occur when investigators match on a potential confounder that is strongly associated with the exposure but either weakly or not associated with the disease. Overmatching is problematic because it makes the matched analysis very inefficient. This occurs because information on the large number of matched sets with concordant exposure histories is lost.

Despite these disadvantages, matching is desirable and even necessary in a number of situations. First, matching is advantageous when the case series in a case–control study is very small, and therefore other options for controlling confounding do not work well. Second, matching is needed when the confounder is a complex nominal variable, such as occupation, neighborhood, or familial characteristic such as sibship. Each of these variables represents a complex web of environmental and occasionally genetic factors that are difficult to measure and control in other ways.

▶ Controlling for Confounding in the Analysis

Even when the study design does not feature randomization, restriction, and matching, it is still possible to achieve excellent control for confounding using methods available during the analysis phase. The three main ways to control for confounding in the analysis of a study are standardization, stratification, and multivariable methods (see Table 11-4). Epidemiologists commonly use standardization to control for demographic variables, such as age, race, gender, and calendar time. The process of direct standardization was described in Chapter 3.

Stratification, which is used both to evaluate and to control for confounding, is defined as "the process of or result of separating a sample into several subsamples according to specified criteria such as age groups, socioeconomic status, etc. The effect of confounding variables may be controlled by stratifying the analysis of results."[12(p272)] With stratification, the investigator evaluates the association within homogeneous categories of the confounder. The homogeneous categories are called strata, and each stratum should be free of confounding by the stratification variable. For example, consider a hypothetical case–control study of dichlorodiphenyldichloroethylene (DDE) (the metabolic by-product of the pesticide dichlorodiphenyltrichloroethane [DDT]) exposure and the risk of breast cancer in which age is a confounder. TABLE 11-5 describes the crude results without stratification by age. Overall, there is a 1.9-fold increased odds of breast cancer among women who were exposed to high DDE levels (odds ratio = $[500 \times 3,400]/[600 \times 1,500] = 1.9$).

Now, let us examine these results stratified into two age groups: women younger than 50 years of age and women 50 years and older (see TABLE 11-6). Note that all of the numbers in the cells of two stratified tables add up to the numbers in the cells of the crude data table (see Table 11-5). Each stratum can be considered a restricted analysis. That is, each stratum restricts the analysis to a narrow range of the confounder. When we stratify the data, we see that there is no association between DDE and breast cancer among women who are younger than 50 years of age and among those who are 50 years and older. The odds ratio is $(50 \times 2,700)/(300 \times 450)$, or 1.0, among women younger than 50 years of age, and it is $(450 \times 700)/(300 \times 1,050)$, or 1.0, among women aged 50 years and older. The magnitude of the association does not differ across the strata, but the stratum-specific odds ratios (1.0) are different from the crude odds ratio (1.9). The appreciable difference between the crude and stratum-specific odds ratios indicates that confounding by age is present.

TABLE 11-5 Crude Data from a Hypothetical Case–Control Study of DDE Exposure and Breast Cancer

DDE level	Cases	Controls
High	500	600
Low	1,500	3,400
Total	2,000	4,000
		Odds ratio = 1.9

TABLE 11-6 Age-Stratified Data from a Hypothetical Case–Control Study of DDE Exposure and Breast Cancer

DDE level	Age younger than 50 years		Age 50 years and older	
	Cases	Controls	Cases	Controls
High	50	300	450	300
Low	450	2,700	1,050	700
Total	500	3,000	1,500	1,000
	Stratum-specific odds ratio = 1.0		Stratum-specific odds ratio = 1.0	

When epidemiologists conduct stratified analyses, they have the option of reporting either the stratum-specific results or calculating a summary measure using standardization or pooling. Standardization involves taking weighted averages of the relevant measures of disease frequency. The weights typically come from the exposed group in the study population. Pooling involves calculating a weighted average of the relative risks instead of the measures of disease frequency. A commonly used method for calculating a pooled estimate of association was first proposed by Mantel and Haenszel.[13] **TABLE 11-7** gives the formulas for the Mantel–Haenszel pooled estimates of relative risk for case–control studies and cohort and experimental studies with count and person-time denominators. In the example in Table 11-6, the Mantel–Haenszel pooled odds ratio is $[(50 \times 2,700/3,500) + (450 \times 700/2,500)]/[(300 \times 450/3,500) + (300 \times 1,050/2,500)] = 1.0$.

Pooling should be conducted only if the stratum-specific estimates are similar to one another. Pooling should not be undertaken if the estimates are appreciably different because this means that effect modification is present. Briefly, effect modification indicates that the strength of the association is modified or differs according to the level of another variable. For example, the relationship between BMI and breast cancer varies according to menopausal status. Higher BMI decreases the risk of breast cancer among premenopausal women and either increases or does not affect risk among postmenopausal women.[14]

It is unusual for stratum-specific measures of association to be exactly the same, even when no effect modification is present. Epidemiologists determine when stratum-specific results are different enough to suggest effect modification by either visually inspecting the results or performing a statistical test, such as the chi-square test for homogeneity.

TABLE 11-7 Formulas for Calculating Mantel–Haenszel Pooled Relative Risks		
Type of study	**Formula**	
Case–control study	$\dfrac{\sum a_i d_i / T_i}{\sum b_i c_i / T_i}$	where a_i, b_i, c_i, and d_i are the cells of each stratified two-by-two table and T_i is the total number of subjects in each stratum.
Cohort or experimental study with count denominators	$\dfrac{\sum a_i (c_i + d_i) / T_i}{\sum c_i (a_i + b_i) / T_i}$	where a_i, b_i, c_i, and d_i are the cells in each stratified two-by-two table and T_i is the total number of subjects in each stratum.
Cohort or experimental study with person-time denominators	$\dfrac{\sum a_i (PT_{0i}) / PT_i}{\sum c_i (PT_{1i}) / PT_i}$	where a_i is the number of exposed cases, c_i is the number of unexposed cases in each stratified two-by-two table, PT_{0i} is the amount of person-time among the unexposed in each stratum, PT_{1i} is the amount of person-time among the exposed in each stratum, and PT_i is the total amount of person-time in each stratum.

Stratified analyses have several advantages. They are straightforward and easy to carry out. Even more important, they allow epidemiologists to view the raw data underlying the complex relationships under study. Their chief disadvantage is that they do not allow investigators to control simultaneously for many variables. This is because they generate a large number of strata relative to the number of study subjects. For example, if investigators wanted to control for four variables simultaneously—gender (two categories: male and female), age (five categories: younger than 50 years, 50–59, 60–69, 70–79, and 80 years and older), race/ethnicity (three categories: White, Black, and Hispanic), and cigarette smoking status (three categories: current smoker, past smoker, and never smoked)—they would need 90 strata ($2 \times 5 \times 3 \times 3 = 90$) to describe all the possible combinations of these four variables. Even if the study size were relatively large, the number of subjects in the cells of some strata would be small or even zero, making the analysis questionable.

Consequently, epidemiologists rely on multivariable analysis when it is necessary to control for many confounding variables. **Multivariable analysis** involves the construction of a mathematical model that describes the association between exposure, disease, and confounders. Numerous multivariable models have been developed for this purpose, each with a certain set of assumptions. The choice of a particular model depends on the relationships among the relevant variables and the study design. For example, multiple linear regression models are used when the dependent variable is continuous; logistic regression models are used when the outcome is dichotomous, as in a case–control study; and Cox proportional hazard and Poisson models are used when rates from a cohort or experimental study are being compared. A disadvantage of multivariable models is that the study data must comport with the model's assumptions. If they do not, the multivariable analysis produces incorrect results. For example, if the model incorrectly assumes that there is a linear relationship between the independent and dependent variables, the results of the multivariable analysis will be skewed. An additional disadvantage is that investigators lose sight of the data when conducting these types of analyses.

Multivariable analyses should never be performed without first conducting a stratified analysis. The stratified analysis should be used to determine which variables are actual confounders that need to be controlled in the multivariable model. Any variable that changes the crude measure of association by an appreciable amount in the stratified analysis should be retained for the multivariable model. For example, consider the hypothetical case–control study of DDE exposure and breast cancer described earlier in this chapter. To identify confounders of this association, investigators should stratify the crude data by each of the following variables one at a time: age at diagnosis, race, age at first birth, religion, socioeconomic status, family history of breast cancer, BMI, prior history of benign breast disease, and prior history of ionizing radiation. These variables are known risk factors for breast cancer and therefore are considered potential confounders. The investigators could later control simultaneously in a logistic regression analysis all variables that changed the crude measure of association by 10% or more and thus were actual confounders in this study population.

▶ Residual Confounding

Residual confounding is a term for the confounding that remains even after many confounding variables have been controlled. Residual confounding arises from several sources. The first source consists of confounders for which data were not collected. For example, a study of risk-taking behaviors following early life exposure to tetrachloroethylene (PCE)-contaminated drinking water found that the risk of using illicit drugs as a teenager was elevated among individuals highly exposed during early life (for example, the risk ratio for using crack/cocaine was 2.1 among highly exposed subjects).[15] Data on other risk factors for substance use during adolescence, such as poor parental supervision and negative peer influences, were not gathered because of limitations in the study questionnaire, and therefore residual confounding by these variables was possible. However, the investigators stated that confounding by these factors was an unlikely explanation for the results because they "would need to be highly correlated with PCE-exposure, an unlikely scenario given the irregular pattern of PCE contamination" in the study communities.[15(p102)] In other words, the investigators thought it was unlikely that these characteristics met the first criterion of a confounder—that it must be associated with the exposure in the underlying population. In contrast, residual confounding from missing information on family history of myopia was the likely reason for the positive association between myopia and early childhood light exposure.[4]

The second source of residual confounding arises from persistent differences in risk within a category of a confounder. It usually occurs when the confounder is classified in very broad categories. For example, if investigators used frequency matching to control for age in 10-year categories, residual confounding might be present if the risk of disease varied within the 10-year age group. The solution for this problem is to categorize the confounder into smaller groups, for example, 5-year age groups.

Third, residual confounding can occur when the confounder is mismeasured, that is, when there is confounder misclassification. **Misclassification** is the "erroneous classification of an individual, a value, or an attribute into a category other than that to which it should be assigned."[12(p186)] Any kind of variable can be mismeasured, including confounders. Misclassification of confounders makes it more difficult to control for that confounder. Greater misclassification leads to greater residual confounding.

▶ Assessment of Mediation

As previously stated, a variable that is a step in the causal pathway is called a mediator and should not be controlled as a confounder in the design or analysis of a study. Instead, a special causal mediation analysis must be conducted to determine its role in the relationship between the exposure and disease.[16] This analysis typically attempts to partition the exposure–disease relationship into natural direct and indirect effects. In other words, the analysis tries to separate the indirect effect of an exposure through the mediating variable(s) from its direct effect without the mediating variable(s). This is typically done by determining the proportion of the overall association that is mediated through the intermediate variable(s). In this way, "mechanisms that underlie an observed relationship between an exposure variable and an outcome variable" are examined.[16] For example, investigators recently examined the effect of exposure to greenness (i.e., natural vegetation) on mortality in a national prospective cohort study of nurses.[17] After controlling for confounding variables, the highest level of greenness around participants' homes was associated with a 12% lower rate of nonaccidental mortality. The investigators also found that the association between greenness and mortality was partly mediated by depression, social engagement, air pollution, and physical activity. In particular, 27% of the association was explained by these four mediating factors, which suggests that greenness is associated with lower mortality in part through lower levels of depression and air pollution and high levels of social engagement and physical activity.

Summary

Confounding may be defined as a mixing of effects between an exposure, an outcome, and a third extraneous variable known as a confounder. Epidemiologists consider confounding a nuisance because it distorts the true association between an exposure and a disease. A study may have a small, moderate, or large amount of confounding. A small degree of confounding may not significantly affect the study results, but a large degree may completely distort the findings. The distortion can either exaggerate or minimize the true association. The former is known as positive confounding, and the latter is known as negative confounding.

A confounding variable has three key features: (1) It is associated with the exposure in the population that produced the cases, (2) it is an independent cause or predictor of disease, and (3) it is *not* an intermediate step in the causal pathway between the exposure and disease. Special types of confounding include confounding by indication, which is confounding between a treatment and the disease for which the treatment is given, and confounding by severity, which is confounding between a treatment and the seriousness of a disease. Both varieties occur in observational studies but not in experimental studies.

Confounding can be controlled in the design, the analysis, or a combination of the two. Unless investigators conduct a study for which randomization is appropriate, they cannot control for confounders without collecting information on them. Crude and adjusted measures of association are compared to determine whether confounding is present. The crude measure is calculated without controlling for confounding, and the adjusted measure is corrected for confounding. If crude and adjusted measures differ appreciably, then the variable is considered a confounder.

Three ways to control for confounding in the design phase are randomization, restriction, and matching. Randomization means that subjects are assigned to the study groups through a random process. It generally ensures that compared groups are balanced on both known and unknown confounders if the sample size is sufficient. Although randomization is an excellent method for controlling confounding, its use is limited to experimental studies. Restriction means that admissibility criteria for enrollment are limited. It is a simple and excellent means to control for confounding, but it limits the generalizability of study results. Matching means that study subjects with identical or nearly identical characteristics are selected. The process is often expensive because it can be difficult to find appropriate matches, particularly when several variables are involved. Thus, matching is typically used to control for complex characteristics (such as neighborhood) that are difficult to control using other methods.

Techniques for controlling for confounding in the analysis include stratified and multivariable analyses. Stratification involves separating the study population into homogeneous categories of a confounder. A meaningful difference between the stratum-specific and crude measures of association indicates the presence of confounding. Stratum-specific or summary measures of association, such as the Mantel–Haenszel pooled estimate, should be used to present results in this situation. Stratified analyses are popular because they are straightforward and easy to carry out; however, they are inefficient for controlling for many confounders simultaneously. Thus, multivariable analysis, which involves specification of a mathematical model, is used in this setting. Although they are powerful, multivariable analyses are conducted in a "black box"(using a computer program whose inner workings are unknown), and therefore the investigator loses sight of the data.

Residual or persistent confounding may be present even after many confounding variables have been controlled. This occurs when data on certain confounders are unavailable, confounders are controlled in overly broad categories, and confounders are collected with measurement error.

A variable that is a step in the causal pathway is called a mediator and should not be controlled as a confounder. Instead, a special causal mediation analysis must be conducted to separate the indirect effect of an exposure through the mediator from its direct effect without the mediating variable.

References

1. Rothman KJ, Greenland S, Lash TL. *Modern Epidemiology.* 3rd ed. Philadelphia, PA: Lippincott Williams and Wilkins; 2008.
2. Hvidtfeldt UA, Tolstrup JS, Jakobsen MU, Heitmann BL, Grønbæk M, O'Reilly E, et al. Alcohol intake and risk of coronary heart disease in younger, middle-aged, and older adults. *Circulation.* 2010;121:1589-1597.
3. Quinn GE, Shin CH, Maguire MG, Stone RA. Myopia and ambient lighting at night. *Nature.* 1999; 399:113-114.
4. Gwiazda J, Ong E, Held R, Thorn F. Myopia and ambient night-time lighting. *Nature.* 2000;404:144.
5. Greenland S, Neutra R. Control of confounding in the assessment of medical technology. *Int J Epidemiol.* 1980;9:361-367.
6. Han L, Brandt C, Allore HG. Antidepressant use and cognitive deficits in older men: addressing confounding by indications with different methods. *Ann Epidemiol.* 2012;22:9-16.
7. Salas M, Hofman A, Stricker BH. Confounding by indication: an example of variation in the use of epidemiologic terminology. *Am J Epidemiol.* 1999;149:981-983.
8. Patel K, Shapiro DE, Brogly SB, Livingston EG, Stek AM, Bardeguez AD, et al. Prenatal protease inhibitor use and risk of preterm birth among HIV-infected women initiating antiretroviral drugs during pregnancy. *JID.* 2010;201:1035-1044.
9. Zota AR, Aschengrau A, Rudel RA, Brody JG. Self-reported chemicals exposure, beliefs about disease causation, and risk of breast cancer in the Cape Cod Breast Cancer and Environment Study: a case-control study. *Environ Health.* 2010;9:40.
10. Meinert CL. *Clinical Trials Dictionary, Terminology and Usage Recommendations.* Baltimore, MD: The Johns Hopkins Center for Clinical Trials; 1996.
11. CAPRIE Steering Committee. A randomized, blinded trial of clopidogrel versus aspirin in patients at risk of ischemic events (CAPRIE). *Lancet.* 1996; 348:1329-1339.
12. Porta M. *A Dictionary of Epidemiology.* 6th ed. New York, NY: Oxford University Press; 2014.
13. Mantel N, Haenszel WH. Statistical aspects of the analysis of data from retrospective studies of disease. *J Natl Cancer Inst.* 1959;22:719-748.
14. van den Brandt PA, Spiegelman D, Yaun S-S, Adami H-O, Beeson L, Folsom AR, et al. Pooled analysis of

prospective cohort studies on height, weight, and breast cancer risk. *Am J Epidemiol.* 2000;152: 514-527.

15. Aschengrau A, Weinberg JM, Janulewicz PA, Romano ME, Gallagher LG, Winter MR, et al. Affinity for risky behavior following prenatal and early childhood exposure to tetrachloroethylene (PCE)-contaminated drinking water: a retrospective cohort study. *Environ Health.* 2011;10:102.

16. Valeri L, VanderWeele TJ. Mediation analysis allowing for exposure-mediator interactions and causal interpretation: theoretical assumptions and implementation with SAS and SPSS macros. *Psych Meth.* 2013;18:137-150.

17. James P, Hart JE, Laden F. Exposure to greenness and mortality in a nationwide prospective cohort study of women. *Environ Health Perspect.* 2016;124:1344-1352.

Chapter Questions

1. Briefly define each of the following terms:
   a. Confounding
   b. Residual confounding
   c. Positive and negative confounding
   d. Directed acyclic graph (DAG)

2. What are the key characteristics of a confounding variable?

3. Consider each of the following scenarios and state whether the variable in question is a confounder. Your choices are yes, no, and can't tell (based on the information given).
   a. A study of the relationship between contact lens use and the risk of eye ulcers. The crude risk ratio is 3.0 and the age-adjusted risk ratio is 1.5. Is age a confounder in this study?
   b. A case–control study of the relationship between cigarette smoking and pancreatic cancer. In this study, coffee drinking is associated with smoking and is a risk factor for pancreatic cancer among both smokers and nonsmokers. Is coffee drinking a confounder in this study?
   c. A study of the relationship between exercise and heart attacks that is conducted among men who do not smoke. Is gender a confounder in this study?
   d. A cohort study of the risk of liver cirrhosis among female alcoholics. Incidence rates of cirrhosis among alcoholic women are compared with those among nonalcoholic women. Nonalcoholics are individually matched to alcoholics on month and year of birth. Is age a confounder in this study?
   e. A study of the relationship between air pollution and asthma among children. The crude and race-adjusted risk ratios are both 2.0. Is race a confounder in this study?
   f. A case-control study of uterine fibroids in relation to use of oral contraceptives (OCs). In this study population, cigarette smoking is associated with uterine fibroids among OC users and nonusers and is not on the causal pathway between OCs and the occurrence of fibroids. Is cigarette smoking a confounder in this study?

4. Draw a directed acyclic graph (DAG) showing the relationship between neighborhood violence and childhood obesity. Potential confounding and mediating variables that should be included in the DAG are race/ethnicity, family income level, diet, and physical activity.

5. Describe three methods for controlling confounding in the study design, and give one advantage and one disadvantage for each method.

6. Describe two methods for controlling confounding during the analysis, and give one advantage and one disadvantage for each method.

7. How do you determine whether a variable confounds an association?

8. State which method to control for confounding is being used in the following scenarios. In each scenario, exercise is the exposure, myocardial infarction is the disease, and gender is the confounder.

   a. A study of exercise and myocardial infarction that is limited to men.

   b. A case–control study of exercise and myocardial infarction that includes men and women. Controls are selected so that the proportions of male and female controls are identical to that among cases.

   c. A study of exercise and myocardial infarction that includes men and women. The study determines the relative risk separately for men and women and compares it with the crude relative risk.

9. Indicate whether the following statements are true or false:

   a. All high-quality epidemiological studies include techniques for controlling confounding.

   b. Mediating variables in a causal pathway are special types of confounders.

   c. The counterfactual ideal is used to guide the selection of a comparison group to minimize confounding.

   d. Epidemiologists can tell whether confounding is present by examining the strength of the crude measure of association.

   e. Experimental studies always have less confounding than observational studies.

   f. If randomization is unsuccessful in an experimental study, investigators may use other options (such as stratified and multivariable analysis) to control for confounding.

   g. Collecting data on potential confounding variables enables multivariable analyses.

CHAPTER 12

Random Error

LEARNING OBJECTIVES

By the end of this chapter the reader will be able to:

- Discuss the key phases in the history of biostatistics.
- Define chance, precision, and random error.
- Describe the process of hypothesis testing, calculate hypothesis testing statistics, and interpret a P value.
- Describe the process of confidence interval estimation, and interpret 95% confidence intervals.
- Calculate measures of central tendency and dispersion for data with normal, binomial, and Poisson distributions.
- Calculate 95% confidence intervals for measures of disease frequency and association.
- Explain the elements of sample size and power calculations.

▶ Introduction

Epidemiologists evaluate whether study results are valid by assessing the presence of three alternative explanations: bias, confounding, and random error. Bias is an error committed by the investigator either in the design or conduct of a study that leads to a false association between the exposure and disease. Confounding stems from the natural mixing of effects between the exposure and disease and a third variable called the confounder. Both bias and confounding are considered systematic errors because they arise from a discernible process.

In contrast, random error leads to a false association between the exposure and disease that arises from chance, an uncontrollable force that seems to have no assignable cause.[1(p309)] Unlike bias and confounding, random errors are considered unsystematic because they arise from an unforeseeable and unpredictable process. Random errors in epidemiological research originate from two sources. First, they can result from measurement errors—that is, mistakes in assessing the exposure and disease. For example, when investigators measure an incidence rate in a particular population, random errors may occur during the process of identifying cases of disease or calculating person-time of follow-up. Second, random errors arise from sampling variability when selecting particular subjects for a study. Sampling variability may cause an unrepresentative sample of the population to be selected "just by chance."

This chapter describes a variety of topics related to random error, including the history of biostatistics in public health; the definition of precision (which is the lack of random error) and factors that influence precision; sampling; hypothesis testing and P values; confidence interval estimation; random variable probability distributions; statistical tests for hypothesis testing; and sample size and power calculations.

▶ History of Biostatistics in Public Health

The evaluation of random error in epidemiological research involves the use of statistics. The field of statistics was first developed in the 19th century as "a science concerned with information that was important to the state."[2(p1932)] Following the Industrial Revolution, various governments supported the collection of a wide variety of statistics on the social, economic, and health conditions of the populace, such as the number and causes of deaths and the number and characteristics of births.

Biostatistics, the branch of statistics that applies statistical methods to medical and biological phenomena, has been used by epidemiologists and other public health practitioners for more than 200 years. Its history, which is inextricably entwined with the history of epidemiology, can be divided into four distinct phases.[2(p1931)] During the first phase in the 19th century, biostatisticians and epidemiologists showed that the patterns of disease followed "law-like" characteristics. These discoveries could not have been made without the pioneering work of individuals such as William Farr, who developed and used statistics to summarize public health information on births and deaths during his 40-year tenure as the compiler of statistical abstracts for the General Register Office in Great Britain. One of the chief epidemiological discoveries of the mid-19th century, John Snow's demonstration that cholera was caused by drinking water contamination, relied on mortality statistics.[2(p1932)]

Although 19th-century pioneers such as Farr and Snow made important discoveries by using descriptive statistics, they placed little emphasis on mathematical reasoning.[2(p1933)] Karl Pearson changed this practice during the second phase of biostatistics in the early 20th century, when he developed a philosophy of statistical reasoning asserting that all scientific reasoning is fundamentally statistical. Pearson became one of the chief architects of the modern theory of mathematical statistics.

During the third phase of biostatistical history, between World Wars I and II, researchers took methods for testing hypotheses used in agricultural research and applied them to medicine and public health.[2(p1934)]

During this period, R. A. Fisher developed theoretical methods for statistical inference, a method for generalizing results from a sample to a population. Fisher also made important contributions to the theory of experimental study design while working as a statistician at an agricultural research station in the United Kingdom. As he discovered the inadequacies of experimental studies of grain productivity, Fisher formulated the principles of randomization, adequate replication, and confounding. These principles, particularly those involving randomization, were later extended to medical research by Sir Austin Bradford Hill in one of the first modern experimental studies of streptomycin treatment of pulmonary tuberculosis.[3]

During the fourth phase, following World War II, researchers extended the statistical techniques developed by Fisher and others to nonexperimental studies, including cohort and case–control designs.[2(pp1934-1935)] During this period, epidemiologists shifted their focus from infectious to noninfectious diseases. This new focus provided the impetus for biostatisticians to solve difficult statistical issues, such as developing appropriate methods for assessing and controlling confounding and for dealing with repeated measurements over time.

Today, biostatisticians and epidemiologists receive professional training in one another's field, and the two groups continue to collaborate closely in the design, conduct, and analysis of epidemiological studies. The emphasis on random error has recently been questioned. Although many epidemiologists and biostatisticians emphasize the role of random error as an explanation for study findings, others believe that it is overemphasized to the point of misinterpreting study results. This misinterpretation typically occurs when investigators mistakenly use statistical significance, a topic covered later in this chapter, as a stringent criterion for judging the presence of an association.

▶ Precision

Precision can be thought of as the lack of random error. It is formally defined as "the state or quality of being precise or exact."[1(p1381)] However, most measurements in epidemiological research are not exact, and epidemiologists use the term *measurement error* to describe these problems.

Consider, for example, a study that uses interviews to measure women's use of vaginal spermicide over the past decade. Although most women would be able to recall whether they ever used spermicides during this period, many would be unable to recall exactly the brand, time, frequency, and duration of use. Inexact recall is a form of measurement error that leads to imprecise data.

There are two schools of thought on the nature of random error.[4(p148)] Epidemiologists known as **probabilists** believe that random error, or chance, is an important, even chief, explanation for events. Probabilists believe that it is impossible to predict the outcome of a coin toss (assuming the coin is fair) because chance rules its unpredictable occurrence.

Epidemiologists known as **determinists** think that every event, act, or decision is the inevitable consequence of prior events, acts, or decisions.[1(p495)] They believe that all events are "predestined to unravel in a theoretically predictable way that follows inexorably from the previous pattern of actions."[4(p148)] Therefore, determinists believe that it would be possible to predict the outcome of a fair coin toss if one could measure accurately all of the antecedent variables that determine its outcome, including the weight of the coin, the force and torque of the throw, the presence of wind, and so forth.

Even determinists acknowledge that it is impossible to measure accurately all variables needed to predict events, even simple ones such as the outcome of a coin toss. This makes it impossible to distinguish determined outcomes from random occurrences, and therefore determinists regard random variation as the equivalent of ignorance about determinants because of its unpredictability.[4(p148)]

In epidemiological research, there are three principal ways to increase precision and reduce random error in a study: (1) increase the sample size of the study, (2) repeat a measurement within a study or repeat the entire study, and (3) use an efficient study design that maximizes the amount of information obtained for a given sample size.[4(pp148-150)]

The absence or reduction of random errors does not guarantee the absence or reduction of systematic errors. In other words, it is possible to have precise but inaccurate findings. **FIGURE 12-1** uses bull's-eye diagrams to depict the relationship between precision and **accuracy**. Consider, for example, a series of scales that are used to weigh a particular individual. This individual's true weight is 123.00 pounds (the center of the bull's-eye). Repeated measurements using a highly accurate and highly precise scale will give weights that are tightly clustered around the bull's-eye (say, 122.90–123.10 pounds). A less precise but accurate scale will give weights more dispersed around the bull's-eye (say, 121.00–125.00 pounds). This could happen if the scale gave weights rounded to whole pounds. In contrast, a highly precise but inaccurate scale will give tightly clustered weights that are skewed away from the bull's-eye (say, 126.90–127.10 pounds). This type of error could occur if the scale were improperly calibrated, and therefore it is considered a systematic error. Lastly, measurements taken with an imprecise and inaccurate scale will give weights that are both dispersed and skewed away from the bull's-eye (say, 125.00–129.00 pounds). Thus, both precision and accuracy are important considerations when epidemiologists select measurement tools for their research.

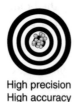

High precision
High accuracy

Low precision
High accuracy

High precision
Low accuracy

Low precision
Low accuracy

FIGURE 12-1 Relationship between precision and accuracy.

▶ Sampling

Random error arises from measurement error and **sampling variability**. Measurement errors stem from inaccuracies in assessing the exposure and disease occurrence, and sampling variability stems from the selection of specific study subjects. Errors in subject selection may lead to an unrepresentative sample of a parent population just by the "luck of the draw." This is another way of saying that the uncontrollable force known as chance caused the sample selection problem.

Samples can be drawn from a parent population either randomly or nonrandomly. In a random (or probability) sample, all individuals have "a fixed and known or equal probability of selection."[5(p238)] To select a **random sample**, investigators first must make a list of individuals in the parent population and then assign a sequential number to each individual. Next, they select a predetermined number of individuals (say 100 or 1,000) using a random number table or another similar process. Tables of random sampling numbers are lists of randomly generated numbers. These tables and more details on the mechanics of their use can be found in most biostatistics textbooks.

There are two main types of random (or probability) samples: simple random samples and stratified random samples.[5(p254)] In a simple random sample, each person has an equal chance of being selected out of the entire parent population. In a stratified random sample, the parent population is first divided into subgroups, or strata, and then a random sample is selected from each stratum. The proportion of the sample drawn from each stratum is weighted according to the population distribution of the stratification variable. For example, if 60% of the parent population consists of men, then 60% of the stratified random sample will also consist of men.

In contrast to a random sample, a nonrandom sample is usually drawn in an ill-defined or haphazard way and therefore does not conform to scientists' definition of random. For instance, a sample of individuals who volunteer for a study or a sample of individuals who happen to use a medical care facility on a particular day are examples of nonrandom samples.

Although not all epidemiological studies involve sampling, particularly random sampling, it is standard practice to consider participants as selected samples.

> In this view, the subjects in a study, whether literally sampled or not, are viewed as a figurative sample of possible people who could have been included in the study or of the different possible experiences the study subjects have had. . . . Conceptually, the actual subjects are always considered a sample of a broader experience of interest.[4(p149)]

Statistical inference is the process of making generalizations from a sample to the source or parent population. The basis for making statistical inferences is the mathematical theory of probability. The probability of an event may be defined as "the event's long-run relative frequency in repeated trials under similar conditions."[6(p63)] Thus, the probability of heads on the toss of a fair coin is 0.5, or 50%. This means that, if one conducts a large number of coin tosses (say 1,000) in exactly the same manner, heads will come up in about half of the tosses.

Probability-based statistics were developed to make inferences beyond actual data. Two commonly used statistics—P values and confidence intervals—are covered in detail in the following sections. Note that these statistics presume that a random sample was taken from the population under study. Because random samples are uncommon in epidemiological research, many epidemiologists question the use of these statistics, particularly P values, in observational studies. At the very least, they encourage cautious interpretation of these statistics.

▶ Hypothesis Testing and P Values

Many epidemiologists use **hypothesis testing** to assess the role of random error in their research. Hypothesis testing is considered a "uniform decision-making criterion" for evaluating random error that is superior to subjective impressions of the data.[7(p211)] The hypothesis testing framework has three main steps. First, investigators specify null and alternative hypotheses. Second, the investigators determine the compatibility of the study results with the null hypothesis using probabilistic methods. Third, they decide whether to reject or not reject the null hypothesis according to the degree of compatibility with the null hypothesis.

The **null hypothesis (H₀)** states that there is no association between the exposure and disease. Thus, a null hypothesis in an epidemiological study might be that the ratio measure of association is equal to 1, or the difference measure of association is equal to 0. The **alternative hypothesis (H_A)** states that there is an association between the exposure and disease. Often, the direction of the alternative hypothesis is specified. For example, there is a positive association between the exposure and disease. Note that the alternative hypothesis contradicts the null hypothesis.

Next, the compatibility of the study data with the null hypothesis is evaluated using a statistical test. The particular test depends on the study design and type of measurement. For example, the **chi-square test**, which is covered later in this chapter, is used to assess random errors in categorical count data. The computation of the test statistic yields a **P value**, which quantifies the compatibility of the study data with the null hypothesis. It is important to note that hypothesis testing assumes that the null hypothesis is true. Accordingly, the P value is defined as the probability of obtaining the observed result and more extreme results by chance alone assuming that the null hypothesis is true. It is also important to assume that there is no bias and confounding when interpreting the P value.

P values can be either one or two sided. A one-sided P value refers to the probability of observing a result at least as extreme as the observed result in one direction or another, but not both. An upper one-sided P value corresponds to the probability of obtaining the observed result or a greater one (see **FIGURE 12-2**). For example, if the observed relative risk is 2.0, the upper one-sided P value refers to the probability of observing relative risks greater than or equal to 2.0. A lower one-sided P value is the probability of obtaining the observed result or a lesser one. For example, if the observed relative risk is 0.5, the one-sided P value refers to the probability of observing relative risks less than or equal to 0.5. In contrast, a two-sided P value corresponds to a probability of seeing either a greater or lesser result. Thus, two-sided P values can be calculated by summing the upper and lower probabilities (areas A and B in Figure 12-2). Two-sided P values are more conservative than one-sided P values and suggest that the true population parameter may be either greater than or less than the null hypothesis value.

Note that the P value is a continuous statistic ranging from 0.0 to 1.0. A small P value indicates a low degree of compatibility between the observed data and null hypothesis because there is only a small chance that a result at least as extreme would have been generated if the null hypothesis were true. Thus, a small P value means that the alternative hypothesis is a better explanation for the results than the null hypothesis. A large P value indicates a high degree of compatibility between the observed data and null hypothesis. Thus, a large P value means that the null hypothesis is a better explanation for the results than the alternative hypothesis. However, no P value (no matter how small) excludes chance, and no P value (no matter how large) mandates chance.

Epidemiologists typically use a cutoff point of 0.05 to determine whether the null hypothesis should or should not be rejected. This cutoff is known as the alpha or **significance level**. Thus, when a P value is less than or equal to 0.05, we reject the null hypothesis in favor of the alternative because random error is an unlikely explanation of the discrepancy between the results and the null hypothesis. When the P value is greater than 0.05, we do not reject the null hypothesis because random

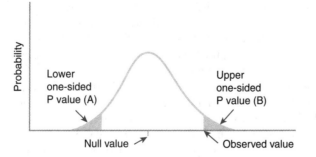

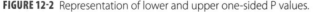

FIGURE 12-2 Representation of lower and upper one-sided P values.

error is a likely explanation for the discrepancy. Results are considered statistically significant when the P value is less than or equal to 0.05 and are considered not statistically significant when the P value is greater than 0.05.

Consider, for example, a hypothetical study on the risk of breast cancer among women who are long-term users of oral contraceptives. Assume that the study measured a 1.8-fold increased risk of breast cancer among long-term pill users and that the P value associated with this relative risk was 0.04. This means that, if the null hypothesis is true and there is no bias or confounding, there is a 4% probability of obtaining the observed result or one more extreme (i.e., a relative risk of 1.8 or greater) by chance alone. Because the P value is less than 0.05, we may conclude that the results are statistically significant and we may reject the null hypothesis.

As another example, consider a hypothetical study on the risk of breast cancer among women who are long-term users of hormone-releasing intrauterine devices (IUDs). Assume that this study found a 1.4-fold increased risk of breast cancer among long-term IUD users and that the P value associated with this relative risk was 0.15. This means that, if the null hypothesis is true and there is no bias or confounding, there is a 15% probability of obtaining the observed result or one more extreme by chance alone. Because the P value is greater than 0.05, we can conclude that the results are not statistically significant and we do not reject the null hypothesis.

The statements "statistically significant" and "not statistically significant" do not indicate the probability that the null hypothesis is true. It does not mean that the null hypothesis has been proven when results are not statistically significant. In fact, it is impossible to prove that the null hypothesis (or any other hypothesis) is true. The most that can be said about results that are not statistically significant is that the data fail to provide sufficient evidence to doubt the null hypothesis. This means that the null hypothesis remains viable until evidence to the contrary is obtained.

This line of reasoning comports with the hypothetico-deductive philosophy of causal inference proposed by Karl Popper in the 1930s.[8] According to Popper's philosophy, hypotheses are formed using creativity and imagination. Predictions are made on the basis of these hypotheses, and observations are collected and compared with predictions. If the observations are incompatible with the predictions, the hypothesis is falsified. Otherwise, the hypothesis remains a reasonable explanation until a better one comes along.

Because the significance level is an arbitrary cutoff, it is possible to incorrectly reject or not reject the null hypothesis. When a significance level of 0.05 is used, there is a 5% chance of erroneously rejecting the null hypothesis when in fact it is true. The incorrect rejection of a null hypothesis is known as a type I, or alpha, error. It is also possible to erroneously fail to reject the null hypothesis when it is false. The incorrect failure to reject a false null hypothesis is called a type II, or beta, error. The complement of the type II, or beta, error (1 minus beta) is known as the power of the statistical test. Thus, statistical power measures the ability of a test to correctly reject the null hypothesis when the alternative hypothesis is true. The differences between the two types of errors are summarized in **TABLE 12-1**. Alpha and beta errors are taken into account when investigators plan the appropriate sample size for a study. This topic is addressed later in this chapter.

In recent years, hypothesis testing, particularly significance testing, has come under criticism for numerous limitations and misuses. In fact, in 2016 the American Statistical Association, the main society that represents U.S. statisticians, issued a strong statement on the misuses and misconceptions of P values.[9] The chief limitation of significance testing is the use of a purely arbitrary cutoff for deciding whether to reject the null hypothesis. For example, it is difficult to argue that there is a meaningful difference between two sets of results whose associated P values are 0.04 and 0.06. Yet significance testing would require that the null hypothesis be rejected on the basis of the former but not the latter. Significance testing has been criticized as a simplistic strategy for studying the complex biological and social phenomena being investigated in epidemiological studies.

Hypothesis testing was originally developed to facilitate decision making in agricultural experiments. Although making decisions is an integral part of public health practice, decisions are rarely based on the results of a single epidemiological study. Furthermore, making decisions on the basis of several studies that have been degraded to being either statistically significant or not statistically significant can give misleading impressions. Consider, for example, five hypothetical studies on the risk of breast cancer among women who lived with smokers during their childhood. Assume that the five studies represent the worldwide literature on the topic and that all of the studies are free from bias and

TABLE 12-1 Possible Outcome of Hypothesis Testing		
		Truth
Conclusion of significance test	**Null hypothesis (H_0) is true**	**Alternative hypothesis (H_A) is true**
Do not reject H_0 (not statistically significant)	Correct conclusion: H_0 is true, and we do not reject H_0	Type II, or beta, error: H_A is true, but we do not reject H_0
Reject H_0 (statistically significant)	Type I, or alpha, error: H_0 is true, but we reject H_0	Correct conclusion: H_A is true and we reject H_0

TABLE 12-2 Results of Five Hypothetical Studies on the Risk of Breast Cancer Following Childhood Exposure to Tobacco Smoke

Study (no. subjects)	Risk ratio	P value	Statistically significant
A (n = 2,500)	1.4	0.02	Yes
B (n = 500)	1.7	0.10	No
C (n = 2,000)	1.6	0.04	Yes
D (n = 250)	1.8	0.30	No
E (n = 1,000)	1.6	0.06	No

confounding. The results of these hypothetical studies are shown in **TABLE 12-2**. Note that the risk ratios are fairly consistent, ranging from 1.4 to 1.8. Thus, on the basis of the measure of association, the studies suggest a modest increase in breast cancer risk among tobacco-exposed women. However, the five studies appear to be inconsistent on the basis of statistical significance: two studies have statistically significant results, and three have statistically nonsignificant results.

Which assessment is correct? We believe that the measure of association (in this case, the risk ratio) gives the most accurate picture of the strength of the relationship between tobacco exposure and breast cancer risk. The P value, on the other hand, gives a sense of the stability of the measure of association. Some studies produce more stable results than others mainly because their size is larger. For example, studies A and C produced more stable results than studies B, D, and E because of larger numbers.

Another reason P values have been criticized is that they mix together two pieces of information: the size of the association and the precision of the association.[10] In other words, P values are confounded statistics because they simultaneously reflect the magnitude of the association and the study size. When study results are summarized with only P values, it is impossible to determine whether a P value is small because the measure of association is strong or the sample size is large. In fact, it is possible to have a trivial increase in the measure of association (say, a risk ratio of 1.1) but a highly significant P value (say, 0.001) just because the study size is large. In addition, it is impossible to determine whether a P value is large because the measure of association is weak or the sample size is small. For example, it is possible to have a study with a large risk ratio (say, 5.0) but a large P value (say, 0.15) because the study size is small.

Statistical testing has led to the dubious practice of "adjusting for multiple comparisons" when examining many hypotheses in a large body of data.[11] The line of reasoning to support this practice is as follows. Under the null hypothesis that there is no association between an exposure and a disease and that any observed association is attributable to chance, a statistically significant association will be observed with a probability of alpha, the significance level. Thus, if alpha is set at the traditional level of 0.05, there is a 5% probability of rejecting a correct null hypothesis.

The theoretical basis for adjusting for multiple comparisons is the "universal null hypothesis," which states that all associations seen in a given body of data reflect only random variation.[11] Thus, when many independent associations are examined for statistical significance, the probability that at least one will be found significant increases in proportion to the number of associations examined, even if all null hypotheses are true. For example, if we test 10 hypotheses within a body of data with an alpha level of 0.05, there is a 40% probability that at least one finding will be statistically significant, assuming that all 10 null hypotheses are true. Thus, to protect against false detection of significant differences that arise when making too many comparisons, statisticians have developed "multiple comparison procedures" that make the criterion for statistical significance more stringent.

However, the assumption of the universal null hypothesis is incorrect because it "undermines the basic premises of empirical research, which hold that nature follows regular laws that may be studied through observations."[11] Making adjustments for multiple comparisons also implies that investigators should not follow up chance or unusual associations with further investigation. However, potentially important findings will be missed if scientists do not follow all possible leads, even those that turn out to be wrong.

Still another reason significance testing has been criticized is that investigators often misinterpret P values. One common misinterpretation is to equate the P value with the probability that the null hypothesis is true. As stated earlier, the P value assumes that the null hypothesis is true and tests the compatibility of the data with the null. Another misinterpretation is to equate a statistically significant association with a causal association. Statistical significance is not one of the suggested guidelines for discriminating between causal and noncausal associations.

Furthermore, statistical significance does not mean that bias and confounding have been ruled out as alternative explanations for study findings. Thus, it is entirely possible to have a statistically significant association that is invalid. Finally, statistical significance does not imply medical, biological, or public health significance. Thus, it is quite possible to have statistically significant findings that are unimportant by all other meaningful criteria. As the American Statistical Association stated, "Scientific conclusions and business or policy decisions should not be based only on whether a p value passes as specific threshold." This process "can lead to erroneous beliefs and poor decision making."[9(p131)]

▶ Confidence Interval Estimation

Another method for quantifying random error in epidemiological studies is **confidence interval** estimation. A confidence interval is typically calculated around a point estimate, which is either a measure of disease frequency or measure of association. The confidence interval quantifies the variability around the point estimate. Several formulas for calculating confidence intervals around measures of disease frequency and association are presented later in this chapter. Note that the width of the confidence interval is determined by (1) random error stemming from measurement error and sampling variability and (2) an arbitrary certainty factor, which is usually set at 95%. Thus, a wider confidence interval indicates a larger amount of random error, and a narrower interval indicates a smaller amount of random error. In other words, a wider interval indicates less precise results, while a narrower interval indicates more precise results. Given a similar degree of measurement error, a narrow confidence interval also indicates that a large sample generated the results, and a wide confidence interval indicates that a small sample produced the results. For example, consider again the five hypothetical studies on the risk of breast cancer among women who lived with smokers during their childhood (see **TABLE 12-3**). Assume that the measurement error involved in assessing smoke exposure was similar across studies. Note that the 95% confidence intervals from the larger studies (A, C) are narrower than those from the smaller studies (B, D, E).

Most epidemiologists use 95% confidence intervals, although some use 90% or 99%. The strict statistical definition of a 95% confidence interval is as follows: If a study were repeated 100 times and 100 point estimates and 100 confidence intervals were calculated, 95 out of 100

TABLE 12-3 Results of Five Hypothetical Studies on the Risk of Breast Cancer Following Childhood Exposure to Tobacco Smoke: Confidence Intervals

Study (no. subjects)	Risk ratio	95% confidence interval	Statistically significant
A ($n = 2{,}500$)	1.4	1.2–1.7	Yes
B ($n = 500$)	1.7	0.7–3.1	No
C ($n = 2{,}000$)	1.6	1.2–2.1	Yes
D ($n = 250$)	1.8	0.6–3.9	No
E ($n = 1{,}000$)	1.6	0.9–2.5	No

confidence intervals would contain the true measure of association. The remaining 5% will exclude the true measure of association.

Although incorrect from a statistical standpoint, there are two other ways that many epidemiologists interpret confidence intervals. First, a confidence interval is often considered the range of possible values within which the true magnitude of effect lies with a stated level of certainty. For example, the 95% confidence interval for study A ranges from 1.2 to 1.7 (see **FIGURE 12-3**). Thus, assuming no bias or confounding, epidemiologists may state that they have 95% confidence that the true measure of association lies somewhere inside the interval from 1.2 to 1.7. Second, epidemiologists often consider a confidence interval as the range of hypotheses that are compatible with the observed data. Thus, epidemiologists may state that, assuming no bias or confounding, the results from study A are consistent with hypotheses that the strength of the association lies between 1.2 and 1.7. Although these two interpretations are incorrect from a statistical viewpoint, they are commonly used alternative explanations.

Confidence intervals may also be used to determine whether results are statistically significant. For example, if the 95% confidence interval does not include the null value (a relative risk of 1.0), the results are considered statistically significant. If the 95% confidence interval does include the null value, the results are not statistically significant. For example, the 95% confidence intervals for studies A and C indicate that these study results are statistically significant, whereas the 95% confidence intervals for studies B, D, and E indicate that these results are not statistically significant (see Table 12-3). However, we strongly discourage the degradation of the confidence interval into the dichotomous designations of statistically significant and not statistically significant because this practice can result in misleading conclusions. Even a cursory examination of the relative risk point estimates and confidence intervals in Figure 12-3 reveals that the results of the five hypothetical studies on the

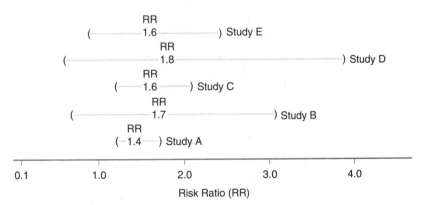

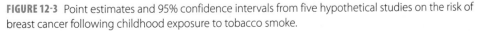

FIGURE 12-3 Point estimates and 95% confidence intervals from five hypothetical studies on the risk of breast cancer following childhood exposure to tobacco smoke.

risk of breast cancer following childhood exposure to tobacco smoke are quite consistent. Not only are the risk ratio point estimates close together, but the confidence intervals are overlapping.

The following analogy about a horse race may help to illustrate the relative importance of the measure of association (e.g., risk ratio) and the measure of statistical stability (confidence interval). A person must answer two questions when betting on the outcome of a horse race: "Which horse should I bet on?" and "How much money should I wager?" In epidemiological studies, investigators should examine the measure of association when deciding on the winning horse. The best choice for the true measure of association is the one that is obtained in a particular study. For example, the results of study A suggest that the best choice for the true risk ratio is 1.4 (see Tables 12-2 and 12-3).

Epidemiologists should examine the confidence interval when deciding how much money to bet. A large amount of money should be wagered when the confidence interval is narrow because this indicates that the results are more precise. Thus, one would wager a large bet on the results of study A (relative risk of 1.4). In contrast, one would wager less money when the confidence interval is wide because this indicates that the results are less precise. Note that this process does not degrade the confidence interval into the dichotomy of statistically significant or not statistically significant. Instead, epidemiologists examine the numerical confidence interval to determine the size of the wager.

Most epidemiologists prefer confidence intervals to P values for evaluating the role of random error. The main reason is that, unlike P values, confidence intervals are not confounded statistics. In other words, confidence intervals do a better job of separating the magnitude of the association from the sample size. First, the width of the confidence interval is mainly influenced by the sample size. For studies with a similar amount of measurement error, a wider interval reflects a smaller sample size, and a narrower interval reflects a larger sample size. In other words, a wider interval indicates less precision, whereas a narrower interval indicates more precision. Note from the data in Table 12-3 and Figure 12-3, that the confidence intervals for studies A and C are much narrower than those of studies B and D because the former are based on many more study subjects than the latter. (Of course, we must assume that the level of measurement error is similar across studies.)

A second reason that confidence intervals are preferable to P values is that the general position of the confidence interval reflects the magnitude of the association. When a confidence interval is high on the risk ratio scale, it means that the point estimate (the measure of association) is large. When the confidence interval is low on the risk ratio scale, it indicates that the point estimate is small. This characteristic stems from the construction of the interval around the point estimate. As can be seen from **FIGURE 12-4**, the point estimate anchors the interval.

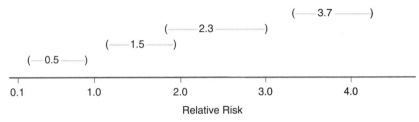

FIGURE 12-4 Point estimates and 95% confidence intervals for associations of different magnitude (the numbers in parentheses indicate the point estimates and the parentheses indicate the ends of the confidence intervals).

Still another reason most epidemiologists prefer confidence intervals to P values is that they are in the same units as the measure of association. Thus, one can "guesstimate" the point estimate by examining the confidence interval. Depending on the measure around which the interval is constructed, the point estimate will be either in the center or very close to the center of the interval. In contrast, one cannot guesstimate the point estimate by examining a P value.

However, confidence intervals have some of the same limitations as do P values. For example, they do not provide information on other explanations for the results, such as bias and confounding, and they do not indicate that the observed association is causal.

▶ P-Value Function

The P value measures the consistency between the observed data and the null hypothesis. This is why the traditional P value is often described as the "null P value." However, it is possible to determine the consistency between the data and other hypotheses by graphing a "P-value function."[4(pp158-159)] For example, the P-value function shown in **FIGURE 12-5** gives the P values for all possible values of a risk ratio. The peak of the P-value function corresponds to the point estimate of the risk ratio, and the width of the function indicates the precision of the data. A narrow function indicates a high degree of precision, and a wide function indicates a low degree of precision.

The P-value function can be used to determine which values of the risk ratio are most likely in light of the study results. For example, the P-value function in Figure 12-5 shows that positive risk ratios are most compatible with the study results because the area under the function is mainly associated with risk ratios greater than 1.0. The P-value function also shows the null P value—the P value for the risk ratio of 1.0 and all possible confidence intervals. Figure 12-5 also shows the null P value and 90% and 95% confidence intervals.

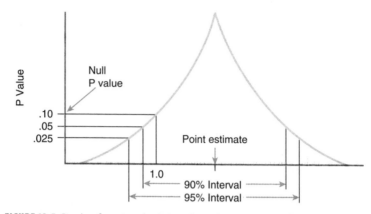

FIGURE 12-5 P-value function depicting the point estimate and 90% and 95% confidence intervals.

▶ Probability Distributions

Mathematical probability theory is the basis for making statistical inferences from a sample to a parent population. To calculate P values and confidence intervals, it is necessary to postulate a particular probability distribution for the data under the null hypothesis. The normal, binomial, and Poisson probability distributions are commonly used in epidemiological research. The normal distribution is used for continuous variables, and the binomial and Poisson distributions are used for discrete events with two mutually exclusive outcomes. These probability distributions are described in the following sections.

Normal Distribution

The **normal distribution**, also known as the Gaussian, or bell-shaped, distribution, is the cornerstone of hypothesis testing and confidence interval estimation for continuous biomedical variables, such as height, blood pressure, and weight. Although many biological variables follow approximately this distribution, variables can be normalized by transforming the data onto a different scale. For example, log transformations of serum triglyceride measurements usually follow a normal distribution.[7(p121)] In addition, an important statistical principle known as the central limit theorem allows us to assume a normal distribution for variables whose underlying distribution of individual observations is not normal. (This principle is discussed later in this chapter.)

Consider, for example, the distribution of heights among the adult residents of Wayland, Massachusetts, a suburban town about 20 miles west of Boston. According to recent data, 14,567 adult men and women live in the town.[12] Let us assume that we visit every home in Wayland and measure the heights of all resident adults. The distribution of heights among these individuals is bell shaped, or normally distributed.

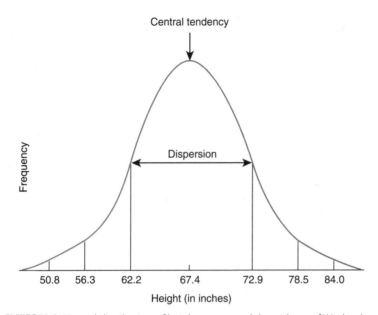

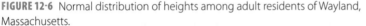

FIGURE 12-6 Normal distribution of heights among adult residents of Wayland, Massachusetts.

Every distribution, including the normal distribution, is typically described by a measure of location, or central tendency, and a measure of dispersion, or spread. The measure of central tendency summarizes the center or middle of the distribution, and the measure of dispersion describes the spread of the distribution (see **FIGURE 12-6**).

The mean, median, and mode are popular measures for describing central tendency. The formula for calculating the population **mean** is as follows:

$$\mu = \sum_{i=1}^{N} \frac{X_i}{N}$$

where μ is the population mean, X_i is each individual's measurement (height), and N is the number of people in the population. The **median** is the middlemost observation of the distribution, that is, the observation in which 50% of the observations fall above it and 50% of the observations fall below it. In particular, if N is the number of observations in a population, the median will be the $(N+1)/2$ th largest observation if N is odd; the median will be the average of $(N/2)$ and $(N/2+1)$ th largest observation if N is even.[7(p10)] The **mode** is the most commonly occurring observation, and distributions with one mode are termed unimodal.

The mean, median, and mode of heights among adults in Wayland are identical at 67.4 inches because the distribution is perfectly symmetrical (see Figure 12-6). If the distribution were skewed or asymmetrical, the three measures would be different. For example, in 2016, the mean annual income among U.S. households was much higher ($81,346) than the median annual income ($57,617) because the distribution is skewed with a tail to the right.[13] The mean is more sensitive to extreme values (in this case, individuals with extraordinarily high incomes) than the median.

Commonly used measures of dispersion are the range, variance, and standard deviation. The **range** is defined as the difference between the highest and lowest values in the distribution. Although range is the simplest measure to calculate, it has a tendency to increase with the number of observations. For this reason, the more stable **variance** and **standard deviation** are generally preferred measures of dispersion.

The formula for the population variance is as follows:

$$\sigma^2 = \sum_{i=1}^{N} \frac{(X_i - \mu)^2}{N}$$

where σ^2 is the population variance, X is each individual's measurement (height), μ is the mean value for the population, and N is the number of individuals in the population.

Because the variance is the square of the original observations, the square root of the variance, known as the population standard deviation, is more commonly used to describe the degree of dispersion. Its formula is as follows:

$$\sigma = \sqrt{\sigma^2} = \sqrt{\sum_{i=1}^{N} \frac{(X_i - \mu)^2}{N}}$$

where σ is the standard deviation, σ^2 is the population variance, X is each individual's measurement (height), μ is the population mean, and N is the number of individuals in the population. The population variance and population standard deviation of heights among adult residents in Wayland are 30.58 inches and 5.53 inches, respectively.

Every normal distribution can be completely described by its mean and standard deviation. For a normal distribution, about 68% of observations in the distribution fall within one standard deviation of the mean, about 95% fall within two standard deviations of the mean, and about 99% fall within three standard deviations of the mean. This is another way of saying that the normal distribution falls off rapidly and has few values in its tails (see Figure 12-5).

Because it is usually impossible or impractical to gather data on an entire parent population to calculate the population mean and variance, investigators commonly collect data from a sample of the population to estimate the population mean and standard deviation. For example, instead of measuring the heights of the entire adult population of Wayland, Massachusetts, we could select a simple random sample of 20 individuals from the population to approximate the population mean

TABLE 12-4 Height (in Inches) for a Simple Random Sample of Adult Residents of Wayland, Massachusetts	
59.0	60.6
60.8	61.0
62.5	63.5
64.1	64.4
64.8	65.4
66.0	66.4
67.6	67.7
67.7	69.2
72.2	75.0
76.6	77.0

and variance. The heights of the 20 individuals selected for this hypothetical sample are listed in **TABLE 12-4**.

The sample mean is calculated using the following formula:

$$\bar{x} = \sum_{i=1}^{N} \frac{x_i}{n}$$

where $\bar{x}$ is the sample mean, x_i is the measurement for each individual in the sample, and n is the number of individuals in the sample. The mean height in the simple random sample of 20 Wayland adults is $(59.0 + 60.6 + 60.8 + 61.0 + 62.5 + 63.5 + 64.1 + 64.4 + 64.8 + 65.4 + 66.0 + 66.4 + 67.6 + 67.7 + 67.7 + 69.2 + 72.2 + 75.0 + 76.6 + 77.0/20)$, or 66.6 inches.

The sample standard deviation is calculated using the following formula:

$$SD = \sqrt{\sum_{i=1}^{N} \frac{(x_i - \bar{x})^2}{n - 1}}$$

where SD is the standard deviation, x_i is each individual's measurement, $\bar{x}$ is the sample mean, and n is the number of individuals in the sample.

Thus, the standard deviation in the Wayland sample is 5.24 inches as calculated from the following:

$$\sqrt{(59.0-66.6)^2+(60.6-66.6)^2+(60.8-66.6)^2 \ldots / 20-1}$$

When the sample mean and standard deviation are computed from a random sample, such as described in Table 12-4, these figures should be good estimates of the mean and standard deviation of the population from which the sample was drawn. However, sampling variability predicts that different random samples will yield slightly different estimates of the population mean and standard deviation.

Another statistic, called the **standard error**, is used to quantify the accuracy of these estimates. For example, the standard error of the mean quantifies the degree to which the sample mean estimates the population mean. Its formula is as follows:

$$\text{SEM}\,(\overline{x}) = \frac{\text{SD}(\overline{x})}{\sqrt{n}}$$

where SEM is the standard error of the sample mean, which is denoted by $\overline{x}$; SD is the standard deviation of the sample mean; and n is the size of the sample.

The standard error and standard deviation are commonly confused. To illustrate the difference between the two, let us suppose that we draw 50 random samples of 20 Wayland residents each and measure the height of all 1,000 participants. Although each sample mean provides a good estimate of the population mean, the mean of the means gives a more accurate estimate than any particular sample mean. According to the statistical principle known as the central limit theorem, when a large number of random samples are drawn, the distribution of the sample means will be approximately normal, regardless of the distribution of the original variables.[6(pp101-102)] The standard error expresses the variation of sample means around the parent population mean, whereas the standard deviation expresses the variation of individual values around a sample mean. The standard error of height measurements from 50 random samples of 20 Wayland residents is 1.17, and the previously calculated standard deviation from one sample of 20 Wayland residents is 5.24.

Binomial Distribution

The **binomial distribution** is another commonly used theoretical probability distribution that describes random variables with two possible discrete outcomes.[7(pp91-97)] In epidemiological settings, it is used to describe dichotomous health outcomes, such as diseased versus not diseased or dead versus alive. One outcome is considered the "success," and the other is considered the "failure." Note that these terms are used arbitrarily; for example, the occurrence of disease might be considered the success, and its nonoccurrence might be considered the failure.

The binomial distribution assumes that the frequencies of success and failure occur with certain probabilities. The probability of success is designated by p, and the probability of failure is designated by $1 - p$, or q. The probabilities of success and failure are evaluated within the context of a **Bernoulli trial**, which is formally defined as a random variable that takes on the value of 1 with a probability of p and the value of 0 with a probability of $1 - p$.[7(p140)] For example, a coin toss can be considered a Bernoulli trial that takes on the value of heads with a probability of 0.5 and the value of tails with a probability of $(1 - 0.5)$, or 0.5. Similarly, each person in an epidemiological study can be considered a Bernoulli trial. For example, each subject in a cohort study can be considered a Bernoulli trial for the occurrence or nonoccurrence of disease. The probability that an individual will develop the disease is p, and the probability that he or she will not develop the disease is q. Likewise, each subject in a case–control study can be considered a Bernoulli trial for the presence or absence of exposure. The probability that the individual is exposed is p, and the probability that he or she is unexposed is q.

Bernoulli trials are based on several assumptions. First, the probabilities of success and failure are assumed to be the same for each trial. Second, the trials are assumed to be independent of one another. This means that the outcome of one trial does not affect the outcome of any other trial. Third, the trials are assumed to be conducted in an identical manner.

The binomial distribution describes the probability of k successes in n independent trials, where p is the probability of success in each trial, k is the number of successes, and n is the number of trials. The mean of the binomial distribution is estimated as follows:

$$\mu = np$$

where μ is the mean, n is the number of Bernoulli trials, and p is the probability of success in each trial. The variance is estimated by

$$\sigma^2 = np(1 - p)$$

where σ^2 is the variance, n is the number of independent Bernoulli trials, and p is the probability of success in a trial. The shape of a binomial distribution for 10 Bernoulli trials when p equals 0.3 is shown in **FIGURE 12-7**. Note that the distribution has a tail to the right. If p were nearer to 0 or 1, the distribution would be more severely skewed.

Because the binomial distribution is very cumbersome to use when the number of trials or sample size is large, the normal distribution is typically used to approximate the binomial in this setting. In fact, the normal distribution is a good approximation of the binomial distribution when n is moderately large and p is not extreme (too near 0 or 1).[7(p139)]

Poisson Distribution

The **Poisson distribution** is a discrete distribution commonly used to describe rare events.[7(p98)] It is frequently used in epidemiological research

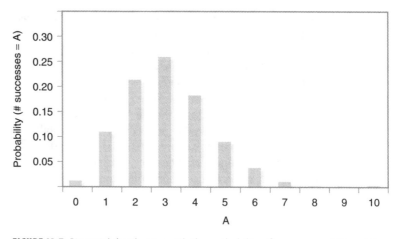

FIGURE 12-7 Binomial distribution with the probability of success, $p = 0.3$, and the number of Bernoulli trials, $n = 10$.

because many diseases are uncommon, particularly if one considers the likelihood of occurrence in a short period of time. Consider, for example, the occurrence of new cases of human immunodeficiency virus (HIV) infection in a population of intravenous drug users over the course of a year. Assuming that (1) the probability of a new HIV infection on any given day is very small, (2) the number of cases occurring on any day is independent of that number on any other day, and (3) the infection rate does not change over time, then the number of HIV infections over a 1-year period follows a Poisson distribution.

Both the mean and variance of a Poisson distribution are equal to μ as defined by the following formula:

$$\mu = \lambda t$$

where λ is the expected number of events per unit time and t is time. Note that μ describes the expected number of events over the time period t.

Not surprisingly, the Poisson distribution is closely related to the binomial distribution. For example, the two distributions are quite similar when the number of Bernoulli trials is large and the probability of success is small. The normal distribution is also used to approximate the Poisson distribution when μ is very large because the Poisson distribution is too unwieldy in this situation.

▶ Hypothesis-Testing Statistics

Many statistical tests are used for hypothesis testing. Commonly used tests in epidemiological research include the **Student *t* test** and the chi-square test. A third type of test is the Z test, which is not described in this chapter. The decision to use a particular statistical test depends on the nature of the data under investigation. For example, the Student *t* test is used to test hypotheses about continuous variables when the variance is unknown or the sample size is small, and the chi-square test is used for discrete data.

The Student t statistic can be used to test a hypothesis about the heights of adult residents in Wayland, Massachusetts (a continuous variable). For example, let us test the null hypothesis that the average height of males is equal to the average height of females by selecting two simple random samples of 20 men and 20 women each. Suppose that we find that the mean height and variance for the male sample are 69.1 and 34.8, respectively, and the mean height and variance for the female sample are 63.7 and 31.4, respectively. The following formula for the two-sample t test can be used to compare these two independent samples:

$$t_{df} = \frac{\overline{x}_1 - \overline{x}_2}{\sqrt{s_p^2(1/n_1 + 1/n_2)}}$$

where t is the test statistic, $\overline{x}_1$ is the mean of the first sample, $\overline{x}_2$ is the mean of the second sample, s_p is the pooled estimate of the common variance, and n_1 and n_2 are the number of individuals in each sample. The degrees of freedom (df), the number of independent comparisons that can be made among members of a sample, equals $n_1 + n_2 - 2$. The result equals the total number of quantities in a series $(n_1 + n_2)$ minus the number of restrictions placed on the series (two, in this case, because two means have been estimated).[6(p32)]

The pooled estimate of the common variance (s^2) estimates the variance of the entire study population (20 males and 20 females) and is calculated as follows:

$$s_p^2 = \frac{(n_1 - 1)s_1^2 + (n_2 - 1)s_2^2}{n_1 + n_2 - 2}$$

where s_p is the pooled variance, n_1 is the number of individuals in the first sample, n_2 is the number of individuals in the second sample, s_1 is the variance of the first sample, and s_2 is the variance of the second sample. Using the data from the samples of men and women, we find that

$$t_{20+20-2} = \frac{69.1 - 63.7}{\sqrt{33.1\,(1/20 + 1/20)}}$$

Thus, the t statistic equals 2.97 and has 38 degrees of freedom. This statistic can be converted into a probability statement, or P value, by looking up its value in a t table (which can be found in most biostatistics textbooks). The t value of 2.97 with 38 degrees of freedom corresponds to a P value of approximately 0.01. Thus, there is about a 1% probability of obtaining the observed height difference between men and women and more extreme differences by chance alone given that the null hypothesis is true.

Now, let us use the chi-square statistic to test a hypothesis about the political affiliations of men and women in Wayland (a discrete variable). In particular, let us test the null hypothesis that the proportion of registered Democrats is identical for men and women by selecting two new simple random samples of 20 men and 20 women each. Suppose that we find that the proportion of Democrats in the male sample is 40% and the proportion of Democrats in the female sample is 50%. The following chi-square formula can be used to compare these two independent samples:

$$X_{df}^2 = \frac{\Sigma(O_i - E_i)^2}{E_i}$$

where X^2 is the chi-square statistic, O_i is the observed count in a category, and E_i is the expected count in the category under the null hypothesis. Again, df stands for the number of degrees of freedom associated with the statistic. **TABLE 12-5** gives the observed counts and the expected values according to the null hypothesis. Note that we expect to see an equal proportion of Democrats among men and women.

Using these data, we calculate the chi-square statistic as follows: $(8-9)^2/9 + (12-11)^2/11 + (10-9)^2/9 + (10-11)^2/11 = 0.40$. The number of degrees of freedom is equal to the product of the number of categories in each variable minus one. Here, there are two categories of each variable (men and women, Democrats and Republicans), and therefore the number of degrees of freedom is $(2-1)(2-1)$, or 1. The chi-square statistic can be converted to a P value by looking up its value in a chi-square table. A chi-square value of 0.40 with one degree of freedom corresponds to a P value of approximately 0.50. Thus, there is a 50% probability of obtaining the observed difference between men and

TABLE 12-5 Observed and Expected Numbers of Democrats and Republicans Among Men and Women in Wayland, Massachusetts

Sex	Democrats	Republicans
Men		
Observed	8	12
Expected	9	11
Women		
Observed	10	10
Expected	9	11

women and more extreme differences by chance alone given that the null hypothesis is true.

▶ Confidence Intervals for Measures of Disease Frequency and Association

Many epidemiologists prefer to quantify random error by estimating confidence intervals. Either approximate or exact methods may be used to calculate confidence intervals. Approximate confidence intervals are easy to calculate because they assume that the point estimate is normally distributed. Exact confidence intervals, which are based on the binomial or Poisson distributions, are difficult to calculate because many values must be tested successively before one arrives at the correct interval value. Thus, epidemiologists primarily use exact intervals when normality cannot be assumed.

This section describes commonly used formulas for calculating approximate 95% confidence intervals around several measures of disease frequency—cumulative incidence, prevalence, incidence rate—and several absolute and relative measures of comparison.

Cumulative Incidence

The cumulative incidence is defined as the proportion of a candidate population that becomes diseased over a specified period of time. Mathematically, it is expressed as follows:

$$\frac{\text{Number of new cases of disease}}{\text{Number in candidate population over a specified time period}}$$

Let us illustrate the calculation of a 95% confidence interval for cumulative incidence. The Six Cities Study was a prospective cohort study that investigated the association between air pollution and mortality. Investigators followed a sample of adults from six locations around the United States to measure the cumulative incidence of mortality.[14] The six locations provided a wide range of pollution levels from the highly polluted city of Steubenville, Ohio, to the relatively unpolluted city of Portage, Wisconsin.

The investigators observed an increased risk of death in the polluted areas. In particular, the cumulative incidence of mortality was 291/1,351 (or 21.5%) among subjects from Steubenville and 232 per 1,631 (or 14.2%) among subjects from Portage. Exact confidence intervals for cumulative incidence are calculated using the binomial distribution. However, when the sample size is large, the following normal distribution approximation formula can be used to quantify random error around these measurements:

$$\text{CI}_{\text{L,U}} = \frac{A}{N} \pm 1.96 \sqrt{\frac{A/N(1 - A/N)}{N}}$$

where $CI_{L,U}$ is the lower and upper bounds of the confidence interval, A is the number of cases of disease (the numerator of the cumulative incidence), and N is the number of individuals in the group (the denominator of the cumulative incidence). This formula works best when the sample size is large and the outcome frequency is fairly high. Because these conditions are met in the Six Cities Study, we can calculate the approximate 95% confidence interval for the cumulative incidence of mortality in Steubenville as follows:

$$CI_{L,U} = \frac{291}{1,351} \pm 1.96 \sqrt{\frac{291/1,351(1-291/1,351)}{1,351}}$$

Thus, the 95% confidence interval ranges from 20.4% to 22.6%. This means that our best estimate for the true cumulative incidence of mortality in Steubenville is 21.5%; however, we are 95% confident that the true cumulative incidence rate lies between 20.4% and 22.6%.

Prevalence

Prevalence is defined as the proportion of the total population that is diseased at a point or during a period of time. Mathematically, it is expressed as follows:

$$\frac{\text{Number of existing cases of disease}}{\text{Number of total population}}$$

The confidence interval formula for cumulative incidence is also appropriate for prevalence measures. For example, let us assume that we measure a prevalence of diabetes among a random sample of adults in Steubenville, Ohio, at 25 per 1,000 people. We calculate the approximate 95% confidence interval for the diabetes prevalence as follows:

$$CI_{L,U} = \frac{25}{1,000} \pm 1.96 \sqrt{\frac{25/1,000(1-25/1,000)}{1,000}}$$

Thus, the 95% confidence interval ranges from 15.3 per 1,000 to 34.7 per 1,000. This means that our best estimate for the true prevalence of diabetes among adults in Steubenville is 25 per 1,000, but we are 95% confident that the true prevalence lies between 15.3 and 34.7 per 1,000.

Incidence Rate

The incidence rate is defined as the occurrence of new cases of disease arising during at-risk person-time of observation. Mathematically, it is expressed as follows:

$$\frac{\text{Number of new cases of disease}}{\text{Person-time of observation}}$$

Let us use incidence rate data from the Six Cities Study to illustrate calculation of the approximate 95% confidence interval for this measure of disease frequency. The incidence rate of death was 291 per 17,914 person-years (or 16.24/1,000 person-years) in Steubenville, Ohio.[14] Exact confidence intervals for incidence rates are calculated using the Poisson distribution. However, when the sample size is large, the following normal distribution approximation formula can be used to quantify the random error around this type of measurement:

$$CI_{L,U} = \frac{A}{R} \pm 1.96\sqrt{\frac{A}{R^2}}$$

where $CI_{L,U}$ is the lower and upper bounds of the confidence interval, A is the number of cases, and R is the time at risk in the study population. Thus, we calculate the 95% confidence interval for the incidence rate of mortality in Steubenville as follows:

$$CI_{L,U} = \frac{291}{17,914} \pm 1.96\sqrt{\frac{291}{17,914^2}}$$

Thus, we are 95% confident that the true mortality rate among adults in Steubenville lies in the range from 14.37 to 18.11 per 1,000 person-years.

Absolute Measures of Comparison

Now, let us calculate an approximate 95% confidence interval for an absolute measure of comparison. Absolute comparisons are calculated for either exposed individuals or the total population. When exposed individuals are the focus, the absolute difference measure is as follows:

$$RD = R_e - R_u$$

where RD equals rate or risk difference (incidence rate difference, cumulative incidence difference, or prevalence difference), R_e equals rate or risk (incidence rate, cumulative incidence, or prevalence) in the exposed group, and R_u equals rate or risk (incidence rate, cumulative incidence, or prevalence) in the unexposed group. The particular formula for the 95% confidence intervals for risk or rate differences depends on the underlying measure of disease frequency and sample size. The following formula for an approximate 95% confidence interval may be used to quantify the random error around an incidence rate difference when the sample size is large:

$$CI_{L,U} = RD \pm 1.96\sqrt{\frac{A_1}{R_1^2} + \frac{A_0}{R_0^2}}$$

where $CI_{L,U}$ is the lower and upper bounds of the confidence interval, RD is the rate or risk difference, A_1 is the number of exposed cases, A_0 is the number of unexposed cases, R_1 is the time at risk in the exposed group, and R_0 is the time at risk in the unexposed group.

Let us use results from the Six Cities Study to illustrate calculation of a 95% confidence interval for an incidence rate difference between Steubenville (the most polluted city) and Portage (the least polluted city). The incidence rates of mortality among subjects in these cities were 291 per 17,914 person-years (or 16.2 per 1,000 person-years) and 232 per 21,618 person-years (or 10.7 per 1,000 person-years), respectively.[14] Thus, the incidence rate difference is equal to 5.5 per 1,000 person-years, and we calculate the corresponding 95% confidence interval as follows:

$$CI_{L,U} = 5.5 \text{ per } 1,000 \text{ person-years} \pm 1.96 \sqrt{\frac{291}{17,914^2} + \frac{232}{21,618^2}}$$

Thus, we are 95% confident that the true incidence rate difference among adults from the two cities ranges from 3.2 to 7.8 per 1,000 person-years.

Relative Measures of Comparison

The relative measure of comparison is based on the ratio of two measures of disease frequency. Mathematically, the relative measure is expressed as follows:

$$RR = \frac{R_e}{R_u}$$

where RR equals rate or risk ratio; R_e equals incidence rate, cumulative incidence, or prevalence in the exposed group; and R_u equals incidence rate, cumulative incidence, or prevalence in the unexposed group. The following normal approximation formula may be used for a 95% confidence interval for a relative risk based on incidence rates when the sample size is large:

$$\ln RR_{L,U} = \ln RR \pm 1.96 \sqrt{\frac{1}{A_1} + \frac{1}{A_0}}$$

where L and U are the lower and upper bounds of the confidence interval, ln RR is the natural log of the rate ratio, A_1 is the number of cases in the exposed group, and A_0 is the number of cases in the unexposed group. Because this formula gives the confidence interval for the natural log of the rate ratio, it is necessary to take the antilog of the two bounds to obtain the confidence interval for the rate ratio itself. Using the incidence rate data from the Six Cities Study, we measure the incidence rate ratio at

16.24 per 1,000 person-years/10.73 per 1,000 person-years, or 1.51,[14] and we calculate the approximate 95% confidence interval as follows:

$$\ln RR_{L,U} = \ln 1.51 \pm 1.96\sqrt{\frac{1}{291} + \frac{1}{232}}$$

Thus, taking the antilog of the two bounds, we are 95% confident that the true relative risk comparing adults from the two cities lies between 1.27 and 1.79.

It is usually impossible to calculate the rate or risk of disease in exposed and unexposed groups in a case–control study, and therefore the odds ratio must be used as the relative measure of comparison in this setting. Either the disease odds ratio (the odds of being a case [a/b] among the exposed versus the odds of being a case among the unexposed [c/d]) or the exposure odds ratio (the odds of being exposed among cases [a/c] versus the odds of being exposed among controls [b/d]) may be calculated.

Consider the following hypothetical case–control study of dichlorodiphenyldichloroethylene (DDE) exposure and the risk of breast cancer (see **TABLE 12-6**).

According to these data, women with high serum DDE levels have a 1.9-fold increased risk of breast cancer as compared with women with low serum DDE levels $\left(\text{odds ratio} = [500 \times 3,400]/[600 \times 1,500] = 1.9\right)$. The following formula for an approximate 95% confidence interval may be used to quantify the random error around an odds ratio:

$$\ln OR_{L,U} = \ln OR \pm 1.96\sqrt{\frac{1}{a} + \frac{1}{b} + \frac{1}{c} + \frac{1}{d}}$$

where ln OR is the natural log of the odds ratio, and a, b, c, and d are the cells of the two-by-two table that refer to the number of exposed

TABLE 12-6 Crude Data from a Hypothetical Case–Control Study of DDE Exposure and Breast Cancer

	Breast cancer	
DDE level	**Cases**	**Controls**
High	500	600
Low	1,500	3,400
Total	2,000	4,000

cases (a), the number of exposed controls (b), and so forth. Using this formula, we calculate the 95% confidence interval as follows:

$$\ln OR_{L,U} = \ln 1.9 \pm 1.96 \sqrt{\frac{1}{500} + \frac{1}{600} + \frac{1}{1,500} + \frac{1}{3,400}}$$

Thus, after taking the antilog of the calculated numbers, we can say that we are 95% confident that the true odds ratio ranges from 1.7 to 2.2. The formulas for approximate 95% confidence intervals are summarized in **TABLE 12-7**.

TABLE 12-7 Approximate 95% Confidence Intervals for Measures of Disease Frequency and Comparison

Point estimate	Definition	95% confidence interval formula
Prevalence (P)	Number of existing cases (A)/ number in total population (N)	$A/N \pm 1.96 \sqrt{\dfrac{A/N(1 - A/N)}{N}}$
Cumulative incidence (CI)	Number of new cases (A)/ number in candidate population (N)	$A/N \pm 1.96 \sqrt{\dfrac{A/N(1 - A/N)}{N}}$
Incidence rate (IR)	Number of new cases (A)/ person-time at risk (R)	$A/R \pm 1.96 \sqrt{A/R^2}$
Incidence rate difference (IRD)	Incidence rate$_{exp}$ (A_1/R_1) − incidence rate$_{unexp}$ (A_0/R_0)	$IRD_{L,U} \pm 1.96 \sqrt{A_1/R_1^2 + A_0/R_0^2}$
Incidence rate ratio (IRR)	Incidence rate$_{exp}$ (A_1/R_1)/ incidence rate$_{unexp}$ (A_0/R_0)	$\ln RR_{L,U} = \ln RR \pm 1.96 \sqrt{1/A_1 + 1/A_0}$
Odds ratio (OR)	Exposure odds among cases (a/c)/ exposure odds among controls (b/d), or disease odds among exposed (a/b)/ disease odds among unexposed (c/d)	$\ln OR_{L,U} = \ln OR \pm 1.96 \sqrt{1/a + 1/b + 1/c + 1/d}$

▶ Sample Size and Power Calculations

Epidemiologists often use sample size calculations to plan the appropriate size of a study because they believe that correct inferences about the parent population can be made only with a sufficient sample size. But exactly what constitutes a "sufficient" sample size? To answer this question, investigators often turn to sample size formulas. These formulas, which can be found in most biostatistics textbooks, take into account the following factors: (1) the expected magnitude of the association, (2) the outcome rate in the comparison group (if a cohort or experimental study is being planned) or the exposure prevalence in the control group (if a case–control study is being planned), (3) the probability of rejecting the null hypothesis when it is true (known as the type I, or alpha, error), (4) the probability of missing a true association (known as the type II, or beta, error), and (5) the relative size of the compared groups.[15(p79)] In general, a large sample size is needed when alpha and beta errors are small, when the expected magnitude of the association is small, and when the outcome rate in the comparison group of a cohort or experimental study or exposure prevalence in the control group of a case–control study is either very small or very large.

The information needed for the formula is gathered from several sources. The expected magnitude of the association comes from prior research. A scientifically important association is used, say, a relative risk of 1.5 or 2.0, when prior studies are absent or ambiguous. The outcome rate in the comparison group (in a cohort or experimental study) or the exposure prevalence in the control group (in a case–control study) comes from pilot data from the actual study population or other populations. For example, a cohort study was designed to investigate the relationship between drinking water contaminants and reproductive and developmental abnormalities in the Cape Cod area of Massachusetts.[16] Outcome rates for the power calculations were gathered from national statistics on low birth weight, prematurity, and birth defects among demographically similar individuals during the years under study. The alpha and beta errors are assigned arbitrarily; usually the alpha error is set at 0.05, and the beta error is set at 0.20 or less. The latter implies that investigators aim for a sample size with at least 80% power (power is equal to 1 minus beta) to detect an association, if one truly exists.

Although sample size formulas are helpful, the information that goes into their calculations is either arbitrary (e.g., alpha and beta errors) or educated guesses (such as expected magnitude of association). Furthermore, sample size calculations fail to account for numerous other factors, including the value of the information gained from a study; the balance between precision and cost; and many unquantifiable social, political, and biological factors.[4(pp149-150)] Thus, these estimates should not be cast in stone but rather should be considered ballpark figures of a sufficient sample size.

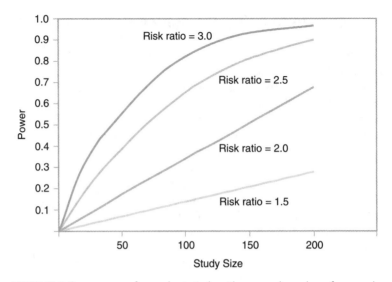

FIGURE 12-8 Power curves for a cohort study with an equal number of exposed and unexposed subjects (alpha error is 0.05; outcome frequency is 0.10).

Some epidemiologists believe that power curves are more informative than sample size calculations for determining the needed study size.[15(pp79-80)] Power refers to the ability of a test to correctly reject the null hypothesis when the alternative hypothesis is true. When an association is present, the power of a study will increase as the study size increases. Power curves can be constructed that plot power against sample size for various estimates of an association. As displayed in **FIGURE 12-8**, power curves show the degree to which the study size must increase to attain greater power at differing estimates of an association.[14(p80)] These curves share some of the same drawbacks that sample size calculations have. However, because they illustrate the informativeness of a particular sample size, they are more valuable for planning a study than sample size calculations. In the end, however, "the question of the most appropriate study size is not a technical decision . . . but a judgment to be determined by experience, intuition, and insight."[15(pp81-82)]

Summary

Random error is considered an unsystematic error because it arises from an unforeseeable and unpredictable process known as chance. Precision is a term for the lack of random error. Two sources of random error are measurement error and sampling variability. Measurement error stems from inaccuracies in assessing the exposure and disease, and sampling variability stems from the selection of specific study subjects. Errors in subject selection lead to an unrepresentative sample of a parent population just by the "luck of the draw." This is another way of saying the uncontrollable force known as chance caused the sample selection problem.

Epidemiologists commonly use hypothesis testing to assess the role of random error and to make statistical inferences, that is, generalizations from a study sample to the parent population. In hypothesis testing, investigators specify the null and alternative hypotheses, evaluate the compatibility of the study results with the null hypothesis using statistical tests and P values, and decide whether to reject or not reject the null hypothesis. Commonly used statistical tests include the chi-square test and Student *t* test. The decision to use a particular test depends on the nature of the data under investigation (e.g., continuous or discrete).

An integral part of hypothesis testing is the calculation of a P value, which is defined as the probability of obtaining the observed result (or a more extreme result) by chance alone assuming that the null hypothesis is true and that there is no bias or confounding. Although the P value is a continuous statistic, epidemiologists commonly use a cutoff of 0.05 (known as the alpha, or significance, level) to determine whether the null hypothesis should be rejected. In recent years, hypothesis testing, particularly the use of P values, has come under criticism. Critics argue that the significance level of 0.05 is a purely arbitrary cutoff that can lead to incorrect interpretations of study results and that the P value is confounded (i.e., it mixes together the effect of the magnitude of the association with the effect of the sample size).

Today, most epidemiologists prefer to use confidence intervals for quantifying random error. A confidence interval is calculated around a point estimate, which is typically a measure of disease frequency or association. Typically, 95% confidence intervals are calculated, and particular formulas for calculating them vary according to the point estimate. Epidemiologists prefer confidence intervals mainly because they are not confounded like P values, which means they can better separate the magnitude of the association from the sample size. The width of the confidence interval is influenced by the sample size, and the general position of the interval reflects the magnitude of the association. The strict statistical definition of a 95% confidence interval is as follows: If a study were repeated 100 times and 100 point estimates and confidence intervals were obtained, 95% of the intervals would contain the true measure of association. Although incorrect from a statistical viewpoint, two other ways to interpret confidence intervals are (1) the range of possible values within which the true magnitude of effect lies with a certain level of certainty, and (2) the range of possible hypotheses that are compatible with the observed data with a certain level of certainty. Both of these interpretations require the assumption that there is no bias or confounding.

Mathematical probability theory is the basis for making statistical inferences from a study sample to a parent population. In fact, it is necessary to postulate a particular probability distribution for the data under the null hypothesis to calculate a P value and confidence interval. The normal, binomial, and Poisson distributions are commonly employed in epidemiological research. The normal distribution is used for continuous variables, and the binomial and Poisson distributions are used for discrete events with two mutually exclusive outcomes. Each probability distribution is described by measures of central tendency and dispersion. The mean, median, and mode are commonly used central tendency measures; range, variance, standard deviation, and standard error of the mean are measures of spread. Formulas to calculate these measures vary according to the probability distribution.

Because correct inferences about the parent population can be made only with a sufficient sample size, epidemiologists use sample size calculations, power curves, experience, and intuition to plan the appropriate size for a study. Sample size formulas take into account the expected magnitude of the association, the outcome rate in the comparison group, and the alpha and beta levels. Power curves plot statistical power against sample size for various estimates of association.

References

1. Pickett JP (ed.). *The American Heritage Dictionary of the English Language.* 4th ed. Boston, MA: Houghton Mifflin Co.; 2000.

2. Armitage P, Colton T (eds.). *Encyclopedia of Biostatistics.* Vol 3. Chichester, England: John Wiley and Sons; 1998.

3. Medical Research Council. Streptomycin in Tuberculosis Trials Committee. Streptomycin treatment of pulmonary tuberculosis. *Brit Med J.* 1948;2:769-782.

4. Rothman KJ, Greenland S, Lash TL. *Modern Epidemiology.* 3rd ed. Philadelphia, PA: Lippincott Williams and Wilkins; 2008.

5. Porta M. *A Dictionary of Epidemiology.* 6th ed. New York, NY: Oxford University Press; 2014.

6. Colton T. *Statistics in Medicine.* Boston, MA: Little, Brown and Co.; 1974.

7. Rosner B. *Fundamentals of Biostatistics.* 5th ed. Pacific Grove, CA: Duxbury Thompson Learning; 2000.

8. Popper KR. *The Logic of Scientific Discovery.* New York, NY: Basic Books; 1959 (reprint of 1935 ed.).

9. American Statistical Association. ASA Statement on Statistical Significance and *P*-Values. *Am Stat.* 2016;70(2):129-133.

10. Lang JM, Rothman KJ, Cann CI. That confounded P-value. *Epidemiology.* 1998;9:7-8.

11. Rothman KJ. No adjustments are needed for multiple comparisons. *Epidemiology.* 1990;1:43-46.

12. Vital statistics. Wayland, Massachusetts, Web site. www.wayland.ma.us/about-us/pages/vital-statistics. Accessed December 2017.

13. Income in the past 12 months: 2016 American Community Survey 1-year estimates. U.S. Census Bureau American FactFinder Web site. https://factfinder.census.gov/faces/nav/jsf/pages/search results.xhtml?refresh=t#acsST. Accessed December 2017.

14. Dockery D, Pope CA, Xu X, Spengler JD, Ware JH, Fay ME, et al. An association between air pollution and mortality in six U.S. cities. *New Engl J Med.* 1993;329:1753-1759.

15. Rothman KJ. *Modern Epidemiology.* 1st ed. Boston, MA: Little, Brown and Co.; 1986.

16. Aschengrau A, Weinberg J, Rogers S, Gallagher LM, Winter M, Vieira V, et al. Prenatal exposure to tetrachloroethylene-contaminated drinking water and the risk of adverse birth outcomes. *Environ Health Perspect.* 2008;116:814-820.

Chapter Questions

1. Define each of the following terms:
   a. Chance
   b. Precision
   c. Statistical inference

2. What is the main assumption involved in hypothesis testing and the calculation of P values?
3. What is the main limitation of significance testing?
4. Why are P values considered confounded statistics?
5. Why has the American Statistical Association recently cautioned against the reliance on P values for making scientific conclusions and policy decisions?
6. A case–control study was conducted in Europe to determine the association between dietary factors and coronary heart disease. The investigators found an odds ratio of 1.8 for coronary heart disease among subjects who cooked with margarine (the exposed group) compared with those who cooked with olive oil (the reference group). The 95% confidence interval for this odds ratio was 0.8 to 4.3, and the upper one-sided P value was 0.10.
   a. State in words your interpretation of the odds ratio.
   b. State in words your interpretation of the 95% confidence interval.
   c. Do you think that this confidence interval is relatively wide or narrow?
   d. State in words your interpretation of the P value.

7. Give one reason many epidemiologists prefer to use confidence intervals instead of P values to assess the role of random error.
8. State the probability distributions that are commonly used in epidemiological research, and describe the settings in which they are used.
9. Indicate whether the following statements are true or false:
   a. Unlike bias and confounding, random errors are unsystematic.
   b. Reducing random error also reduces errors from bias and confounding.
   c. Precise exposure data can be achieved by repeating the exposure measurements.
   d. Precise results are always more accurate than imprecise results.
   e. Increasing the sample size decreases the chance of selecting an unrepresentative sample.
   f. A statistically significant finding always has public health significance.

10. State which of the following studies is more precise; that is, which has a smaller amount of random error?

	Rate ratio	95% confidence interval
Study A	1.04	0.9–1.2
Study B	1.44	0.8–2.0

11. Epidemiologists plan the appropriate size for a study by:
    a. Using judgment, experience, and intuition
    b. Performing sample size calculations
    c. Both A and B
    d. Neither A nor B

12. A follow-up study of the relationship between recent alcohol consumption (measured as "yes" or "no") and boating accidents found a risk ratio of 2.0 and a P value of 0.15. The best interpretation of this finding is:

 a. There was no association between alcohol consumption and boating accidents because the P value indicates that the results were not statistically significant.

 b. There was a 30% risk of having a boating accident among people who drank recently as compared with a 15% risk of having a boating accident among people who did not drink recently. The P value indicates that there is a 15% probability of obtaining this result or a more extreme result, assuming that the null hypothesis is true and that there is no bias or confounding.

 c. People who drank recently were twice as likely to have a boating accident as compared with people who did not drink recently. The P value indicates that there is a 15% probability of obtaining this result or a more extreme result, assuming that the null hypothesis is true and that there is no bias or confounding.

 d. None of the above

CHAPTER 13

Effect Measure Modification

LEARNING OBJECTIVES

By the end of this chapter the reader will be able to:
- Define and provide examples of effect measure modification, including synergy and antagonism.
- Distinguish between confounding and effect measure modification.
- Describe the methods for evaluating effect measure modification.
- State the relationship between the measure of association and effect measure modification.

▶ Introduction

Epidemiologists evaluate whether a study result is valid by assessing the presence of **bias**, confounding, and **random error**. **Confounding** is a mixing of effects between an exposure, an outcome, and a third variable known as the confounder.[1(p129)] Epidemiologists control for confounding using a variety of methods in the design and analysis of a study. While assessing and controlling for confounding during the analysis, investigators also determine whether the magnitude of the association between an exposure and a disease is changed or modified by a third variable. If the size of the association changes according to the level of a third variable, then effect measure modification is present. Unlike bias and confounding, which are problems that the investigator needs to eliminate, effect modification is a natural phenomenon of scientific interest that the investigator aims to describe and understand. This chapter defines and describes effect measure modification, explains how it differs from confounding, and describes the principal ways to evaluate its presence.

▶ Definitions and Terms for Effect Measure Modification

Effect measure modification, also known as **heterogeneity of effect**, means that the strength of the association between an exposure and a disease differs according to the level of another variable. This other variable is called the effect modifier. For example, a notable study found that gender was a modifier of the association between high ambient temperature and mortality.[2] The harmful effect of hot weather was 20 times greater among women than among men.

The term *homogeneity of effect* is used when effect modification is absent. An example of homogeneity of effect is the relationship between religion, age, and breast cancer. Jewish women have a higher risk of breast cancer than do women who belong to other religious groups at both young and old ages.[3] Furthermore, older women have a higher risk of breast cancer than younger women, regardless of their religious affiliation.

Epidemiologists often use the term *effect modification* instead of *effect measure modification* to describe the change in an association according to the level of the third variable. However, this simplification leads to ambiguity because effect measure modification depends on the particular measure of association describing the relationship between the exposure and disease.[1(pp61-62)] That is, effect measure modification depends on whether a ratio measure or a difference measure is being used. When effect modification is absent using a ratio measure of association, it will usually be present when a difference measure of association is used and vice versa. (This concept is discussed later in the chapter.) Consequently, it is important to describe the presence of effect measure modification as specifically as possible, for example, by stating "heterogeneity of the risk ratio was observed." The expression *statistical interaction* is also commonly used to describe effect measure modification. It too should be avoided because the term is too vague.

Effect measure modification should not be considered merely an arbitrary statistical phenomenon, but rather it should be regarded as a causal framework for gaining insight into a natural phenomenon.[1(pp71-83)] For example, menopausal status modifies the relationship between a woman's weight and her risk of breast cancer.[4] The risk of breast cancer increases with body mass index among postmenopausal women but not among premenopausal women. These different associations likely reflect biological differences, such as differences in circulating hormone levels between pre- and postmenopausal women, and therefore provide important clues to the pathological mechanism whereby a normal breast cell is transformed into a cancerous one.

Epidemiological literature contains many well-known examples of effect measure modification that have both helped epidemiologists to understand the biology of a particular disease and led to important medical and public health policy recommendations. One example is the modification of the relationship between cigarette smoking and bronchogenic cancer (cancer of the lung, bronchus, and trachea) by asbestos exposure.[5] In a landmark study, Selikoff and colleagues found that asbestos insulation workers in general had a 10-fold increased risk of dying from bronchogenic cancer. However, they also found that asbestos insulation workers who smoked had 92 times the risk of dying from bronchogenic cancer as compared with men who did not smoke and were not exposed to asbestos. This tremendous increased risk among individuals with both exposures reflects the pathological process whereby the carcinogens in cigarette smoke and asbestos fibers exacerbate one another to transform normal cells into malignant ones. These data have also been used to guide occupational and safety health recommendations to reduce workplace exposure to chemical and physical agents such as asbestos and to initiate smoking cessation campaigns among working groups, especially those exposed to asbestos.[6]

Another well-known example of effect measure modification is the modification of the relationship between oral contraceptives and myocardial infarction by the presence of other factors such as cigarette smoking and obesity.[7] For example, Mann and colleagues found that women who had recently used oral contraceptives had about a threefold increased risk of myocardial infarction as compared with women who did not use oral contraceptives. However, women who had at least two additional risk factors for myocardial infarction (such as high lipid levels, cigarette smoking, and obesity) had a 78-fold increased risk of myocardial infarction compared with women who did not have any of these risk factors. Again, the heterogeneity of the risk ratio has helped us understand the biological basis of myocardial infarction and provided a rational basis for physician recommendations that certain women avoid using oral contraceptives.[8] In addition, it may have prompted manufacturers to produce safer formulations of oral contraceptives.

▶ Effect Measure Modification Versus Confounding

Confounding and effect measure modification are sometimes confused. This is because effect measure modification, like confounding, involves a third variable in addition to the exposure and disease and is evaluated by conducting stratified analyses. However, one has nothing to do with the other. In fact, examples of a particular variable may be (1) a confounder but not an effect modifier, (2) an effect modifier but not a confounder, (3) both a confounder and an effect modifier, or (4) neither a confounder nor an effect modifier. The key difference is that confounding is a problem that epidemiologists aim to eliminate and effect measure modification is an interesting occurrence that epidemiologists aim to describe. The occurrence of interest is the change in the relation of an exposure and a disease according to the level of another variable. Thus, we pose two different questions when we consider confounding and effect measure modification in stratified analyses. For confounding, we are asking whether the crude measure of association is distorted and whether the stratum-specific and adjusted summary estimates are different from the crude estimate. For effect modification, we are asking whether the association differs according to the level of a third variable, that is, whether the stratum-specific estimates are different from one another.

▶ Evaluation of Effect Measure Modification

To explain effect measure modification, it is helpful to return to the crude and stratified analyses that examined the hypothetical relationship between dichlorodiphenyldichloroethylene (DDE) exposure and the odds of breast cancer. Let us first examine the crude data (see **TABLE 13-1**). There is a 1.9-fold increased odds of breast cancer among women who were exposed to high DDE levels $\big(\text{odds ratio} = [500 \times 3,400]/[600 \times 1,500] = 1.9\big)$.

Now, let us examine these results stratified into two age groups—women younger than 50 years of age and women aged 50 years and older (see **TABLE 13-2**). Note that there is no association between DDE and

TABLE 13-1 Crude Data from a Hypothetical Case–Control Study of DDE Exposure and Breast Cancer

	Breast cancer	
DDE level	**Cases**	**Controls**
High	500	600
Low	1,500	3,400
Total	2,000	4,000
	Odds ratio = 1.9	

TABLE 13-2 Age-Stratified Data from a Hypothetical Case–Control Study of DDE Exposure and Breast Cancer

DDE level	Age younger than 50 years		Age 50 years and older	
	Cases	Controls	Cases	Controls
High	50	300	450	300
Low	450	2,700	1,050	700
Total	500	3,000	1,500	1,000
	Stratum-specific odds ratio = 1.0		Stratum-specific odds ratio = 1.0	

TABLE 13-3 Data from a Hypothetical Case–Control Study of DDE Exposure and Breast Cancer Stratified According to Lactation History

DDE level	Never breastfed		Breastfed	
	Cases	Controls	Cases	Controls
High	140	300	360	300
Low	550	2,600	950	800
Total	690	2,900	1,310	1,100
	Stratum-specific odds ratio = 2.2		Stratum-specific odds ratio = 1.0	

breast cancer among women who are younger than 50 years or among those who are 50 years and older. Each stratum-specific odds ratio is 1.0. Thus, the magnitude of the odds ratio does not differ across the strata, but the stratum-specific odds ratio (1.0) is different from the crude odds ratio (1.9). The noticeable difference between the crude and stratum-specific odds ratios indicates that confounding by age is present. On the other hand, the lack of a difference between the two stratum-specific odds ratios indicates that effect measure modification by age (in this case, heterogeneity of the odds ratio) is absent.

Now, let us consider the effect of lactation history on the relationship between DDE levels and breast cancer risk (see **TABLE 13-3**). The women are divided into two groups: those who never breastfed and those who breastfed at least one child before their diagnosis or index year. (The index year is a cutoff date for controls that is comparable to the diagnosis year for cases. Only exposures and effect measure modifiers that occur before the index or diagnosis year are etiologically relevant.)

Here, the association varies according to a woman's lactation history. The odds ratio among women who never breastfed is 2.2, and the odds ratio among those who breastfed at least one child is 1.0. In other words, women who have high DDE exposure levels and never breastfed have a 2.2-fold increased odds of breast cancer, and women who have high DDE levels but did breastfeed have no elevation in disease odds. The heterogeneity of the stratum-specific odds ratio indicates that lactation history is an effect modifier of the relationship between DDE exposure level and breast cancer. These data support two possible underlying physiological mechanisms: (1) breastfeeding may reduce the susceptibility of the breast tissue to environmental carcinogens through tissue differentiation[9] or (2) breastfeeding may reduce breast tissue exposure to environmental carcinogens through excretion.[10]

Epidemiologists generally use two methods to determine whether the stratum-specific results are different from one another: visual inspection or a statistical test. In the example in Table 13-3, simple visual inspection indicates clearly that the two odds ratios are different. If a more formal assessment is desired, numerous statistical tests are available to test the null hypothesis that the differences in the stratum-specific measures of association reflect merely random variation. In this example it is appropriate to use the **chi-square test** for homogeneity of the odds ratios over different strata with the Woolf method.[11(pp603-604)] This analysis tests the **null hypothesis (H$_0$)** that the stratum-specific odds ratios are equal versus the **alternative hypothesis (H$_A$)** that at least two of the stratum-specific odds ratios are different. The number of stratum-specific odds ratios depends on the number of strata. There are only two strata in the example in Table 13-3, but there can be more.

The test is based on the following chi-square test statistic:

$$X^2_{\text{HOM}} = \sum_{i=1 \text{ to } k} w_i (\ln OR_i - \ln OR)^2$$

where $\ln OR_i$ is the log odds ratio relating disease to exposure in the ith stratum of the potential effect modifier, $\ln OR$ equals the weighted average log odds ratio over all strata, and w_i is the weight that is inversely proportional to the variance of $\ln OR_i$.

More specifically, $\ln OR_i = \log$ odds ratio in the ith stratum $= \ln\left[(a_i d_i)/(b_i c_i)\right]$, where a_i, b_i, c_i, and d_i are the cells of the two-by-two table relating disease to exposure in the ith stratum, weight $= w_i = \left[1/a_i + 1/b_i + 1/c_i + 1/d_i\right]^{-1}$, and $\ln OR = \sum_{i=1 \text{ to } k} w_i \ln OR \Big/ \sum_{i=1 \text{ to } k} w_i$.

Note that the purpose of the weighting is to weight strata with lower variances more than strata with higher variances. This is done because low-variance strata have more subjects than high-variance strata. The weighted differences between $\ln OR_i$ and $\ln OR$ are summed over all of the strata (1 to k). Once the chi-square statistic is calculated, a **P value** may be obtained from a table of chi-square values. This chi-square test has $k - 1$ degrees of freedom, where k is the total number of strata.

The null hypothesis (H_0) in the hypothetical example described in Table 13-3 is as follows: The odds ratio among women who never breast-fed is equal to the odds ratio among women who breastfed at least one child. In addition, the alternative hypothesis (H_A) is that the odds ratio among women who never breastfed is different from the odds ratio among women who did breastfeed. Using the formula just given, we perform the following calculations:

$$X^2_{HOM} = \sum_{I=1 \text{ to } k} w_i (\ln OR_i - \ln OR)^2$$

where $\ln OR_1$ among women who never breastfed equals $\ln[(140 \times 2{,}600/300 \times 550)] = 0.791$, w_1 among women who never breastfed equals $[1/140 + 1/2{,}600 + 1/300 + 1/550]^{-1} = 78.927$, $\ln OR_2$ for a positive breast-feeding history equals $\ln[(360 \times 800/300 \times 950)] = 0.010$, w_2 for a positive history of breastfeeding equals $[1/360 + 1/800 + 1/300 + 1/950]^{-1} = 118.906$, and $\ln OR = [(0.79) \times (62.15) + (0) \times (118.91)]/(62.15 + 118.91) = 0.322$.

Thus, the test statistic is given as follows:

$$X^2_{HOM} = 78.927(0.791 - 0.322)^2 + 118.906(0.010 - 0.322)^2 = 28.94$$

with one degree of freedom

Referring to a chi-square table, we note that the corresponding P value is less than 0.001. This indicates that we can reject the null hypothesis that the odds ratios are the same across breastfeeding history strata and we can conclude that effect measure modification of the odds ratio is present. Thus, the visual inspection and statistical test lead us to the same conclusion.

Now, let us turn to a real-life example of effect measure modification from the Boston Partners Study, a classic cohort study of biological and behavioral risk factors for the transmission of human immunodeficiency virus (HIV) among infected men and their partners. Investigators conducted this analysis to clarify the risk of HIV infection from unprotected receptive anal intercourse, with and without the use of the drug amyl nitrite.[12] This example illustrates another method for assessing the presence of effect measure modification.

The investigators hypothesized that amyl nitrite inhalation relaxed the smooth muscles and dilated the blood vessels around the anal sphincter, thereby allowing for more traumatic sexual activity and facilitating entry of HIV into the bloodstream during anal intercourse. Thus, they compared the odds ratios for the four possible exposure categories: (1) a history of nitrite use and a history of unprotected receptive anal intercourse, (2) no history of nitrite use and a history of unprotected receptive anal intercourse, (3) a history of nitrite use and no history of unprotected receptive anal intercourse, and (4) no history of nitrite use and no history of unprotected receptive anal intercourse. The last exposure category—a negative history of both exposures—served as the referent category for all the comparisons. The results are provided in **TABLE 13-4**.

Note that, compared with men with a negative history of both unprotected receptive anal intercourse and nitrite use, the risk of HIV infection was higher among men with a positive history of unprotected receptive anal intercourse and nitrite use (RR = 10.1) than among men with a positive history of unprotected receptive anal intercourse and a negative history of nitrite use (RR = 4.1) and among men with a positive history of nitrite use and a negative history of unprotected anal intercourse (RR = 2.7).

Now, let us compare the excess risk ratios to determine whether effect measure modification is present on the additive scale. The excess risk ratio is defined as the risk ratio minus one. Thus, the excess risk ratio associated with having both factors is 9.1 (10.1 − 1.0), the excess risk ratio associated with only unprotected receptive anal intercourse is 3.1 (4.1 − 1.0), and the excess risk ratio associated with only nitrite use is 1.7 (2.7 − 1.0). Because the excess risk ratio associated with having both factors together (9.1) is larger than the sum of the excess risk ratio associated with each factor alone (3.1 + 1.7 = 4.8), we may conclude

TABLE 13-4 Risk Ratios for HIV Infection According to History of Nitrite Use and Unprotected Receptive Anal Intercourse

Exposure category	Number of persons	Risk ratio
Nitrite use/unprotected receptive anal intercourse	317	10.1
No nitrite use/unprotected receptive anal intercourse	102	4.1
Nitrite use/no unprotected receptive anal intercourse	31	2.7
No nitrite use/no unprotected receptive anal intercourse	31	1.0

Data from Seage GR III, Mayer KH, Horsburgh CR, Holmberg SD, Moon MW, Lamb GA. The relation between nitrite inhalants, unprotected receptive anal intercourse, and the risk of human immunodeficiency virus infection. *Am J Epidemiol.* 1992;135:1-11.

that there is effect measure modification known as "the departure from additivity."

It is possible to have a stronger level of effect measure modification known as "the departure from multiplicity." This occurs when the risk ratio associated with having both factors together is larger than the product of the risk ratio associated with each factor alone. In fact, supplemental data from the Boston Partners Study found that men who always used nitrite inhalants when participating in unprotected receptive anal intercourse had a 33.8-fold increased risk of HIV infection as compared with men who never used inhalants and never engaged in unprotected receptive anal intercourse. The risk ratio associated with such frequent nitrite use (33.8) represents a departure from multiplicity because it is greater than the product of the risk ratios associated with each factor alone ($4.1 \times 2.7 = 11.1$). Note that departure from additivity represents a low to moderate level of effect measure modification and departure from multiplicity represents a high level.

▶ Synergy and Antagonism

The terms *synergy* and *antagonism* are used to describe effect measure modification. **Synergy**, which is also known as positive interaction, is said to occur when the excess risk ratio among individuals with both factors is greater than the sum of the excess risk ratios of each factor considered alone. Thus, synergy occurs when two factors work in concert to produce more disease than one would expect based on the action of either factor working alone. Synergy is a more general term for "departure from additivity or multiplicity." Several examples of synergy have been given in this chapter, including the relationship between nitrite use, unprotected anal intercourse, and the risk of HIV infection; the relationship between smoking, asbestos exposure, and lung cancer; and the relationship between oral contraceptives, smoking and other risk factors, and myocardial infarction.

Antagonism, which is also known as negative interaction, is said to occur when the excess risk ratio among individuals with both factors is less than the sum of the excess risk ratios of each factor considered alone. It means that one factor reduces or even cancels out the effect of the other factor. Consider, for example, a hypothetical study of the risk of gastroenteritis following the ingestion of contaminated shellfish. Individuals who ate the shellfish were three times more likely to develop gastroenteritis during the 24-hour follow-up period than those who did not eat the shellfish. However, when the consumption of other food items was taken into account, the investigators found that individuals who consumed an alcoholic beverage along with the contaminated shellfish had only a 1.5-fold increased risk of gastroenteritis and those who did not consume any alcoholic beverages with the contaminated fish had a 5-fold

TABLE 13-5 Hypothetical Risk Ratios for Gastroenteritis According to Consumption of Contaminated Fish and Alcoholic Beverages

Exposure category	Risk ratio
Ate contaminated fish/drank alcoholic beverage	1.5
Ate contaminated fish/did not drink alcoholic beverage	5.0
Did not eat contaminated fish/drank alcoholic beverage	1.0
Did not eat contaminated fish/did not drink alcoholic beverage	1.0

increased risk of gastroenteritis (see **TABLE 13-5**). Of course, there was no increased risk of gastroenteritis among individuals who did not eat contaminated shellfish, regardless of their alcohol consumption. Thus, the excess risk ratio for individuals with both exposures $(1.5 - 1.0 = 0.5)$ was less than the sum of the excess risk ratios for individuals with only one of the exposures $[(5.0 - 1.0) + (1.0 - 1.0) = 4.0]$. A plausible explanation for these results is that the alcoholic beverage killed the pathogenic bacteria in the subject's gastrointestinal tract.

▶ Choice of Measure

Effect measure modification depends on the measure of association that is being used, that is, whether a ratio measure (rate, risk, or odds ratio) or difference measure (risk or rate difference) is being used. Thus, when effect modification is present using a ratio measure, it will necessarily be absent when a difference measure is used, and vice versa.

Consider a hypothetical example of the risk of breast cancer following exposure to radiation according to the age at which the radiation exposure occurred (see **TABLE 13-6**). When the incidence rate ratio is constant at 2.5, the incidence rate difference changes according to the age at exposure. In this hypothetical example, the incidence rate difference increases because the incidence rate increases with age more dramatically among exposed women. In addition, when the incidence rate difference is constant at 140 cases per 100,000 person-years, the incidence rate ratio decreases with age. The higher rate ratios at younger ages may reflect the lower baseline rate of breast cancer at younger ages. In fact, effect measure modification seen on the ratio scale may represent nothing more than different levels of baseline risk.

TABLE 13-6 Hypothetical Incidence Rates, Rate Ratios, and Rate Differences of Breast Cancer Following Radiation Exposure According to the Age at Which the Exposure Occurred

Constant incidence rate ratios/changing incidence rate differences

Age of exposure (years)	Incidence rate (per 100,000 person-years)	Rate ratio	Rate difference
20	125 among exposed/50 among unexposed	2.5	75
30	300 among exposed/120 among unexposed	2.5	180
40	450 among exposed/180 among unexposed	2.5	270

Constant incidence rate differences/changing incidence rate ratios

20	210 among exposed/70 among unexposed	3.0	140
30	310 among exposed/170 among unexposed	1.8	140
40	420 among exposed/280 among unexposed	1.5	140

▸ Evaluating Effect Measure Modification and Confounding in Stratified Analyses

Epidemiologists conduct stratified analyses to evaluate simultaneously the presence of effect measure modification and confounding. FIGURE 13-1 contains a decision tree for evaluating data for both of these issues and provides information on the proper presentation of the results.

First, investigators conduct a crude analysis of the relationship between the exposure and disease. Next, they conduct a stratified analysis that separates the crude data according to levels of the potential confounder/effect modifier. Effect measure modification is evaluated either by examining the stratum-specific estimates visually or by performing a statistical test. Effect measure modification is considered present if the stratum-specific estimates are sufficiently different from one another and absent if

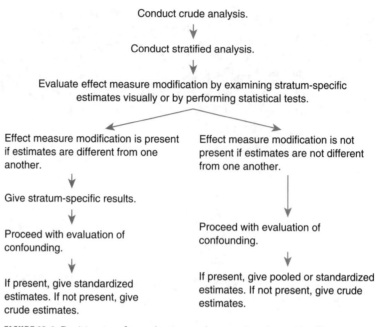

Conduct crude analysis.

↓

Conduct stratified analysis.

↓

Evaluate effect measure modification by examining stratum-specific estimates visually or by performing statistical tests.

Effect measure modification is present if estimates are different from one another.

↓

Give stratum-specific results.

↓

Proceed with evaluation of confounding.

↓

If present, give standardized estimates. If not present, give crude estimates.

Effect measure modification is not present if estimates are not different from one another.

↓

Proceed with evaluation of confounding.

↓

If present, give pooled or standardized estimates. If not present, give crude estimates.

FIGURE 13-1 Decision tree for evaluating and presenting data with effect measure modification and confounding.

the stratum-specific estimates are not different enough. The results of the visual inspection and statistical test may differ, and therefore investigators must judge which results are more likely to be correct. Next, investigators evaluate confounding by comparing the stratum-specific estimates with the crude estimate. If both confounding and effect measure modification are present, stratum-specific and standardized estimates should be presented. If effect measure modification is present but confounding is absent, crude and stratum-specific estimates should be presented. If effect measure modification is absent but confounding is present, the pooled or standardized results should be presented. If neither confounding nor effect measure modification is present, the crude results alone are sufficient.

Summary

Effect measure modification is defined as a change in the strength of an association between an exposure and a disease according to the level of a third variable. Other commonly used terms for this phenomenon include heterogeneity of effect and (less preferable) statistical interaction. Unlike confounding, which is considered a nuisance that epidemiologists aim to eliminate, effect measure modification is an interesting scientific phenomenon that epidemiologists aim to describe. Because its presence depends on the particular measure of association, effect measure modification should be described using terms that specify the measure (e.g., heterogeneity of the risk ratio). Furthermore, when effect measure modification is present using a ratio measure, it will usually be absent when a difference measure is used. Departure from additivity represents a low to moderate degree of modification, and departure from multiplicity represents a high degree. Synergy occurs when two factors work together to produce more disease than one would expect based on the action of either factor alone. In contrast, antagonism occurs when one factor reduces the effect or even cancels out the effect of another factor. Effect measure modification is evaluated in stratified analyses through visual inspection, statistical tests, or evaluation of excess relative risks.

References

1. Rothman KJ, Greenland S, Lash TL. *Modern Epidemiology.* 3rd ed. Philadelphia, PA: Lippincott Williams and Wilkins Publishers; 2008.
2. Yu W, Vaneckova P, Mengersen K, Pan X, Tong S. Is the association between temperature and mortality modified by age, gender and socioeconomic status? *Sci Total Environ.* 2010;408:3513-3518.
3. Egan KM, Trichopoulos D, Stampfer MJ, Willett WC, Newcomb PA, Trentham-Dietz A, et al. Jewish religion and risk of breast cancer. *Lancet.* 1996;347:1645-1646.
4. Wang J, Yang DL, Chen ZZ, Gou BF. Associations of body mass index with cancer incidence among populations, genders and menopausal status: a systematic review and meta-analysis. *Cancer Epidemiol.* 2016;42:1-8.
5. Selikoff IJ, Hammond EC, Churg J. Asbestos exposure, smoking, and neoplasia. *JAMA.* 1968;204:104-110.
6. Robbins A. Adverse Health Effects of Smoking and the Occupational Environment. NIOSH pub. no. 79-122. Cincinnati, OH: National Institute for Occupational Safety and Health; 1979.
7. Mann JI, Vessey MP, Thorogood M, Doll R. Myocardial infarction in young women with special reference to oral contraceptive practice. *Brit Med J.* 1975;2:241-245.
8. Estrogen and progestin (oral contraceptives). MedlinePlus Web site. https://medlineplus.gov /druginfo/meds/a601050.html. Updated September 15, 2014. Accessed February 2017.
9. Russo J, Russo IH. Development of the human breast. *Maturitas.* 2004;49:2-15.
10. Murrell TG. Epidemiological and biochemical support for a theory on the cause and prevention of breast cancer. *Med Hypotheses.* 1991;36:389-396.
11. Rosner B. *Fundamentals of Biostatistics.* 5th ed. Pacific Grove, CA: Duxbury Thompson Learning; 2000.
12. Seage GR III, Mayer KH, Horsburgh CR, Holmberg SD, Moon MW, Lamb GA. The relation between nitrite inhalants, unprotected receptive anal intercourse, and the risk of human immunodeficiency virus infection. *Am J Epidemiol.* 1992;135:1-11.

Chapter Questions

1. Define each of the following terms:
   a. Effect measure modification
   b. Heterogeneity and homogeneity of effect
   c. Synergy
   d. Antagonism

2. Briefly describe the key difference between confounding and effect measure modification.

3. Briefly describe how epidemiologists determine whether a variable is an effect modifier. Be sure to describe how this differs from the assessment of confounding.

4. A case–control study was conducted to determine whether the relationship between cigarette smoking and lung cancer is modified by the presence of asbestos exposure. The following results were obtained:

Exposed to	Odds ratio for lung cancer
Both smoking and asbestos	50.0
Only smoking	10.0
Only asbestos	5.0
Neither	1.0

   a. Is asbestos an effect measure modifier of the relation between smoking and lung cancer?
   b. State the reason for your answer.

5. The association between heavy alcohol consumption and the risk of oral cancer was investigated in a case–control study with 475 cases and 400 controls. The following results were seen:

Heavy alcohol consumption	Cases	Controls
Yes	350	200
No	125	200
Total	475	400

   a. Calculate the crude odds ratio based on these data.
   b. Sex was considered a potential confounder and/or effect measure modifier in this study. The data were stratified into males and females to assess these issues. Calculate the stratum-specific odds ratios among males and females using the following data:

Heavy alcohol consumption	Males		Females	
	Cases	Controls	Cases	Controls
Yes	300	150	50	50
No	50	50	75	150

c. Is sex a confounder in this study?

d. Is sex an effect measure modifier in this study?

e. Briefly justify your answers to parts C and D.

6. State whether each of the following statements is true or false:

a. If effect measure modification is present using a ratio measure of comparison, then it will also be present using a difference measure.

b. Statistical tests are sometimes useful for assessing the presence of effect measure modification.

c. Departure from additivity is a higher degree of effect measure modification than departure from multiplicity.

CHAPTER 14

Critical Review of Epidemiological Studies

LEARNING OBJECTIVES

By the end of this chapter the reader will be able to:

- Describe a method for critically evaluating the published literature.
- Apply the critique outline to published articles.

▶ Introduction

One of the most useful outcomes of studying epidemiology is learning how to critically evaluate the scientific literature. Critical assessment of this literature is an important skill for public health professionals because the findings of epidemiological research inform so many activities. For example, the application of epidemiological research methods have helped determine the effect of state laws requiring universal background checks in reducing firearm-related deaths in the United States,[1] the effectiveness of taking a low-dose aspirin during the preconception period to prevent pregnancy loss,[2] the interaction between nitrite inhalants and unprotected receptive anal intercourse on the risk of human immunodeficiency virus (HIV) infection,[3] the scientific basis for setting permissible pollutant levels,[4] the safety of home-based vaginal births after cesarean delivery,[5] the effectiveness of folic acid fortified flour in reducing certain birth defects,[6] and methods for improving patient decision making.[7] Epidemiological research has helped us understand the pattern of occurrence and etiology of diseases throughout the world, including HIV infection, tuberculosis, Lyme disease, Chlamydia infection, cardiovascular disease, stroke, cancer, diabetes, Alzheimer's disease, osteoarthritis, and depression.

Publishing in scientific journals is a major avenue for communicating the results of epidemiological studies. The major public health and epidemiology journals include *American Journal of Public Health, American Journal of Epidemiology, Epidemiology, Annals of Epidemiology*, and *International Journal of Epidemiology*. Medical and subspecialty journals also publish the results of epidemiological studies. Some of the best known general medicine journals are *New England Journal of Medicine, Journal of the American Medical Association*, and *Lancet*.

Journal articles are typically organized in the following format: abstract, introduction, materials and methods, results, discussion, conclusions, and references. The purpose of the abstract is to provide a short summary of the goals, methods, main findings, and conclusions of the study. The introduction describes the context and motivation for the study. The materials and methods section reports on the setting, design, data collection procedures, and analysis of the study. In our opinion, this section is the most important part of the article because it provides critical information about the study's validity. The results section describes the characteristics of the study population and the study findings. It typically includes text, several tables, and figures. The findings of epidemiological studies are quantitative in nature and usually include measures of disease frequency and association. The discussion section provides the scientific interpretation of the findings, places the findings in the context of other research, and acknowledges the study's limitations. The conclusions, which are either part of the discussion or in a separate section, briefly summarize the findings and their implications. The conclusions often include recommendations for future research and public health policy; however, some epidemiologists have discouraged the latter practice.[8] The article concludes with references for all cited scientific facts.

The critique outline shown in **EXHIBIT 14-1** has been adapted from an outline originally developed by Richard Monson of Harvard University's T.H. Chan School of Public Health.[9(p94)] We believe that it is a useful guide for learning how to evaluate a study, and we have used it extensively in our teaching. The outline helps "disentangle the skeins of serendipity, bias, and intent that run throughout epidemiologic research."[10(p556)] In other words, it provides a framework to help epidemiologists assess (1) whether the methods used to select the study subjects and collect and analyze the data were comparable across groups; (2) whether any errors were committed in the design, conduct, or interpretation of the study; and (3) what effect these errors had on the reported findings.[9(p94)]

The critique outline is organized into three sections: data collection, analysis, and interpretation. All well-written articles published in reputable journals should contain the information needed to answer the critique questions. If an article does not contain most of this information, one can assume that the study quality is poor. If an article is silent

---

EXHIBIT 14-1 Outline for Critiquing Epidemiological Studies

A. Collection of data
1. What was the context of the study?
2. What were the objectives of the study?
3. What was the primary exposure of interest? Was this accurately measured?
4. What was the primary outcome of interest? Was this accurately measured?
5. What type of study was conducted?
6. Describe the source of the study population, process of subject selection, sample size, and ratio of **propositi** to comparison subjects. (Propositi are exposed subjects in an experimental or cohort study and cases in a case–control study.)
7. Could there have been bias in the selection of the study subjects? How likely was this bias?
8. Could there have been bias in the collection of information? How likely was this bias?
9. What provisions were made to minimize the influence of confounding factors prior to the analysis of the data? Were these provisions sufficient?

B. Analysis of data
1. What methods were used to control confounding during data analysis? Were these methods sufficient?
2. What measures of association were reported in this study?
3. What measures of statistical stability were reported in this study?

C. Interpretation of data
1. What were the major results of this study?
2. How is the interpretation of these results affected by information bias, selection bias, and confounding? Discuss both the direction and magnitude of any bias.
3. How is the interpretation of these results affected by nondifferential misclassification? Discuss both the direction and magnitude of this misclassification.
4. Did the discussion section adequately address the limitations of the study?
5. What were the authors' main conclusions? Were they justified by the findings?
6. To what larger population can the results of this study be generalized?

Adapted from Monson RR. *Occupational Epidemiology.* 2nd ed. Boca Raton, FL: CRC Press; 1990:94.

on a particular issue, it is usually safe to assume that the issue was not addressed. For example, if an article does not mention that the interviewers were masked to the subjects' disease status, one can assume that no masking occurred.

▶ Guide to Answering the Critique Questions

The following section provides guidelines for answering the critique questions. We advise students to read an article twice before attempting to answer the questions. The purpose of the first reading is to become familiar with the article. The second reading should be done with the critique questions in mind. Note that the answers to many of these questions can be found in the introduction and materials and methods sections of an article. One last piece of advice—a critique should be brief. A long critique defeats an important benefit of the review process, and the production of a brief, easy-to-read summary makes future readings of the article unnecessary.

Collection of Data

What was the context of the study? This question deals with the investigators' motivation for the study. For example, the observations that stimulated the study may have come from laboratory research, clinical reports, or other epidemiological studies. The answer to this question gives the reader a sense of the particular contribution made by the study at hand. For example, the study may be the first of its kind, or it may be replicating results of an earlier study in a different population but with larger numbers or using more refined methods. For example, Zierler and Rothman conducted a case–control study of congenital heart disease and maternal use of Bendectin in early pregnancy because a study that they had conducted earlier found an association that they suspected was the result of recall bias.[11] The new study was designed "expressly to evaluate and remove any bias that might have arisen when exposure histories obtained from mothers of affected offspring were compared with exposure histories obtained from mothers of healthy controls."[11(p347)]

What were the objectives of the study? This question deals with the purpose of the study, that is, the hypothesis being tested. Hypotheses are suppositions about an exposure–disease relationship that lead to refutable predictions.[12(p139)] Examples of hypotheses are as follows:

- Following American Cancer Society cancer screening guidelines reduces the incidence of colon cancer.
- Unprotected receptive anal intercourse increases the risk of HIV transmission among homosexual men.
- Removal of lead-contaminated soil accessible to children decreases their blood lead levels.

Whenever possible, the hypothesis should quantify the relationship between the exposure and disease. For example, a reduction of 1,000 ppm or more of lead in soil accessible to children will decrease their blood lead levels by at least 3 mg/dL.[13] Specific hypotheses are easier than nonspecific ones to test and refute.

What was the primary exposure of interest? Was this accurately measured? The exposure of interest is the factor that either causes, prevents, or treats the outcome. It is important to consider whether the exposure was accurately defined and measured because exposure misclassification stems from broad definitions and inaccurate measurements. Thus, when evaluating the accuracy of exposure data, one should also compare the exposure's conceptual and operational definitions. For example, the conceptual exposure definition in a study conducted to investigate the breast cancer risk associated with tetrachloroethylene-contaminated drinking water was simply "exposure to tetrachloroethylene-contaminated drinking water." An ordinal estimate of exposure to tetrachloroethylene-contaminated water was operationally defined as "the estimated mass of tetrachloroethylene that entered the home through the drinking water during a specified period."[4] Exposure to contaminated water was estimated using an algorithm based on information about the water pipe that supplied each subject's home. This information included the pipe length, diameter, installation date, and number of homes served by the water pipe. Note that this operational definition omits important behavioral data on water use and therefore may lead to exposure misclassification.

When reviewing an article, the reader should look for steps that were taken to ensure the accuracy of the exposure data, such as use of exposure biomarkers, use of sensitive and specific exposure definitions, and verification of one information source with another. Also, it is important to note how broadly the exposure categories were defined. For example, several exposure categories were compared in the tetrachloroethylene-contaminated drinking water study: ever versus never exposed, low versus never exposed, high versus never exposed, and very high versus never exposed.[4]

Clearly, the ever-exposed category was quite broad, and the three exposure level categories were narrower. It is possible to get different results with different exposure definitions. For example, investigators in the contaminated drinking water study reported increases in the risk of breast cancer among very highly exposed individuals (odds ratio = 1.6–1.9) but not among ever-exposed individuals (odds ratio = 1.1).[4]

What was the primary outcome of interest? Was this accurately measured? The outcome of interest is the end point being studied, such as a precursor of disease; disease incidence, prevalence, and recurrence; symptom improvement; side effects; length of survival; and mortality. It is important to consider whether the outcome was accurately defined and measured because loose definitions and inaccurate measurement can result in misclassification. Thus, when evaluating the accuracy of an outcome variable, one should compare its conceptual and operational definitions. For example, the conceptual outcome definition in the study on the cancer risk associated with tetrachloroethylene-contaminated drinking water was breast cancer, which is defined as a malignant neoplasm of the breast tissue.[4] However, as required by the operational definition, all cases of breast cancer were reported to the state cancer registry, pathologically confirmed, and diagnosed at stages 1 through 4. These requirements helped ensure that all the cases in the study truly had breast cancer.

When reviewing an article, the reader should look for measures taken to improve the accuracy of the outcome data, such as use of a combination of signs and symptoms, examinations, and tests to define cases of disease; verification of information from one source with another; use of sensitive and specific biomarkers of disease or its precursors as outcome measures; use of the likely causal mechanism to define and group cases of disease; and use of reputable registries (such as cancer registries) to identify or corroborate disease reports.

What type of study was conducted? The main epidemiological study designs are experimental, cohort (prospective and retrospective), case–control, cross-sectional, and ecological studies. It is important to know which design was used because certain designs are more prone to bias than others. The following paragraph briefly reviews the key features of each design.

Experimental studies examine preventions and treatments for disease. Their hallmark is the investigator's assignment of participants to compared groups. Random assignment is recommended but not required. Observational (cohort, case–control, cross-sectional, and ecological) studies investigate causes, preventions, and treatments for disease. Observational study participants become exposed without the investigator's intervention. Subjects in a cohort study are defined according to their exposure level and are followed for disease occurrence. In contrast, subjects in a case–control study are defined as either cases or controls, and their exposure histories are examined. Cross-sectional studies examine the relationship between an exposure and a disease in a well-defined population at a single point in time. Their main limitation is that they do not allow investigators to infer the temporal sequence between exposure and disease if the exposure is a changeable characteristic. Ecological studies examine rates of disease in relation to a population-level factor and use groups—not individuals—as units of analysis. Their main limitation is known as the ecological fallacy, an inability to apply the group-level relationship to the individual level.

Describe the source of the study population, process of subject selection, sample size, and ratio of propositi to comparison subjects. This information allows the reader to evaluate many important topics including the potential for selection bias and confounding, the statistical power of the study, and the generalizability of the results. The source of the study population is the underlying population from which the subjects were drawn. For example, the underlying population of a hospital-based case–control study is the catchment area of the hospital. Cases and controls will be comparable, and confounding will be reduced if the catchment areas (and underlying populations) for cases are similar to those for controls. Furthermore, the source population and actual study population greatly influence to whom the study results are applicable.

The process of subject selection should be carefully examined for evidence of selection bias, which is described in more detail in the next question. The sample size and ratio of propositi to comparison subjects provides information on the statistical power of the study—that is, the ability of the study to detect an association that is truly present. The ratio of propositi to comparison subjects is the ratio of exposed to unexposed subjects (e.g., for a cohort study) or the ratio of cases to controls (for a case–control study). These ratios are often one to one, but they may be as high as one to three or one to four. High ratios and a large sample size improve the statistical power of the study.

Could there have been bias in the selection of the study subjects? How likely was this bias? Selection bias is an error that arises from systematic differences in selecting the study groups or in following the selected groups. These differences lead to an effect estimate among subjects in the study that is different from the estimate obtainable from the entire underlying population. Selection bias can cause the true measure of association to be either over- or underestimated. Selection bias is more likely in case–control studies and retrospective cohort studies because both the exposure and disease have occurred by the time of subject selection. However, it can also occur in prospective cohort and experimental studies if there are differential losses to follow-up.

When reviewing an article, the reader should look for evidence of the specific types of selection bias, including control selection bias in case–control studies; the healthy worker effect in occupational cohort studies; self-selection bias; differential surveillance, diagnosis, and referral of subjects according to exposure and disease status; and differential losses to follow-up. It is particularly important to consider selection bias when different criteria are used to select cases and controls and these criteria are related to the exposure; when participation rates or follow-up rates are low and different across compared groups; when diagnostic practices and referral patterns are not taken into account; and when self-referrals are accepted into a study.

Losses to follow-up occur when subjects can no longer be located or they no longer want to participate in the study. It can bias the study results when subjects who are lost differ from those who remain with respect to the exposure and outcome. When evaluating a study, the reader should note the proportions and any available demographic information on subjects lost to follow-up. Losses greater than 20%, especially if they occur among different types of subjects than those who remain, call the validity of the study into question.

Could there have been bias in the collection of information? How likely was this bias? Information bias is an error that arises from systematic differences in the way that information on the exposure and disease is obtained from the study groups. It results in incorrect classification of participants as either exposed or unexposed or as diseased or not diseased. This type of bias arises after the subjects have been selected for study. When reviewing an article, the reader should look for evidence of the specific types of information bias, including recall bias, interviewer bias, and differential and nondifferential misclassification. Except for nondifferential misclassification of a dichotomous exposure and nondifferential loss to follow-up, these biases can pull the measure of association either toward or away from the null.

Recall bias can occur when individuals with particular adverse health events remember or report their previous exposure differently than do individuals who are not affected. Thus, recall bias can occur only in retrospective studies that gather data from study subjects. When evaluating a study, the reader should look for methods that may have been used to avoid recall bias, such as development of a carefully designed questionnaire, use of closed-ended questions, comparison of diseased cases to diseased controls (in case–control studies), use of a prospective study, collection of study data that is not based on interviews and questionnaires, or use of participants who are masked to the study hypothesis. The reader should also note whether the investigators undertook a direct assessment of recall bias, such as asking participants about their knowledge of the hypothesis and stratifying the results on the basis of their responses.

Interviewer bias occurs when there are systematic differences in soliciting, recording, or interpreting information from in-person and telephone interviews. This bias can occur when interviewers lack training in appropriate interview techniques (such as nondirective probing) or are aware of the study hypothesis and the disease or exposure status of subjects or when questionnaires are unstructured. Epidemiologists can request to receive the study questionnaire from the corresponding author to assess its structure.

Misclassification occurs when the subject's exposure or disease status is erroneously classified. Misclassification can be either nondifferential or differential. Nondifferential misclassification means that inaccuracies with respect to disease are independent of exposure or that inaccuracies with respect to exposure are independent of disease. This type of misclassification, which is probably the most common form of bias in epidemiological research, biases the results toward the null if the misclassified exposure variable is dichotomous. Differential misclassification means that inaccuracies with respect to disease are dependent on exposure status and vice versa. When evaluating a study for misclassification, the reader should carefully examine the operational exposure and disease definitions. Misclassification should be considered when single (instead of multiple) measurements are used to define the exposure or disease, data are not validated using alternate information sources, or subjects are required to recall information from long ago.

What provisions were made to minimize the influence of confounding factors prior to the data analysis? Were these provisions sufficient? Confounding is a bias in the crude measure of association between an exposure and a disease that is the result of a third factor that is associated with the exposure and is an independent risk factor for the disease. Confounding can bias results either toward or away from the null. The methods to control for confounding prior to data analysis include randomization, restriction, matching, and using the same source population for the compared groups. Collecting information on potential confounders is an important provision to control for confounding prior to data analysis because (except for randomization) it is impossible to control for a confounder at any stage without data. When evaluating a study, the reader should review the information on confounders that was collected. If data on key confounders are missing, residual confounding may have occurred.

It is also important to determine the methods used to address confounding. Randomization is the "act of assigning or ordering that results from a random process."[14(p222)] Random methods include flipping a coin or using a random number table or a computerized random number generator. A unique advantage of randomization is that it will control for variables that the study investigator is unable to measure if the sample size is sufficient. Restriction means that admissibility criteria for study subjects are limited. Thus, a study that is restricted to women has no confounding by gender. Restriction limits the generalizability of the findings. Matching means that the investigator selects study subjects so that the potential confounders are distributed in an identical manner. Closer matches control for confounding better than broader matches. For example, matching by age within 2 years will control for confounding better than matching within 10 years. Note that matching in the design phase of a case–control study requires a matched analysis. If this analysis is not done, the measure of association will be biased toward the null.

Analysis of Data

What methods were used to control confounding during the data analysis? Were these methods sufficient? During analysis, the main ways to control for confounding are standardization, stratification, matched analysis (for case–control studies), and multivariable analysis. Standardization involves taking weighted averages of the relevant measures of disease frequency. The weights typically come from the exposed group in the study population. This method is commonly used to control for demographic characteristics such as age. Stratification is "the process of or result of separating a sample into several subgroups according to specific criteria."[12(p272)] Thus, it enables the investigator to evaluate an association within homogeneous categories of a variable. The narrower the category is, the better the control of confounding. Multivariable analysis involves the construction of a mathematical model that describes the association between the exposure, disease, and confounders. Commonly used methods of multivariable analysis include multiple linear regression, logistic regression, Poisson regression, and Cox proportional hazard models. The main advantage of multivariable models is that they allow investigators to control for many confounders simultaneously.

What measures of association were reported in this study? Commonly used measures of association in epidemiological studies are rate ratios, risk ratios, rate differences, risk differences, odds ratios, standardized mortality ratios, and standardized proportional mortality ratios. Note that the alternative terms—attributable and relative risk and rate—are also commonly used. Other measures of association, such as mean differences, are used when the data are continuous. It is important to distinguish the measure of association from the measure of statistical stability, described in the next question. Sometimes, authors incorrectly interpret the measure of statistical stability as the measure of association.

What measures of statistical stability were reported in this study? Hypothesis testing and interval estimation are used to assess the precision of study findings and to evaluate the role of chance in epidemiological studies. Chance refers to the likelihood that an unrepresentative sample was drawn because of "the luck of the draw." P values and confidence intervals are the two main ways to assess the role of chance in epidemiological research. The null P value and 95% confidence interval are most commonly used. The P value is defined as the probability of observing the study results or more extreme results given that the null hypothesis is true. Thus, it measures the compatibility of the data with the null hypothesis. The 95% confidence interval is defined as follows: if one repeats a study 100 times, the true measure of association will lie inside the confidence interval in 95 out of 100 studies. Although incorrect from a statistical viewpoint, a 95% confidence interval can also be conceptualized as follows: assuming no bias or confounding, one has 95% confidence or assurance that the true measure of association lies somewhere inside the interval. A statistically significant result has been arbitrarily defined as a P value less than 0.05 or a 95% confidence interval that does not include the null. Statistical significance has been overemphasized in epidemiological research.

Interpretation of Data

What were the major results of this study? A critique should describe the main results of the study using words and numbers. Qualitative statements such as "The study found a relationship between the exposure and disease" are inadequate because it is necessary to know how strong the relationship was.

How is the interpretation of these results affected by information bias, selection bias, and confounding? Discuss both the direction and magnitude of any bias. The reader should gather all the relevant information from the other sections of the critique to determine the net effect of any information bias, selection bias, and confounding that may be present in the study. It is important to assess the likelihood of bias and confounding and their magnitude and direction. A small amount of bias or confounding will usually not have a major effect on the study results, but a large amount of bias or residual confounding could completely alter the findings. The effect of bias and confounding will also depend on the true size of the association. They can account entirely for a weak association, but they are unlikely to account entirely for a strong one.

It may be useful to conduct a sensitivity analysis to determine the magnitude of the bias. This analysis determines the robustness of the results by examining the extent to which they are affected by assumptions about the amount of bias.[12(p259)] Both likely and extreme scenarios should be considered. For example, how would the results be altered if one assumed that 0%, 20%, and 100% of the people lost to follow-up had the disease of interest?

How is the interpretation of these results affected by nondifferential misclassification? Discuss both the direction and magnitude of this misclassification. Nondifferential misclassification is a common form of bias that pulls the results toward the null under certain circumstances. Null results need to be carefully examined for nondifferential misclassification to determine whether mismeasurement caused the findings. In addition, mismeasurement causes positive results to be weaker than they otherwise would have been.

Did the discussion section adequately address the limitations of the study? A self-critical examination of the study methods and findings should be included in the discussion section of the article. For example, the discussion section of the article on breast cancer risk associated with tetrachloroethylene-contaminated drinking water made the following statements:

> These results are likely affected by exposure misclassification because we used the Webler-Brown method to estimate the historical PCE [an abbreviation for tetrachloroethylene] exposures. Incorrect model assumptions or errors in determining the model's input variables would have led to errors in estimating . . . the amount of pollutant that entered the

home. . . . However, because the PCE exposure assessments were conducted blindly, we think that these errors are likely nondifferential, and so associations . . . are likely biased toward the null.[4(pp171–172)]

What were the authors' main conclusions? Were they justified by the findings? The conclusions are a brief summary of the findings and their implications. In addition, the authors sometimes include recommendations for future research and public health policy. All conclusions should be supported by the study findings. For example, the conclusion of the breast cancer and tetrachloroethylene-contaminated drinking water article was as follows: "The results of the present study . . . suggest that women with the highest RDDs of PCE-contaminated drinking water have small to moderate increases in the risk of breast cancer compared with unexposed women."[4(p171)] The authors went on to say that more research on the relationship between solvent exposure and breast cancer should be conducted because data on this topic are scarce and more preventable causes of breast cancer need to be identified.

To what larger population can the results of this study be generalized? The internal validity of a study must be established before the study results can be generalized to populations beyond the study subjects. If a study is invalid, its results cannot be generalized to any population. The evaluation of generalizability, or external validity, requires review of the study methods (e.g., whether restriction was used to control for confounding); the composition of the study population (e.g., whether minorities were included); and subject matter knowledge, such as the biological basis of the association (e.g., whether the same results would be expected among men and women).

▶ Sample Critiques of Epidemiological Studies

This section provides critiques for three published articles. The first article deals with an early, interesting study of the risk of HTLV-III/LAV (now known as HIV) infection among household contacts of AIDS patients[15] (see **EXHIBIT 14-2**). The second article deals with a study of the long-term effects of childhood lead exposure on the central nervous system[16] (see **EXHIBIT 14-3**). And the third article evaluates a new preventive drug for breast cancer[17] (see **EXHIBIT 14-4**). Because all these studies present interesting issues regarding their quality and interpretation, they provide useful examples for practicing the critique process.

EXHIBIT 14-2   Summary of "Prevalence of HTLV-III/LAV in Household Contacts of Patients with Confirmed AIDS and Controls in Kinshasa, Zaire"

Background and Objectives: Because of concern that HTLV-III/LAV can be transmitted in close-contact settings, a seroprevalence study was conducted among household contacts of individuals with confirmed acquired immunodeficiency syndrome (AIDS) as well as household contacts of control subjects who were seronegative for HTLV-III/LAV.

Methods: Household members of 46 patients with AIDS and 43 seronegative controls from Kinshasa, Zaire, were identified and tested for serologic testing for evidence of HTLV-III/LAV infection. Eligible household members were required to live in the same household as the AIDS patient or control subject for at least 6 months.

Results: A total of 9.8% of 204 case household members and 1.9% of 155 control household members were seropositive (relative risk = 5.1; 95% confidence interval, 1.7 to 15.2). In addition, 61.1% of spouses of AIDS patients were positive for HTLV-III/LAV compared with 3.7% of spouses of control subjects (relative risk = 16.5; 95% confidence interval, 3.7 to 75.0). Except for spouses, the prevalence of HTLV-III/LAV seropositivity was not significantly different between household contacts of AIDS cases and seronegative controls.

Conclusions: Nonsexual transmission of HTLV-III/LAV is probably very rare. These data from Zaire confirm the results of studies from the United States and Europe, which suggest that horizontal transmission of HTLV-III/LAV is unlikely to occur.

Adapted from Mann JM, Quinn TC, Francis H, Nzilambi N, Bosenge N, Bila K, et al. Prevalence of HTLV-III/LAV in household contacts of patients with confirmed AIDS and controls in Kinshasa, Zaire. *JAMA*. 1986;256:721-724.

Critique of a Study on the Prevalence of HIV in Household Contacts of AIDS Patients in Kinshasa, Zaire

A. Collection of data

1. **What was the context of the study?** At the time of the study, the virus that causes AIDS (HTLV-III/LAV, now known as HIV) was known to be transmitted sexually, through contact with blood, and to infants. However, epidemiologists were concerned that it could also be transmitted in close-contact settings through other fluids. This study of household contacts appears to be the first of its kind in Zaire, where the epidemiological pattern of AIDS is considerably different from that in the United States and Europe.

2. **What were the objectives of the study?** The purpose of the study was to "examine the possibility of household transmission of HTLV-III/LAV in Kinshasa, Zaire."

3. **What was the primary exposure of interest? Was this accurately measured?** The exposed subjects were

household members of AIDS patients who were diagnosed at Mama Yemo Hospital and met a modified Centers for Disease Control and Prevention definition of AIDS based on clinical criteria and laboratory tests, including repeated testing by enzyme-linked immunosorbent assay (ELISA) and Western blot. Unexposed subjects were household members of HTLV-III/LAV seronegative individuals who were the same gender and age as the AIDS patients. Seronegative individuals were selected from patients in the orthopedic and surgical wards of Mama Yemo Hospital or were identified as former Mama Yemo patients by four Zairian physicians. A household member was defined as a person who lived in the same household as the AIDS patient or the seronegative patient for at least 6 months during 1983 or 1984. The exposure appears to be accurately measured through the use of clinical symptoms, multiple laboratory tests, and sensitive and specific definitions.

4. **What was the primary outcome of interest? Was this accurately measured?** The primary outcome was a positive antibody test of HTLV-III/LAV. It was accurately measured because it was based on two positive ELISA results and one positive Western blot assay.

5. **What type of study was conducted?** A cross-sectional study was conducted. The authors' use of the terminology "case-households" and "control-households" is misleading because a case–control study was not conducted.

6. **Describe the source of the study population, process of subject selection, sample size, and ratio of propositi to comparison subjects.** The source population consisted of household members of AIDS patients and seronegative patients from Mama Yemo Hospital in Kinshasa, Zaire. The study enrolled 46 patients with AIDS and 45 apparently seronegative patients. Two supposedly seronegative patients were subsequently excluded when they were found to be seropositive. The authors provided no information on the number of AIDS patients and seronegative patients who were approached but refused to participate. The authors attempted to enroll all household members who met the eligibility criteria. They enrolled 204 household members of AIDS patients and 155 household members of seronegative patients. This represented 65% and 54% of the household contacts of AIDS and seronegative patients, respectively, who were approached. The ratio of propositi to comparison subjects was 204 to 155, or 1.3 to 1.

7.   **Could there have been bias in the selection of the study subjects? How likely was this bias?** Although similar selection criteria for exposed and unexposed subjects minimized the possibility of certain types of selection bias, self-selection bias is possible given the low and slightly different participation rates among exposed and unexposed subjects (65% and 54%, respectively). However, this would have led to bias only if the decision to participate was related both to the exposure (being a household member of an AIDS or seronegative patient) and to the outcome (being seropositive or seronegative). The authors stated, "Not all household members participated in this study. If HTLV-III/LAV infections in case-household members led to failure to participate because of ill health or death, a bias against detection of household clusters would have occurred."

8.   **Could there have been bias in the collection of information? How likely was this bias?** The investigators obtained the outcome data through laboratory tests, and therefore recall bias and interviewer bias were not possible. The authors did not state whether the laboratory personnel who performed the serological tests were aware of the exposure status of subjects, but these tests are fairly objective and therefore it is unlikely that this knowledge would have influenced the serologic test results. Exposure data were obtained through interviews and laboratory tests. For example, the interviews identified the household members and each household member's relationship to the index patient (e.g., spouse, parent, or child). The authors did not state whether the interviewers were masked, but it is unlikely that the key interview data were influenced by interviewer or recall bias.

9.   **What provisions were made to minimize the influence of confounding factors prior to the analysis of the data? Were these provisions sufficient?** The AIDS and seronegative index patients came from the patient population of Mama Yemo Hospital. These two groups were selected to be of similar age and gender, and therefore it appears that some matching occurred. However, it is unknown whether the catchment areas are exactly the same for these two groups of patients. The authors collected information on some confounders. For example, they collected information on household size, age, gender, religion, marital status, educational level, and occupation. Patients with AIDS and seronegative patients were similar for almost all demographic variables. The only difference between AIDS and seronegative patients

was that the former were more likely to have a high-level occupation. No differences were seen among household contacts for length of residence and total household size. However, the household contacts of AIDS patients were more likely to be women than were the household contacts of seronegative patients. No information was collected on many other risk factors for infection, including sexual practices, blood transfusions, scarifications, or medical injections, and therefore residual confounding by these unmeasured factors may be present.

B.   Analysis of data

1.   **What methods were used to control confounding bias during data analysis? Were these methods sufficient?** Investigators used no methods to control for confounding in the analysis, and therefore residual confounding may be present.

2.   **What measures of association were reported in this study?** The study reported prevalence ratios.

3.   **What measures of statistical stability were reported in this study?** The study reported 95% confidence intervals.

C.   Interpretation of data

1.   **What were the major results of this study?** The prevalence of seropositivity among household contacts of AIDS patients and seronegative patients was 9.8% (20/204) and 1.9% (3/155), respectively (relative risk = 5.1; 95% confidence interval, 1.7 to 15.2). When these data were stratified by the relationship to the index patient, the prevalence of seropositivity was 61.1% (11/18) among spouses of AIDS patients and 3.7% (1/27) among spouses of seronegative patients (relative risk = 16.5; 95% confidence interval, 3.7 to 75.0). In addition, 4.8% (9/186) of nonspousal household contacts of AIDS patients and 1.6% (2/128) of nonspousal contacts of seronegative patients were seropositive (relative risk = 3.1; 95% confidence interval, 0.7 to 13.3). Although the prevalence of seropositivity was higher among parents, children, and sibling household contacts of AIDS patients than among household contacts of seronegative patients, the number of seropositive household contacts was quite small, and therefore the relative risk estimates were highly imprecise.

2.   **How is the interpretation of these results affected by information bias, selection bias, and confounding? Discuss both the direction and magnitude of any bias.** Information bias is unlikely in this study; however, selection bias and confounding were quite possible. Selection bias probably resulted from the low and slightly differential participation rates of exposed and unexposed

subjects. In fact, the authors presented the results of a 1984 seroprevalence study from Kinshasa that suggested that the seroprevalence rate among exposed subjects was as expected but that the rate among unexposed subjects was less than expected. Missing data on key confounders (such as other sources of infection) also make the results difficult to interpret because the magnitude of the residual confounding may be large and its direction is difficult to predict.

3. **How is the interpretation of these results affected by nondifferential misclassification? Discuss both the direction and magnitude of this misclassification.** Although nondifferential laboratory errors were possible, they were not likely given that two ELISA and one Western blot were used to define seropositive subjects. Furthermore, these tests are known to have a high level of sensitivity and specificity. In addition, interview data on subjects' relationship to the index patients were objective and easy to determine. Thus, nondifferential misclassification of exposure and outcome were unlikely to have affected the study results.

4. **Did the discussion section adequately address the limitations of the study?** The authors acknowledged the possibility of selection bias and residual confounding.

5. **What were the authors' main conclusions? Were they justified by the findings?** The authors concluded that the data do not support the hypothesis that nonsexual transmission occurs among household members. However, the authors' conclusions are not justified by their findings. Although the numbers were small, the risk of infection was 3.1 times higher among nonspousal household contacts of AIDS patients than among nonspousal contacts of seronegative patients. The 95% confidence interval for this association ranged from 0.7 to 13.3, and therefore the data are consistent with a wide range of values for the relative risk, not just the null value. The main error that the authors made was "equating the lack of statistical significance with the lack of effect."[18]

6. **To what larger population can the results of this study be generalized?** If valid, the study results could be generalized to persons in other developing countries with living conditions similar to those in Zaire (e.g., crowded housing, lack of modern sanitary systems, and substantial numbers of mosquitos). However, given the possibility of selection bias and confounding and the low level of precision, it would be unwise to generalize these results to any population.

EXHIBIT 14-3 Summary of "Low-Level Environmental Lead Exposure in Childhood and Adult Intellectual Function: A Follow-Up Study"

Background and Objectives: While many prior studies support an association between early life exposure to lead and the risk of neurocognitive impairment in childhood, it is unclear if the increased risk of impaired intellectual function extends into adulthood.

Methods: The investigators recruited adults who had participated as newborns and young children in a prospective cohort study that assessed the relationship between early life exposure to lead and intellectual function as measured by the Wechsler Abbreviated Scale of Intelligence (WASI). The relationship between lead levels and intelligence quotient (IQ) scores was examined using linear regression models.

Results: A total of 43 young adults (average age was 29.0 years) participated in the IQ testing. Average blood lead concentration during late childhood had the strongest relationship with IQ ($\beta = -1.89 \pm 0.70$, $p = 0.01$). Reduced IQ was also associated with blood lead concentration at age 6 months ($\beta = -1.66 \pm 0.75$, $p = 0.03$), 4 years ($\beta = -0.90 \pm 0.41$, $p = 0.03$), and 10 years ($\beta = -1.95 \pm 0.80$, $p = 0.02$).

Conclusions: The results of this study suggest that lead exposure in childhood predicts IQ in young adulthood and that school-age exposure may be a period of special vulnerability. However, the small sample size made it difficult to rule out confounding by maternal IQ. Thus, a larger follow-up study is warranted.

Adapted from Mazumdar M, Bellinger DC, Gregas M, Abanilla K, Bacic J, Needleman HL. Low-level environmental lead exposure in childhood and adult intellectual function: a follow-up study. *Environ Health*. 2011;10:24.

Critique of a Study on the Low-Level Lead Exposure During Childhood and Adult Intellectual Function

A.   Collection of data

1.   **What was the context of the study?** Low doses of lead exposure are known to have toxic effects on the central nervous system of infants and children; however, it is unknown whether these effects persist into adulthood. A previous assessment of the same population found that early childhood blood lead levels were associated with cognitive function (as measured by IQ) in adolescence. This study extends follow-up through to ages 28 to 30 years.

2.   **What were the objectives of the study?** The purpose of the study was to evaluate the intellectual function in adulthood among a sample of 28- to 30-year-olds who were first recruited in 1979–1981 as newborns.

3.   **What was the primary exposure of interest? Was this accurately measured?** The primary exposure was the blood lead levels from samples obtained at birth; 6, 12, and 18 months; and 2, 4, and 10 years. Lead concentrations were quantified using graphic furnace atomic absorption spectrometry. The accuracy of the assay method was not described. Investigators computed overall mean blood lead concentration, maximum blood lead concentration, mean early childhood (0–2 years)

blood lead concentration, and mean late childhood (2–4 years) blood lead concentration.

4. **What was the primary outcome of interest? Was this accurately measured?** A single masked child neurologist administered the WASI to all subjects to obtain estimates of Full-Scale IQ, Verbal IQ, and Performance IQ. A 25% subset was selected to confirm that the administration and scoring were accurate.

5. **What type of study was conducted?** A retrospective cohort study was conducted.

6. **Describe the source of the study population, process of subject selection, sample size, and ratio of propositi to comparison subjects.** This study reexamined adults who were initially studied as children. The initial source population consisted of 249 infants born at the Brigham and Women's Hospital in Boston, Massachusetts, between August 1979 and April 1981. Names and last known addresses were available for only the 148 subjects who participated in the 10-year follow-up. Only 89 were located in the United States, and 43 of those (48%) enrolled in the current follow-up study completed a questionnaire and neuropsychological testing.

7. **Could there have been bias in the selection of the study subjects? How likely was this bias?** Given the low participation rate, there is the potential for selection bias. However, nonparticipants were similar to participants for many characteristics, including lead levels in childhood and maternal IQ, thus providing some reassurance that the likelihood of differential participation according to exposure and outcome was small.

8. **Could there have been bias in the collection of information? How likely was this bias?** The individual performing the neuropsychological tests was masked to exposure status, and therefore observer bias (which is akin to interviewer bias) was eliminated. It is unknown whether subjects themselves were aware of their exposure status, but it is unlikely that they would purposely alter their test performance on the basis of this information.

9. **What provisions were made to minimize the influence of confounding factors prior to the analysis of the data? Were these provisions sufficient?** Investigators collected data on numerous potential confounders, including maternal educational level and IQ.

B. Analysis of data
   1. **What methods were used to control confounding bias during data analysis? Were these methods sufficient?** Because of the small sample size, all potential

confounders could not be controlled for simultaneously. Multiple linear regression analyses were used to control for each confounder one at a time. These confounders included gender, birth weight, gestational age, birth order, history of concussion, current smoking status, mother's educational level and IQ, race, socioeconomic status, maternal alcohol use during pregnancy, and maternal smoking during pregnancy.

2. **What measures of association were reported in this study?** Mean differences in IQ test scores were used as the measures of association.

3. **What measures of statistical stability were reported in this study?** P values and 95% confidence intervals were reported.

C. Interpretation of data

1. **What were the major results of this study?** Reduced intellectual functioning in adults was related to blood lead levels measured in childhood. In particular, a 1 μg/dL increase in mean late childhood blood lead concentration was associated with a 1.89 point reduction in Full-Scale IQ in adulthood (95% confidence interval: −3.30, −0.47). Following the adjustment for maternal IQ, mean late childhood blood lead concentration was associated with a 1.11 point reduction in Full-Scale IQ in adulthood (95% confidence interval: −2.29, 0.06).

2. **How is the interpretation of these results affected by information bias, selection bias, and confounding? Discuss both the direction and magnitude of any bias.** Because the exposure data were accurate laboratory measures and the outcome data were generated using a masked neurologist with some verification, it is unlikely that information bias affected the results. In addition, although only a small portion of the original sample participated in this follow-up study, the characteristics of participants and nonparticipants were similar, making selection bias unlikely. Following adjustment for confounding by maternal IQ, the association between late childhood blood lead levels and adult IQ was weaker and no longer statistically stable. In addition, the small sample size made it difficult to control adequately for confounding. Thus, there may be residual confounding.

3. **How is the interpretation of these results affected by nondifferential misclassification? Discuss both the direction and magnitude of this misclassification.** Nondifferential misclassification of exposure and outcomes was possible but unlikely to be large because

exposure and outcome measurements were fairly accurate (e.g., laboratory measurements of blood lead levels). Nondifferential misclassification probably biased associations for the continuous measures toward the null.

4. **Did the discussion section adequately address the limitations of the study?** The discussion section acknowledges the small sample size and potential residual confounding by maternal IQ.

5. **What were the authors' main conclusions? Were they justified by the findings?** The authors concluded that the associations reported earlier between lead exposure in childhood intellectual functioning persist into adulthood but cautioned that confounding by maternal IQ cannot be ruled out as an alternative explanation for the observed association. These conclusions are supported by the findings.

EXHIBIT 14-4 Summary of "Effects of Tamoxifen Versus Raloxifene on the Risk of Developing Invasive Breast Cancer and Other Disease Outcomes"

Background and Objectives: Tamoxifen is a selective estrogen receptor modulator (SERM) that has been approved for the reduction of both invasive and noninvasive breast cancer risk among high-risk women. Raloxifene is a second-generation SERM that has been shown to reduce the risk of breast cancer among older women with osteoporosis. The purpose of the current study was "to compare the relative effects and safety of raloxifene and tamoxifen on the risk of developing invasive breast cancer and other disease outcomes."

Methods: The current trial was a double-masked, randomized experimental study conducted among high-risk postmenopausal women from approximately 200 clinical institutions in North America. Study subjects included 19,747 women whose mean age was 58.5 years at enrollment. Women were randomized to receive either oral tamoxifen (20 mg/d) or raloxifene (60 mg/d) for a maximum of 5 years. The primary outcome was the incidence of invasive breast cancer. Secondary outcomes included the incidence of uterine cancer, noninvasive cancer, bone fractures, and thromboembolic events.

Results: A total of 163 cases of invasive breast cancer occurred in the tamoxifen group as compared with 168 cases in the raloxifene group (incidence, 4.30 per 1,000 versus 4.41 per 1,000, risk ratio [RR], 1.02; 95% confidence interval [CI], 0.82–1.28). Only 57 cases of noninvasive breast cancer occurred in the tamoxifen group as compared with 80 raloxifene group (incidence, 1.51 versus 2.11 per 1,000; RR, 1.4; 95% CI, 0.98–2.00). A total of 36 cases of uterine cancer occurred in the tamoxifen group while 23 cases occurred in the raloxifene group (RR, 0.62; 95% CI, 0.35–1.08). No differences were seen for other invasive cancers, ischemic heart disease, or stroke. Thromboembolic events and cataracts occurred less often in the raloxifene group (RR, 0.70; 95% CI, 0.54–0.91 for thromboembolic events and RR, 0.79; 95% CI, 0.68–0.92 for cataracts). The frequency of osteoporotic fractures was similar in both groups.

Conclusions: Raloxifene and tamoxifen are equally effective in reducing the risk of invasive breast cancer but raloxifene does not reduce the risk of noninvasive breast cancer. Raloxifene has a lower risk of thromboembolic events and cataracts and a similar risk of osteoporotic fractures as tamoxifen.

Adapted from Vogel VG, Constantino JP, Wickerham DL, Cronin WM, Cecchini RS, Atkins JN, et al. Effects of tamoxifen vs raloxifene on the risk of developing invasive breast cancer and other disease outcomes. *JAMA*. 2006;2727-2741.

6. **To what larger population can the results of this study be generalized?** These results can be generalized to other children in developed countries of similar socio-economic status and with similar lead levels.

Critique of a Study on Tamoxifen Versus Raloxifene on the Risk of Developing Invasive Breast Cancer and Other Disease Outcomes

A. Collection of data

1. **What was the context of the study?** Tamoxifen has been approved by the FDA for the reduction of breast cancer risk. However, concern about its side effects has prompted testing other similar drugs. Recent clinical trials have suggested that raloxifene, a drug used to prevent and treat osteoporosis, may reduce risk of breast cancer in postmenopausal women. The current study was launched to compare the two drugs among postmenopausal women at increased risk of breast cancer.

2. **What were the objectives of the study?** The purpose of the study was "to compare the relative effects and safety of raloxifene and tamoxifen on the risk of developing invasive breast cancer and other disease outcomes."

3. **What was the primary exposure of interest? Was this accurately measured?** The experimental treatment group received raloxifene (60 mg/d) for up to 5 years. The comparison group received tamoxifen (20 mg/d) for up to 5 years. The observed rate of nonadherence to the protocol regimen was less than the planned level, and therefore it is likely that these exposures were measured fairly accurately.

4. **What was the primary outcome of interest? Was this accurately measured?** The investigators studied several endpoints, including invasive breast cancer, noninvasive breast cancer, uterine cancer, bone fractures, and thromboembolic events. All endpoints were accurately measured because they were verified by the collection of pathology reports, surgical reports, discharge summaries, and other medical record documents.

5. **What type of study was conducted?** A randomized clinical trial (experimental study) was conducted.

6. **Describe the source of the study population, process of subject selection, sample size, and ratio of propositi to comparison subjects.** From July 1999 through December 2005, a total of 184,460 women were screened for

predicted breast cancer risk at nearly 200 clinical centers throughout North America. A total of 19,747 women who were at high risk of breast cancer, were medically eligible, and agreed to participate were enrolled and randomized to either raloxifene ($n = 9,875$) or tamoxifen ($n = 9,872$). Therefore, the source population consisted of the patient populations of the clinical centers. The ratio of propositi to comparison subjects was one to one.

7. **Could there have been bias in the selection of the study subjects? How likely was this bias?** Selection bias was unlikely because a prospective study was conducted and the outcomes were unknown at enrollment. In addition, losses to follow-up were low and similar in both groups (1.3% in the raloxifene group and 1.5% in the tamoxifen group).

8. **Could there have been bias in the collection of information? How likely was this bias?** Clinicians and subjects were masked to the treatment group, and therefore this type of bias is unlikely. The main outcomes were verified by record review, and therefore interviewer bias and recall bias were unlikely. Noncompliance with the assigned treatment regimen (as measured by study dropouts and women who permanently discontinued therapy) was also lower than expected.

9. **What provisions were made to minimize the influence of confounding factors prior to the analysis of the data? Were these provisions sufficient?** Randomization was used to control for confounding. It appears to have been successful because participant characteristics, including age, race, and family history of breast cancer, were quite similar between compared groups.

B. Analysis of data
1. **What methods were used to control confounding bias during data analysis? Were these methods sufficient?** An intent-to-treat analysis was performed. This type of analysis preserves the benefits of randomization. Stratified analyses were also conducted according to age, race, family history of breast cancer, tumor size, nodal status, and other variables.

2. **What measures of association were reported in this study?** Relative risks were reported.

3. **What measures of statistical stability were reported in this study?** The authors reported 95% confidence intervals and P values.

C. Interpretation of data
1. **What were the major results of this study?** A total of 173 cases of invasive breast cancer developed among

patients assigned to tamoxifen as compared with 168 cases among patients assigned to raloxifene. Thus, compared with women who were assigned to tamoxifen, there was similar risk of invasive breast cancer (relative risk, 1.02; 95% confidence interval, 0.8 to 1.3) among women who were assigned to raloxifene. There were fewer thromboembolic events, cataracts, and cases of uterine cancer but more cases of noninvasive breast cancer in the raloxifene group. Rates of other invasive cancers, ischemic heart disease events, osteoporotic fractures, and total deaths were similar in both groups.

2. **How is the interpretation of these results affected by information bias, selection bias, and confounding? Discuss both the direction and magnitude of any bias.** These results do not appear to be influenced by selection bias, information bias, or confounding. This was primarily because the study was a large, randomized, and double-masked trial and because follow-up rates were high and outcome measures were verified.

3. **How is the interpretation of these results affected by nondifferential misclassification? Discuss both the direction and magnitude of this misclassification.** The rate of noncompliance was similar and less than planned in the two groups. However, only 68% of women in the tamoxifen group and 72% of women in the raloxifene group were compliant with the protocol by the end of the follow-up (mean follow-up, 3.9 years). Thus, it is possible that the findings would have been stronger had all women received their assigned treatments. The authors chose to conduct an intent-to-treat analysis to preserve the benefits of randomization and to determine the effectiveness of the treatment under everyday practice conditions. They also could have conducted an efficacy analysis to determine the effects of treatment under ideal conditions. The efficacy analysis would have excluded the noncompliers.

4. **Did the discussion section adequately address the limitations of the study?** The discussion section did not describe any study limitations. However, the authors do discuss their results in relation to those from other studies.

5. **What were the authors' main conclusions? Were they justified by the findings?** The authors conclude that raloxifene and tamoxifen are equally effective in reducing the risk of invasive breast cancer but that raloxifene does not reduce the risk of noninvasive breast cancer.

These conclusions were justified by the results seen in this population.

6. **To what larger population can the results of this study be generalized?** These results can be generalized to other postmenopausal women at high risk of breast cancer. Stratified analyses also showed that raloxifene benefited minority participants, and therefore the results may also be generalized to Blacks and other minorities.

Summary

The ability to critically evaluate the results of published epidemiological studies is an important skill for public health professionals. The critique outline presented in this chapter is a useful framework for conducting such an assessment. The outline helps the reader to assess (1) whether the methods used to select the study subjects and collect and analyze the data were comparable across groups; (2) whether any errors were committed in the design, conduct, and interpretation of the study; and (3) what effect these errors had on the reported findings.

The critique outline is divided into three sections that address data collection, analysis, and interpretation. The section on data collection poses questions about the context and objectives of the study; the primary exposure and outcome definitions; the study design; selection of the study population; and likelihood for selection bias, information bias, and confounding. The section on data analysis deals with the methods for handling confounding and the measures of association and statistical stability. The section on data interpretation covers the major results and how the interpretation of the results might be influenced by bias, confounding, and nondifferential misclassification. This section closes with questions about the authors' conclusions and whether they were justified by the study data and a question on the generalizability of the findings.

References

1. Kalesan B, Mobily ME, Keiser O, Fagan JA, Galea S. Firearm legislation and firearm mortality in the USA: a cross-sectional, state-level study. *Lancet.* 2016;387:1847-1855.

2. Mumford SL, Silver RM, Sjaarda LA, Wactawski-Wende J, Townsend JM, Lynch AM, et al. Expanded findings from a randomized controlled trial of preconception low-dose aspirin and pregnancy loss. *Hum Reprod.* 2016;31:657-665.

3. Seage GR III, Mayer KH, Horsburgh CR, Holmberg SD, Moon MW, Lamb GA. The relation between nitrite inhalants, unprotected receptive anal intercourse, and the risk of human immunodeficiency virus infection. *Am J Epidemiol.* 1992;135:1-11.

4. Aschengrau A, Rogers S, Ozonoff D. Perchloroethylene-contaminated drinking water and the risk of breast cancer: additional results from Cape Cod, Massachusetts, USA. *Environ Health Perspect.* 2003;111:167-173.

5. Tilden EL, Cheyney M, Guise JM, Emeis C, Lapidus J, Biel FM, et al. Vaginal birth after cesarean: neonatal

outcome and United States birth setting. *Am J Obstet Gynecol.* 2017;216:403.e1-403.e8.

6. Wang H, DeSteur H, Cheng G, Zhang X, Pei L, Gellynck X, et al. Effectiveness of folic acid fortified flour for prevention of neural tube defects in a high risk region. *Nutrients.* 2016;8:152.

7. Leighl NB, Shepherd HL, Butow PN, Clarke SJ, McJannett M, Beale PJ, et al. Supporting treatment decision making in advanced cancer: a randomized trial of decision aid for patients with advanced colorectal cancer considering chemotherapy. *J Clin Oncol.* 2011;29:2077-2084.

8. Rothman KJ. Policy recommendations in epidemiology research papers. *Epidemiology.* 1993; 4:94-95.

9. Monson RR. *Occupational Epidemiology.* 2nd ed. Boca Raton, FL: CRC Press; 1990.

10. Walker AM. Reporting the results of epidemiologic studies. *Am J Public Health.* 1986;76:556-560.

11. Zierler S, Rothman KJ. Congenital heart disease in relation to maternal use of Bendectin and other drugs in early pregnancy. *New Engl J Med.* 1985;313:347-352.

12. Porta M. *A Dictionary of Epidemiology.* 6th ed. New York, NY: Oxford University Press; 2014.

13. Weitzman M, Aschengrau A, Bellinger D, Jones R, Hamlin JS, Beiser A. Lead-contaminated soil abatement and urban children's blood lead levels. *JAMA.* 1993;269:1647-1654.

14. Meinert CL. *Clinical Trials Dictionary: Terminology and Usage Recommendations.* 2nd ed. Hoboken, NJ: John Wiley and Sons, Inc.; 2012.

15. Mann JM, Quinn TC, Francis H, Nzilambi N, Bosenge N, Bila K, et al. Prevalence of HTLV-III/LAV in household contact of patients with confirmed AIDS and controls in Kinshasa, Zaire. *JAMA.* 1986;256:721-724.

16. Mazumdar M, Bellinger DC, Gregas M, Abanilla K, Bacic J, Needleman HL. Low-level environmental lead exposure in childhood and adult intellectual function: a follow-up study. *Environ Health.* 2011; 10:24.

17. Vogel VG, Costantino JP, Wickerham DL, Cronin WM, Cecchini RS, Atkins JN, et al. Effect of tamoxifen vs raloxifene on the risk of developing invasive breast cancer and other disease outcomes. *JAMA.* 2006;2727-2741.

18. Rothman KJ. Zaire: nonsexual household transmission of AIDS [letter]. *JAMA.* 1986;256:3091.

CHAPTER 15

The Epidemiological Approach to Causation

LEARNING OBJECTIVES

By the end of this chapter the reader will be able to:

- Define and state the important characteristics of a cause.
- Describe the historical development of disease causation theories, including the germ theory and the web of causation.
- Discuss the causal guidelines proposed by Sir A.B. Hill, including their limitations.
- Distinguish between a risk factor and a cause.
- Describe the key elements of the sufficient-component cause model.
- Discuss why most scientists believe that the human immunodeficiency virus (HIV) is the cause of HIV infection and acquired immune deficiency syndrome (AIDS).

▶ Introduction

In his book *When Bad Things Happen to Good People*, Rabbi Harold Kushner tries to explain why God allows ordinary people to face extraordinary pain and tragedy.[1(pp1-5)] The idea for the book originated with Kushner's own attempt to make sense of the death of his 14-year-old son. Kushner states that sometimes there is no reason and that it is just a case of bad luck. To those who ask "Why did this happen to me?" Kushner answers that it was not part of God's fixed plan but rather that "randomness" from the "corners of the universe where God's creative light has not yet penetrated" is accountable.[1(p53)]

Whether randomness or a fixed plan causes events—good and bad—is a matter of debate among theologians and epidemiologists. Some epidemiologists, called **probabilists**, believe that randomness or chance is an explanation for events. Others, known as **determinists**, think that everything has a cause and that chance is merely a term that we use when we cannot explain something because of limitations in our knowledge.[2(p116)]

At times, Kushner also seems to support the deterministic view. For example, he states,

> I don't know why one person gets sick, and another does not, but I can only assume that some natural laws which we don't understand are at work. . . . As we have learned more about how the human body works, as we understand more of the natural laws built into the world, we have some answers. . . . The man who smokes two packs of cigarettes a day for twenty years and develops lung cancer faces problems which deserve our sympathy but he has no grounds for asking "How could God do this to me?"[1(pp60,65)]

Certainly, epidemiologists, probabilists and determinists alike, would agree that their goal is to learn about what causes and prevents disease. How epidemiologists determine causative and preventive factors involves a process known as causal inference. The scientific philosophy of causal inference began in ancient times and has changed considerably over the centuries. First, the doctrine of rationalism predominated. This philosophy states that knowledge accumulates through reason rather than observation.[3(p278)] For example, if the statements "All robins have red breasts" and "This bird is a robin" are correct, then the rationalist would conclude that "This bird has a red breast" without looking at any birds.

The philosophy of empiricism has prevailed since the Scientific Revolution of the 1700s. Empiricism emphasizes inductive inference—the formulation of explanatory hypotheses from making observations.[3(pp97-98)] For example, if the empiricist observes 100 robins and finds that they all have red breasts, he would hypothesize that all robins have red breasts, thereby making a generalization from a set of observations.

In the early 1930s, Karl Popper challenged the inductivist philosophy with his proposal that knowledge accumulates by deductive reasoning and by falsifying hypotheses that are already in one's mind.[4] According to Popper's hypothetico-deductive approach, hypotheses are formed using creativity and imagination, and no data are needed. Predictions are made on the basis of these hypotheses, and observations are collected and compared with predictions. If the observations are incompatible with the predictions, the hypothesis is falsified. Otherwise, the hypothesis remains a reasonable explanation until a better one comes along. According to this philosophy, the scientific value of a hypothesis increases with the degree to which testable and falsifiable predictions can be made from it.[5] Falsifiability increases with the empirical content of the hypothesis. For example, it is easier to falsify the precise hypothesis "Children living in homes with floor and window-well dust lead levels above 1,000 parts per million have five times the risk of becoming lead poisoned as compared with children who do not live in such conditions" than it is to falsify the general hypothesis "Lead-contaminated dust causes childhood lead poisoning."

Today, most practicing epidemiologists use a combination of inductive and deductive reasoning to learn about the factors that cause and prevent disease. However, many have adopted Popper's thesis that causal relationships can never be proven. Instead, they acknowledge that causal inference involves judgments that are made using accumulated knowledge. This knowledge comes from many fields of study in addition to epidemiology, including medicine, biology, physics, chemistry, and toxicology.

Because causal inference is a judgment, epidemiologists often have different views about the causality of certain relationships. In fact, disagreement is the rule rather than the exception. For example, even though mainstream scientists believe that the human immunodeficiency virus (HIV) is the cause of HIV infection and acquired immunodeficiency syndrome (AIDS), virologist Peter Duesberg and his colleagues think that HIV is harmless. Instead, they believe that HIV/AIDS can be caused by many different agents, such as illicit drug use, antiretroviral drugs used to treat HIV/AIDS, and malnutrition.[6]

This chapter further develops the concepts of causation and causal inference by providing the definition and characteristics of a cause, the historical development of disease causation theories, the popular model of assessing causation proposed by Sir Austin Bradford Hill, and a more recent conceptual model of causation known as the sufficient-component cause model. The chapter concludes with a description of why mainstream scientists believe that HIV is the cause of HIV/AIDS.

▶ Definitions of a Cause

According to the *American Heritage Dictionary*, a **cause** is that which produces "an effect, result, or consequence" or "the one, such as a person, event, or condition, that is responsible for an action or result."[7(p296)] The dictionary's synonyms for cause include "reason" and "occasion." For example, the reason for the car accident was the icy road conditions, or the occasion for the robbery was the absence of the night watchman. This present-day dictionary's definitions of causation follow the canons of causation first proposed by the 19th-century philosopher John Stuart Mill. One of his tenets known as "the method of difference" states that *A* causes *B* if, all else being held constant, a change in *A* is accompanied by a subsequent change in *B*.[3(p215)]

Modern epidemiologists have restated this definition in several ways. For example, Rothman, Greenland, and Lash have defined a cause as "an event, condition, or characteristic that preceded the disease onset and that, had the event, condition or characteristic been different . . . the disease would not have occurred at all or would not have occurred until some later time."[2(p6)] In contrast, Susser opted for the following simple, pragmatic definition: "something that makes a difference."[8(p637)]

How do we know when something makes a difference? How can we tell the difference between real causes and their imposters?[8] The principles of epidemiological research provide some answers. Epidemiological research involves generating and testing specific hypotheses about factors that cause and prevent disease. A hypothesis is defined as "a tentative explanation for an observation, phenomenon, or scientific problem that can be tested by further investigation."[7(p866)] Epidemiologists test hypotheses by making comparisons, usually within the context of a formal study. For example, an epidemiologist might compare the death rate among people exposed to high levels of air pollution to the rate among people exposed to low levels. In this setting, the epidemiologist is starting with the potential cause and searches for its effects. On the other hand, an epidemiologist could start with the disease and search for its causes. For example, he or she might compare prenatal cocaine use among women who gave birth to an infant with a congenital malformation with those who gave birth to a normal infant.

These types of comparisons are usually quantified in terms of absolute and relative measures of comparison. For example, people exposed to high levels of air pollution might have death rates from lung diseases that are twice the rates of people exposed to low levels of pollution. This increased death rate in the highly exposed group indicates that there is a modest association between air pollution levels and mortality.

However, the presence of an association does not necessarily imply that there is a causal relationship between the two factors. For example, there is an association between roosters crowing at dawn and the rising of the sun. This does not mean that the rooster causes the sun to rise. Thus, there are both causal and noncausal associations, and the science of **causal inference** is a method for distinguishing between the two.

Epidemiologists typically follow a two-step process when practicing causal inference. First, they determine whether the observed result is valid or true. An association is considered valid only when three alternative explanations have been eliminated: bias, confounding, and random error. **Bias** is a systematic error in the way the study subjects were selected or the data were gathered. For example, diseased people who live in highly polluted areas may be more willing to participate in studies than those living in less polluted areas. **Confounding** is a distortion in the results that arises from comparing dissimilar groups. For example, the association between air pollution and mortality may not be attributable to air pollution but to a higher prevalence of cigarette smoking among the people living in highly polluted areas as compared with those living in less polluted areas. **Random error** is the probability that the observed results are attributable to **chance**. Thus, the twofold increase in deaths from lung disease among people living in highly polluted areas may be attributable to "the luck of the draw."

If systematic bias, confounding, and random error are considered unlikely alternative explanations of an association, epidemiologists believe that the association is real, and therefore they begin the second step in the process of causal inference: assessing whether the exposure has actually caused the outcome. Causal inference is a complicated process with no hard and fast rules. In fact, there is considerable disagreement among epidemiologists about the appropriate way to make causal inferences, ranging from the use of causal "criteria" to the evaluation of competing hypotheses with "crucial" observations.

▶ **Characteristics of a Cause**

According to Susser, true causes have three essential attributes: association, time order, and direction.[8] **Association** means that "a causal factor *(X)* must occur together with the putative effect *(Y)*." In other words, there must be a "statistical dependence" between the causal factor and effect. If no association is found, causality can be rejected. Epidemiologists quantify associations by making absolute or relative comparisons between two or more groups.

Time order means that the cause must precede the effect. A cause may antedate the effect by either a long or short period of time. The former is termed a *distant cause*, and the latter is called a *proximate cause*. For chronic diseases such as cancer, distant causes often precede the cancer diagnosis by decades, and proximate causes precede it by months or years. For example, diethylstilbestrol (DES) exposure in utero is considered a distant cause of adenocarcinoma of the vagina because this exposure occurs on average 20 years before the cancer diagnosis among the affected women.[9] In contrast, hormone replacement therapy is considered a proximate cause of breast cancer because only current exposures and not past ones carry an increased risk.[10]

Direction, the third essential attribute of a cause, means that there is an asymmetrical relationship between the cause and effect. In other words, one must demonstrate that "a change in an outcome is a consequence of change in an antecedent factor" so that a symmetrical relationship is noncausal.[8] A symmetrical relationship is one where X leads to Y *and* Y leads to X. The arrow in the diagram below would go in both directions in a symmetrical relationship. For example, there is an asymmetrical relationship between exposure to cigarette smoke during pregnancy and the occurrence of low birth weight in the offspring. Prenatal exposure to cigarette smoke causes low birthweight,[11] but low birth weight does not cause prenatal smoke exposure. This type of relationship can be diagrammed as follows:

$$X \rightarrow Y$$

TABLE 15-1 Key Characteristics of Causes

■ Essential attributes include association, time order, and directionality.

■ Causes include host and environmental factors.

■ Causes include active agents and static conditions.

■ Causes may be either positive (presence induces disease) or negative (absence induces disease).

Several other characteristics of a cause are also worth noting. First, causes include both host and environmental factors. Host characteristics include a person's genetic makeup, sex, age, immunity level, diet, behaviors, and existing diseases. These factors typically affect a person's susceptibility to disease. Environmental factors pertain to determinants that are external to the individual and thereby encompass a wide range of natural, social, and economic events and conditions. For example, the presence of infectious agents, reservoirs in which the organisms multiply, vectors that transport the agent, poor and crowded housing conditions, and political instability are environmental factors that cause communicable diseases.

Causes can also be characterized as being active or passive. According to Susser,

> If the determinant is an active agent, it produces a change; the determinant is an intended or unintended intervention or a natural force or an accident, or the removal or absence of something needed, like vitamins for example. If the determinant is a static condition, it is an unchanging antecedent in a given set of circumstances: outcomes differ as the nature or quality of the condition differs. Usually, conditions are fixed attributes or circumstances like sex, heritage, or geography.[8(p637)]

Causes can also be considered positive or negative. The presence of a positive cause results in disease, and the absence of a negative cause (which is also known as a preventive exposure) causes disease. Examples of positive causes include cigarette smoking, exposure to DES, hormone replacement therapy, and ionizing radiation. Negative causes include vitamins, vaccines, a nutritious diet, and adequate exercise. The key characteristics of causes are summarized in **TABLE 15-1**.

▶ Risk Factors Versus Causes

Epidemiologists often use the term *risk factor* instead of cause. Although this term partially reflects epidemiologists' caution about making causal

TABLE 15-2 Risk Factors for Breast Cancer

Characteristic	High-risk group	Low-risk group
Country of birth	North America, Northern Europe	Asia, sub-Saharan Africa
Socioeconomic status	High	Low
Marital status	Never married	Ever married
Religion	Ashkenazi Jewish	Seventh Day Adventist, Mormon

Adapted from *Breast Cancer Facts & Figures, 2017-2018*. cancer.org. https://www.cancer.org/content/dam/cancer-org/research/cancer-facts-and -statistics/breast-cancer-facts-and-figures/breast-cancer-facts-and-figures-2017-2018.pdf; and Jemal A, Bray F, Center M, Ferlay J, Ward E, Forman D. Global cancer statistics. *CA Cancer J Clin*. 2011;61(2):69-90.

inferences, it is useful to discuss its meaning in the context of causal inference. Consider, for example, the following well-known factors that increase a woman's risk of breast cancer: living in North America, having a high socioeconomic status, never marrying, and being of Ashkenazi Jewish descent (see **TABLE 15-2**). These are considered distal risk factors for breast cancer that can be used to identify more proximate causes. For example, women who have never married have an increased risk of breast cancer because they are more likely to be childless. Childlessness in turn is associated with less differentiated breast tissue that is more susceptible to carcinogens.[12] Note that risk factors such as these, although often a few steps upstream from the proximate causes of disease, are no less important.

In contrast, consider the causes of an automobile fatality. The direct causes include the speed of the car, presence of hazardous road conditions, the time of day, level of traffic, and mental state of the driver. These factors are more proximate to "that which produces an effect, result, or consequence" than the previously described breast cancer risk factors.

▶ Historical Development of Disease Causation Theories

During ancient times, concepts of causation were influenced mainly by people's religious beliefs. For example, people believed that illnesses occurred because of divine retribution for committing sins. Around the 4th century BCE, Hippocrates introduced the idea that people became ill because of an imbalance in the four body humors: phlegm, yellow bile, blood, and black bile.[13(pp767-768)] He hypothesized that these imbalances were caused by changes in season, air, winds, water, and stars as well as personal habits.

Although Hippocrates had many ideas that were correct, his misconceptions about disease causation predominated for the following 2,000 years. Even in the 1800s, people thought that disease arose spontaneously or from foul clouds called miasmas. In the mid-1800s, Louis Pasteur, Miles Berkeley, and others revolutionized the concept of causality with the germ theory of disease.[14(pp5-6)] This theory states that specific transmissible pathogens are responsible for disease.

In the mid- to late 1800s, Jakob Henle and his student Robert Koch developed a set of postulates of disease causation that were based on the germ theory. These postulates are summarized as follows: (1) The microorganism will occur in every case of the disease and can explain the pathology and clinical changes associated with the disease; (2) the microorganism must be shown to be distinct from any others that might be found with the disease; and (3) if the microorganism is isolated and repeatedly grown in culture, it will induce a new case of disease in a susceptible animal.[15] The first postulate is particularly important because it embodies the idea of causal specificity, that is, the one-to-one relationship between a microorganism and the occurrence of disease. This is a concept that works well for infectious diseases but not for noninfectious diseases. It is important to note that Henle and Koch did not consider these rigid criteria for causation.[16]

In the 1960s, another causal paradigm—the web of causation—gained popularity because it was more useful than the Henle–Koch postulates for understanding the causes of noninfectious diseases. Consider, for example, lead poisoning, which is a disease that is defined by an elevated blood lead level and affects children's cognitive and behavioral development, growth, blood pressure, and hearing.[17(p21)] The causal web shows that its occurrence can be explained by a complex web of many interconnected factors, including both host and environmental determinants (see **FIGURE 15-1**). It illustrates that there are many ways to become lead poisoned and that these pathways or causes may differ from person to person. For example, a young child may become lead poisoned by ingesting dust that has been contaminated with lead from crumbling paint, industrial pollution, or automobile traffic. On the other hand, an adult may become lead poisoned from workplace exposures, such as bridge work, or a hobby, such as stained-glass work. Thus, the causal web paradigm represented a fundamental shift in thinking about disease causation because it incorporates the idea of multiple causes of disease. In addition, the paradigm implies that cases of disease can be prevented by cutting a few strands of the web. Usually, those factors that are closest to the disease are targeted.

In the early 1990s, Krieger criticized the use of the web because of its "hidden reliance on biomedical individualism to guide the choice of factors incorporated in the web." She proposed an alternative approach that incorporates an ecosocial framework.[18] This approach focuses on the origins of the web, including the social, political, and economic determinants of health, instead of individual-level determinants.

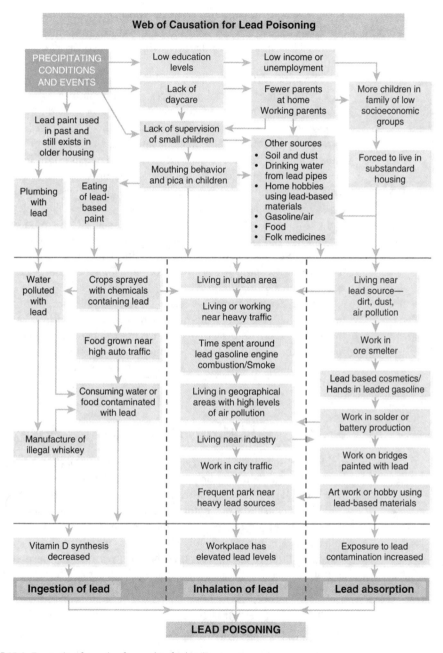

Web of Causation for Lead Poisoning

FIGURE 15-1 Example of a web of causality for lead poisoning.

Thus, for lead poisoning, such an approach would focus research questions on the reasons for particular web components, such as substandard housing, lack of daycare, workplace exposure to lead, and so forth.

During the 1950s and 1960s, epidemiologists also developed a new set of postulates for causal inferences regarding noninfectious diseases of entirely unknown etiology.[8] They were first proposed after the discovery of the association between smoking and lung cancer. From the start, many established scientists debated whether this association was causal. Thus, it became important to find a new paradigm for judging the causes of noninfectious diseases. Many individuals contributed to what are now known as "causal criteria," and five criteria were identified in the 1964 Report of the Advisory Committee to the U.S. Surgeon General on Smoking and Health to support the claim that smoking causes lung cancer. The best known criteria for assessing causation were proposed in 1965 by Sir Austin Bradford Hill.[8] Hill's nine "criteria"—or as they are more appropriately termed, *guidelines*—are described in the next section.

In the 1970s, Rothman presented a view of causation that has come to be known as the sufficient-component theory of causation.[19] Although the theory was an outgrowth of the ideas of earlier epidemiologists, Rothman was the first to present the "causal pies," a pictorial representation for thinking about causes.[20(p39)] This model of causation is described later in this chapter.

▶ Hill's Guidelines for Assessing Causation

In his much-cited 1965 publication, Sir A.B. Hill (**FIGURE 15-2**) suggested a set of nine guidelines to help determine whether associations are causal (see **TABLE 15-3, Hill's Guidelines for Assessing Causation**).[21]

Like Henle and Koch before him, Hill never intended his guidelines to be used as rigid criteria. He considered them to be imperfect guides to help epidemiologists decide what aspects of an association should be considered before concluding that the most reasonable interpretation is causal.

Strength of Association

True causes must exhibit the attribute of association.[8] Hill's first guideline—**strength of association**—takes this idea further by proposing that large associations are more likely to be causal than small ones. For example, there is a strong association between smoking and the risk of developing lung cancer. The risk among smokers is about 20 times greater than that among those who never smoked.[22] In addition, the risk further increases with the number of cigarettes smoked per day and the duration of smoking. Such strong associations are likely to be

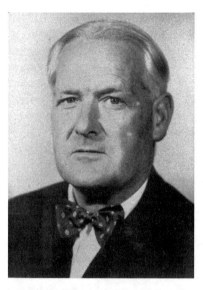

FIGURE 15-2 Sir Austin Bradford Hill suggested guidelines for assessing causation.
© Wellcome Library, London

TABLE 15-3 Hill's Guidelines for Assessing Causation
◼ Strength of association
◼ Consistency
◼ Specificity
◼ Temporality
◼ Biological gradient
◼ Plausibility
◼ Coherence
◼ Experiment
◼ Analogy

causal because they are unlikely to be accounted for entirely by alternative explanations such as bias and confounding.

Even though he emphasized this guideline, Hill stated, "We must not be too ready to dismiss a cause-and-effect hypothesis merely on the grounds that the observed association appears to be slight. There are many occasions in medicine when this is in truth so."[21(p296)] Thus, it is quite possible for weak associations to be causal. However, it is harder to rule out the effect of undetected biases on these associations. For example, many studies have found a weak association (i.e., 31% excess risk) between exposure to environmental tobacco smoke and lung cancer.[23] Although it is quite possible that the association resulted from bias or confounding, most scientists believe that it is causal.

Consistency

Hill asserted that associations are more likely to be causal if they are observed repeatedly "by different persons, in different places, circumstances and times." This is because replication and **consistency** increase our confidence that the association is not attributable to an error or fallacy. For example, one of the reasons that epidemiologists believe that smoking causes lung cancer is that this association has been observed in so many different studies conducted by different investigators, in different locations, with different types of populations, and in different time periods.

However, Hill also stated, "There will be occasions when repetition is absent or impossible and yet we should not hesitate to draw conclusions."[21(p297)] In fact, there may be reasonable explanations for differing study results. For example, one study may have examined low-level exposures, whereas another examined high-level exposures. Or one study may have enrolled only men, whereas another enrolled only women. Given the numerous biological and cultural differences between the genders, it is perfectly reasonable to think that the strength of an association differs by gender. Thus, it is important to remember that, although the presence of consistency may provide evidence of causality, its absence does not preclude causation.

Specificity

The concept of **specificity**, which was first developed for infectious diseases, means that a cause should lead to a single effect and vice versa. Although Hill stated that specific associations enabled investigators to draw conclusions about causation without hesitation, he also acknowledged that the lack of specificity did not necessarily leave investigators "sitting irresolutely on the fence." In fact, most practicing epidemiologists consider this guideline useless because it has so many well-known exceptions. For example, smoking is a cause not only of cancer of the lung but also cancer of the liver and colon–rectum as well as many noncancerous conditions, such as chronic obstructive pulmonary disease.[24(pp8-11)] Furthermore, many diseases have more than one cause. For example, the causes of lung cancer include tobacco smoke (both active and passive exposure), arsenic, silica, asbestos, and ionizing radiation.[22(pp255-268)]

Temporality

Time order, or **temporality**, means that the cause must precede the disease. Temporality is the only one of Hill's guidelines about which there is complete agreement among epidemiologists. Prospective study designs are best for providing evidence of temporality because epidemiologists are usually sure that the cause preceded the occurrence of the disease in this type of study.

Biological Gradient

Hill stated, "If the association is one which can reveal a **biological gradient**, or dose-response curve, then we should look most carefully for such evidence."[21(p298)] In other words, an association is more likely to be causal if its strength increases as the exposure level increases. Hill gives as an example the linear rise in lung cancer death rates with the number of cigarettes smoked, stating that this evidence "adds a very great deal to the simpler evidence that cigarette smokers have a higher death rate than non-smokers."[21(p298)]

However, even Hill acknowledged that there may be other or more complex dose–response relationships between a particular exposure and disease (see **FIGURE 15-3**). For example, it is possible for an exposure to exhibit a threshold effect below which there are no adverse outcomes.

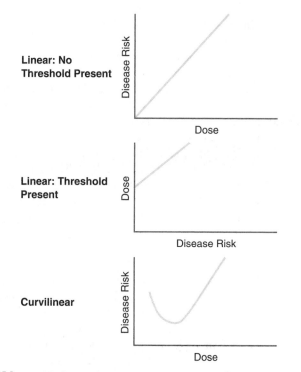

FIGURE 15-3 Possible forms of dose–response relationships.

In a study on the risk of miscarriage among pregnant women exposed to trihalomethanes (common contaminants of chlorinated drinking water that form when chlorine reacts with naturally occurring compounds in the raw water), investigators found no meaningful increase in the risk of miscarriage until contaminant levels reached 75 mg per liter.[25] These results support the idea of a threshold effect at this exposure level. It is also possible that there is a curvilinear relationship between an exposure level and the risk of disease. For example, diets that have either too few or excessive amounts of certain vitamins can lead to illness. The absence of a particular dose–response relationship (such as linear, threshold, or curvilinear) means only that the causal hypothesis that predicts that specific dose–response curve has been disputed.[2(p28)]

Plausibility

Hill asserted that there should be an existing biological or social model to explain the association. For example, it is biologically plausible that smoking causes lung cancer because cigarettes contain many carcinogenic substances. On the other hand, Hill conceded, "This is a feature I am convinced we cannot demand. . . . In short, the association we observe may be one new to science or medicine and we must not dismiss it too light-heartedly as just too odd."[21(p298)] In fact, many epidemiological studies have identified cause–effect relationships before biological mechanisms were identified. For example, researchers discovered the carcinogenic substances in cigarette smoke many years after the initial epidemiological studies linking smoking to cancer.

Despite Hill's reservations, many practicing epidemiologists believe that biological **plausibility** is an important consideration when judging the nature of an association. Consider, for example, an unusual study that compared the outcomes of hospitalized cardiac patients, half of whom were prayed for by Christian strangers who volunteered for the study.[26] In this double-masked experiment, the prayed-for patients had fewer heart attacks and contracted pneumonia less often than those who were not prayed for. Many epidemiologists have difficulty believing that this association was causal because of the lack of a biological model to explain it. Instead, they speculate that factors other than divine powers were at work, such as baseline differences in the level of illness between the two groups.

Coherence

Coherence is very close to biological plausibility. According to Hill, it means that "the cause-and-effect interpretation of our data should not seriously conflict with generally known facts of the natural history and biology of the disease."[21(p298)] For example, Hill found that the association between cigarette smoking and lung cancer is coherent with several diverse facts: (1) the temporal rise in both smoking and lung cancer over several decades, (2) the different temporal pattern in lung cancer between men and women because women began smoking later than men, (3) the histopathological evidence from the bronchial epithelium of smokers, and (4) the carcinogenic action of cigarette smoke in laboratory animals. Still, he stated, "The lack of such evidence cannot nullify the epidemiologic observations." For example, biological differences between species may account for differences between man and laboratory animals.

Experiment

Experiment is not a causal guideline in its strictest sense; rather, it is a method for testing a causal hypothesis. This guideline is a reprise of John Stuart Mill's "method of difference" canon, which states that *A* causes *B* if, all else being held uniform, a change in *A* leads to a subsequent change in *B*.[3(p215)] In the context of epidemiological research, this guideline suggests that an intervention initiated by the investigator that modifies the exposure through prevention, treatment, or removal should result in less disease or no disease at all. For example, a study of smoking cessation methods should result in lower lung cancer rates among former smokers, assuming the intervention is effective.

If available, well-designed and well-conducted experimental studies provide strong evidence for or against causation. Unfortunately, it is often infeasible and unethical to conduct experimental studies, and therefore observational studies provide most of the epidemiological data for judging whether an association is causal. Consequently, the absence of experimental evidence should not be taken as evidence against causation.

Analogy

Hill suggested that epidemiologists use an **analogy** or a similarity between the observed association and any other associations. Hill gave the following example for two causes of birth defects: "With the known effects of the drug thalidomide and the disease rubella we would be ready to accept slighter but similar evidence with another drug or another viral disease in pregnancy."[21(p299)] Critics of this guideline state that the absence of an analogy implies only that the investigator is unimaginative, not that the association is noncausal.[2(p30)]

▶ Use of Hill's Guidelines by Epidemiologists

Note that the guidelines offered by Hill have many exceptions and uncertainties. Even Hill concluded,

> Here then are nine different viewpoints from all of which we should study association before we cry causation. . . . none of my

nine viewpoints can bring indisputable evidence for or against the cause-and-effect hypothesis. . . . What they can do . . . is to help us make up our minds on the fundamental question—is there any other way of explaining the set of facts before us, is there any other answer equally, or more likely, than cause and effect?[21(p299)]

We agree with the essence of Hill's conclusion; however, we think that one part of his statement is incorrect—temporality *is* a requirement for causality.

Some epidemiologists support the use of Hill's guidelines for causal inference,[8] and others oppose it, particularly those who follow the Popperian philosophy of falsification.[27(pp153-162)] Some have proposed an alternative approach: testing competing causal theories using "crucial" observations.[2(pp25-26)] This process involves formulating competing hypotheses as specifically as possible, making predictions on the basis of each hypothesis, collecting observations that test each hypothesis, and assessing the compatibility of the observed data with each hypothesis. Ideally, the investigator will find a crucial observation that will be compatible with one hypothesis and will refute the others.

Whichever approach is preferred, we believe that it is important for epidemiologists to follow Hill's advice that public health actions may be taken even when there is insufficient evidence to definitely conclude causation. As Hill states,

All scientific work is incomplete—whether it be observational or experimental. All scientific work is liable to be upset or modified by advancing knowledge. That does not confer upon us a freedom to ignore the knowledge that we already have, or to postpone the action that it appears to demand at a given time.[21(p300)]

▶ Sufficient-Component Cause Model

In 1976, Rothman outlined the conceptual model of causation known as the sufficient-component cause model.[19] He viewed the model as a way to bridge the gap between theoretical ideas of causation and the practice of epidemiology. He defined a **sufficient cause** as a "complete causal mechanism" that inevitably produces disease.[2(p6)] A fundamental feature of this model is that a sufficient cause is not a single factor but rather a minimal set of factors that unavoidably produce disease. For example, a sufficient cause for HIV infection may be composed of the following factors: exposure to a person who is also infected with HIV, participation in a risky activity with that infected person (such as unprotected anal intercourse, shared injection equipment), susceptibility to HIV, and the absence of antiretroviral drugs (drugs that reduce HIV viral load and may reduce the risk of transmission and acquisition). Thus, the set of factors may include the presence of causative exposures and the lack of preventive ones.

Each participating factor in a sufficient cause (such as susceptibility to HIV) is termed a **component cause**. In fact, most "causes" of interest to epidemiologists are actually components of sufficient causes. Note that a single component cause or a subset of component causes does not result in disease—the entire constellation is needed. For example, a person cannot develop AIDS unless he or she is susceptible, *and* is exposed to HIV, *and* has unprotected intercourse, and so on. Merely being exposed to HIV is insufficient to cause HIV infection.

Another important tenet of the sufficient-component cause model is the idea that a disease can originate from several different sufficient causes. Thus, there may be several different causal constellations for HIV infection. For example, one sufficient cause may include exposure to contaminated blood transfusions and another may include practicing unsafe sex with an infected partner. Different sufficient causes may or may not have causal components in common. A causal component that is a member of every sufficient cause is termed a *necessary cause*. For example, exposure to HIV (by whatever route) is a necessary cause of HIV infection.

Most component causes are neither necessary nor sufficient causes of a disease. For example, smoking is neither a necessary nor sufficient cause of lung cancer. Not all smokers get lung cancer, and some non-smokers get lung cancer. Other causal components, such as susceptibility to the carcinogenic effects of cigarette smoke, must be present for an individual to succumb to this disease.

The "causal pies" first presented by Rothman help to illustrate the concepts of sufficient, component, and necessary causes. **FIGURE 15-4** shows a disease with three sufficient causes. In this example, there are three "pathways" for getting the disease. Each sufficient cause in turn has five component causes labeled A through J. Component cause A is

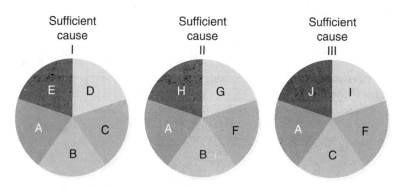

FIGURE 15-4 Conceptual scheme for the causes of a hypothetical disease.

Reprinted from Rothman KJ. Causes. *Am J Epidemiol.* 1976;104:589.

regarded as a necessary cause because it appears as a member of each sufficient cause. In contrast, none of the other component causes (B through J) are considered necessary causes because they do not appear in all three sufficient causes.

The sufficient-component cause model has several important attributes. First, blocking the action of a single causal component stops the completion of the sufficient cause and thereby prevents the disease from occurring by that pathway. This means that it is not necessary to identify all component causes of a particular sufficient cause to prevent the disease. For example, an effective HIV vaccine will prevent cases of HIV infection, even though many causal components remain unknown.

Second, the completion of a sufficient cause is synonymous with the biological onset of disease. Thus, the disease begins when the last component cause "falls into place." Note that the biological onset of the disease process is not necessarily synonymous with the onset of symptoms or the clinical diagnosis. The latter events may occur long after biological onset. For example, the natural progression from HIV infection to an AIDS diagnosis (without treatment) may take more than a decade, during which the virus is infecting and destroying CD4 T lymphocytes and damaging the immune system.[28]

The third important feature of the sufficient-component cause model is that component causes may act far apart in time. Thus, some causal components may be distant causes and others may be proximate causes. For example, consider the following possible causal components of breast cancer: carrying the BRCA1 gene, having an early age at menarche, giving birth at a late age, and taking hormone replacement therapy during menopause. The action of these causal components spans nearly a woman's entire lifetime.

The length of time from the action of a causal component until disease initiation is termed the *induction period*.[2(pp15-16)] For example, assume that the component causes in sufficient cause I of Figure 15-4 act in alphabetical order. Thus, the induction period for A is longer than that for B, which is longer than that for C, and so on. The induction time is zero for E, the component cause that acts last. This is because the disease process begins the instant that the last component cause acts.

Diseases themselves should not be characterized as having either a short or long induction period.[2(p16)] For example, some epidemiologists would say that salmonellosis has a short induction period because it occurs within 3 days of ingesting contaminated food. However, even though the induction period for one causal component—eating contaminated food—is only a few days, the induction period for other causal components (such as the presence of low immune function) may be weeks, months, or even years.

The *latent period*, which is defined as the interval from disease onset to detection, follows the induction period.[2(pp16-17)] This period is commonly known as the preclinical phase of a disease. Diseases are detected

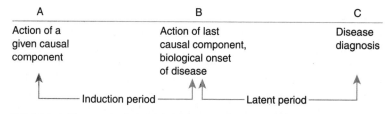

FIGURE 15-5 Temporal relationship between induction and latent periods.

either when abnormal signs and symptoms appear or when screening tests, such as mammograms, are administered. The temporal relationship between the induction and latent periods is depicted in **FIGURE 15-5**.

▶ Why Mainstream Scientists Believe That HIV Is the Cause of HIV/AIDS

HIV/AIDS is an illness that causes the collapse of the immune system, which in turn makes the body vulnerable to numerous deadly infections that the body would otherwise have little difficulty handling. Although the majority of scientists believe that HIV causes HIV/AIDS, a small group of scientists, including virologist Peter Duesberg, still believe that HIV/AIDS is a behavioral rather than an infectious disease. Duesberg and his followers (who include the former president of South Africa, Mbeki) continue to believe that HIV is a harmless virus and that HIV/AIDS is caused by the use of recreational drugs and antiretroviral drugs in the United States and Europe and by malnutrition in Africa.[6,29]

As a way of summarizing the concepts of causal inference described earlier in this chapter, let us examine the evidence that mainstream scientists have used to counter Duesberg's claims. First, scientists have stated that HIV has fulfilled the Henle–Koch postulates for causation for infectious microbes.[30] Several papers from the early 1980s provided the evidence to support the first two postulates, particularly the one-to-one correspondence between HIV and HIV/AIDS. For example, Gallo and colleagues routinely found HIV in people with HIV/AIDS symptoms and failed to find HIV among those who lacked either HIV/AIDS symptoms or associated risk factors.[31]

Henle and Koch's third postulate, which states that the microorganism must be isolated from a diseased host and must induce a new case of disease when given to a susceptible animal, took longer to fulfill because there are no good animal models for HIV/AIDS. Evidence to support this postulate finally emerged in the early 1990s from the accidental infection of three laboratory workers with a pure molecularly cloned strain of HIV.[32] None of the lab workers had any of the typical behavioral risk factors, such as a history of intravenous drug use or homosexual sex, and so these factors could not explain their disease. One worker developed *Pneumocystis carinii* pneumonia, an AIDS-defining disease, 68 months after showing evidence of infection. This individual did not receive any antiretroviral drugs until 83 months after infection, and therefore these drugs, as Duesberg claimed, could not have caused his disease. The other two laboratory workers showed severe declines in immune function over time but no AIDS-defining diseases, and one of them eventually received antiretroviral drugs. Duesberg was not convinced by these data because only one worker developed an AIDS-defining disease. However, Anthony Fauci, the head of the National Institute of Allergy and Infectious Diseases (the federal agency that conducts and funds most research on HIV/AIDS) stated, "As far as I'm concerned, the laboratory workers prove causation."[32(p1647)]

Several other lines of evidence also convinced the general scientific community that HIV causes HIV/AIDS. This evidence typically fulfilled one of Hill's guidelines for causation. Some evidence came from prospective epidemiological studies that followed large numbers of initially healthy individuals. These studies found a consistent relationship between HIV antibody levels and the eventual development of AIDS. (HIV antibodies develop only in response to HIV infection.) For example, a Canadian study followed a group of 715 gay men for almost 9 years. The investigators found 136 cases of HIV/AIDS among men with preexisting HIV antibody and no cases of HIV/AIDS among men who were antibody negative.[33] Another prospective study that followed 1,027 men from San Francisco for 8 years found 215 cases of HIV/AIDS among the men who were antibody positive and no cases of HIV/AIDS among the antibody-negative men.[34]

There are two principal reasons studies such as these have provided persuasive causal evidence. First, the associations were very strong (no HIV/AIDS cases among HIV-negative men versus hundreds of cases among HIV-positive men). Second, the prospective study designs provided evidence that the HIV infection preceded the development of AIDS. In other words, they provided evidence of a clear temporal relationship between the cause and the effect.

Many epidemiological studies have also found a dose–response relationship between measures of infection severity, such as plasma HIV levels, and the risk of progression to AIDS and death. For example, Mellors and colleagues found that only 0.9% of men with low baseline HIV levels died of AIDS, whereas 18.1% of men with moderate HIV levels and 69.5% of men with high HIV levels died during the 10-year follow-up period.[35] Another study among HIV-infected hemophiliacs found that each (log 10) unit increase in baseline viral load was associated with a 2.4-fold increase in AIDS-related illness during the follow-up period.[36]

The absence of a dose–response relationship between factor VIII (the clotting factor used to treat hemophilia) and the risk of dying was used to counter Duesberg's early claim that noninfectious contaminants of factor VIII cause HIV/AIDS. For example, a study following 2,000 individuals with hemophilia in the United States and Europe found that HIV-infected hemophiliacs who received low, medium, and high cumulative doses of factor VIII had similar death rates during the follow-up period (34.5% for low, 39.0% for medium, and 38.8% for high).[37] Most scientists believe that if exposure to contaminants in factor VIII were the cause of HIV/AIDS and subsequent deaths, the death rates would have been higher for those who received higher doses of factor VIII.

Many studies have disproved Duesberg's claim that antiretroviral medications cause HIV/AIDS. In fact, these studies have supported the hypothesis that HIV causes HIV/AIDS because many of these drugs work by attacking unique aspects of HIV replication. Prospective studies of antiretroviral drugs have been shown to treat HIV/AIDS by suppressing HIV levels, causing clinical symptoms to disappear, and improving survival. For example, one study following more than 49,000 participants found that all antiretroviral therapies improve survival in comparison with no treatment and that the more intensive treatments produce the greatest improvements in survival.[38] The fact that many studies have shown similar results despite using different methodologies, different types of patients, and different investigators has been cited as evidence for their credibility. These data have supported Hill's guidelines on experiment and consistency.

Other evidence supporting Hill's guideline on coherence rebutted the idea that antiretroviral drugs cause HIV/AIDS. First, people died of AIDS before antiretroviral drugs were available, and therefore these drugs could not have caused these deaths. Second, there was a sharp decline in AIDS deaths beginning in 1996 when antiretroviral drugs were introduced. In particular, the Centers for Disease Control and Prevention reported that deaths from AIDS in the United States peaked at 51,842 in 1995 and then fell to 38,296 in 1996, down to 18,249 in 1999, and 15,458 in 2015.[39,40] Most scientists believe that these temporal trends are consistent with the idea that antiretroviral drugs have controlled rather than caused HIV/AIDS.

Other studies rebutted Duesberg's claim that the use of illicit drugs causes HIV/AIDS. For example, the San Francisco Men's Health Study followed 812 homosexual/bisexual men and 215 heterosexual men for the development of HIV/AIDS.[34] Heavy drug use involving marijuana, cocaine, and amphetamines was equally common among both groups of men, yet the 215 cases of AIDS that occurred during the 8 years of follow-up were restricted to homosexual participants. Thus, there was strong evidence that these drugs did not have a role in the occurrence of HIV/AIDS among these men.

Additional evidence that HIV/AIDS is not caused by recreational drugs has come from the National Household Survey on Drug Abuse. The survey has charted increases or no change in the use of many of the drugs that Duesberg has claimed to cause HIV/AIDS, including heroin, cocaine, and inhalants.[41,42] It is counterintuitive for purported causes of HIV/AIDS to have remained stable or increased while the number of HIV/AIDS cases and deaths has declined.

Duesberg's theory has another important shortcoming. Its narrowly defined risk groups do not account for everyone who develops HIV/AIDS. For example, this theory does not account for the fact that 61% of reported HIV/AIDS cases among women have occurred among those who have no risk factors other than heterosexual contact with an HIV-infected man.[40] Nor does his theory account for the HIV-infected children born to infected mothers who developed AIDS in contrast to their HIV-negative siblings who remained healthy.

How can Duesberg and his colleagues still maintain their views in light of all of this evidence? According to one science writer, "mainstream AIDS researchers argue that Duesberg's arguments are constructed by selective reading of the scientific literature, dismissing evidence that contradicts his theses, requiring impossibly definitive proof, and dismissing outright studies marked by inconsequential weaknesses."[30] Duesberg's unscientific approach contradicts the tenets of epidemiological research and causal inference as practiced by most scientists. However, it serves to emphasize the notion that causation is ultimately in the eyes of the beholder.

Summary

A cause may be defined as "an event, condition, or characteristic that preceded the disease onset and that, had the event, condition or characteristic been different . . . the disease event either would not have occurred at all or would not have occurred until some later time,"[2(p6)] or more simply, as "something that makes a difference."[8(p637)] The three essential attributes of a cause are association, time order, and direction. Causes include host and environmental factors, active agents and static conditions, and positive and negative factors.

Disease causation theories have changed considerably over time, from divine retribution for committing sins, to foul clouds called miasmas, to imbalances in body humors. In the 1800s, a revolutionary concept called the germ theory was proposed that states that specific transmissible pathogens are responsible for disease. During this period, Jakob Henle and Robert Koch developed a set of postulates of disease causation based on the germ theory. In the 1960s, an important causal paradigm known as the web of causation was developed. This paradigm incorporates the idea of multiple causes of disease and therefore is useful for noninfectious diseases.

During the 1960s, Hill described a set of nine guidelines to help determine whether associations are causal. These guidelines include strength of association, consistency, specificity, temporality, biological gradient, plausibility, coherence, experiment, and analogy. These guidelines have many exceptions and uncertainties, and Hill never meant them to be used as rigid criteria. Both the Henle–Koch postulates and Hill's guidelines have been used by mainstream scientists to support the idea that HIV is the cause of HIV/AIDS.

A more recently developed conceptual model of causation that bridges theoretical ideas of causation with the practice of epidemiology is known as the sufficient-component cause model. In this model, a sufficient cause is a "complete causal mechanism" that "inevitably produces disease."[2(p6)] A sufficient cause includes at least one minimal set of factors (called component causes) that unavoidably causes disease. Blocking the action of a single component cause stops the completion of the sufficient cause and prevents the disease from occurring by that mechanism. This means that it is not necessary to identify all component causes of a sufficient cause to prevent the disease.

References

1. Kushner H. *When Bad Things Happen to Good People*. New York, NY: Avon Books; 1981.
2. Rothman KJ, Greenland S, Lash TL. *Modern Epidemiology*. 3rd ed. Philadelphia, PA: Lippincott Williams and Wilkins; 2008.
3. Flew A. *A Dictionary of Philosophy*. Aylesbury, Great Britain: Laurence Urdang Associates Ltd.; 1979.
4. Popper KR. *The Logic of Scientific Discovery*. New York, NY: Basic Books; 1959 (reprint of the 1935 ed.).
5. Buck C. Popper's philosophy for epidemiologists. *Int J Epidemiol*. 1975;4:159-168.
6. Goodson P. Questioning the HIV-AIDS hypothesis: 30 years of dissent. *Front Public Health*. 2014;2:1-12.
7. Pickett JP (ed.). *The American Heritage Dictionary of the English Language*. 4th ed. Boston, MA: Houghton Mifflin; 2000.
8. Susser M. What is a cause and how do we know one? A grammar for pragmatic epidemiology. *Am J Epidemiol*. 1991;133:635-648.
9. Herbst AL, Ulfelder H, Poskanzer DC. Adenocarcinoma of the vagina: association of maternal stilbestrol therapy with tumor appearance in young women. *New Engl J Med*. 1971;284:878-881.
10. Million Women Study Collaborators. Breast cancer and hormone-replacement therapy in the Million Women Study. *Lancet*. 2003;362:419-427.
11. Inoue S, Naruse H, Yorifuji T, Kato T, Murakoshi T, Doi H, et al. Impact of maternal and paternal smoking on birth outcomes. *J Public Health (Oxf)*. 2016;39(3):1-10. doi: 10.1093/pubmed/fdw050.
12. Russo J, Moral R, Balogh GA, Mailo D, Russo IH. The protective role of pregnancy in breast cancer. *Breast Cancer Res*. 2005;7:131-142.
13. *Dorland's Illustrated Medical Dictionary*. Philadelphia, PA: W.B. Saunders; 1994.
14. Brock TD, Brock KM. *Basic Microbiology with Applications*. 2nd ed. Englewood Cliffs, NJ: Prentice Hall Inc.; 1978.
15. Carter KC. Koch's postulates in relation to the work of Jacob Henle and Edwin Klebs. *Med Hist*. 1985;29:353-374.
16. Evans AS. Causation and disease: a chronological journey: the Thomas Parran Lecture. *Am J Epidemiol*. 1978;108:249-258.
17. *Preventing Lead Exposure in Young Children: A Housing-Based Approach to Primary Prevention of Lead Poisoning*. cdc.gov. https://www.cdc.gov/nceh/lead/publications/primarypreventiondocument.pdf. Published October 2004. Accessed June 26, 2018.
18. Krieger N. Epidemiology and the web of causation: has anyone seen the spider? *Soc Sci Med*. 1994;39:887-903.
19. Rothman KJ. Causes. *Am J Epidemiol*. 1976;104: 587-592.
20. Greenland S (ed.). *Evolution of Epidemiologic Ideas: Annotated Readings on Concepts and Methods*. Chestnut Hill, MA: Epidemiology Resources Inc.; 1987.
21. Hill AB. The environment and disease: association or causation? *Proc Royal Soc Med*. 1965;48:295-300.
22. Adami H-A, Hunter D, Trichopoulos D (eds). *Textbook of Cancer Epidemiology*. New York, NY: Oxford University Press; 2002.
23. Kim CH, Lee YC, Hung RJ, McNallan SR, Cote ML, Lim WY, et al. Exposure to secondhand tobacco smoke and lung cancer by histological type: a pooled analysis of the International Lung Cancer Consortium (ILCCO). *Int J Cancer*. 2014;135:1918-1930.
24. *The Health Consequences of Smoking: 50 Years of Progress: A Report of the Surgeon General: Executive Summary*. stacks.cdc.gov. https://stacks.cdc.gov/view/cdc/21586/. Published 2014. Accessed April 2018.
25. Waller K, Swan SH, Delorenze G, Hopkins B. Trihalomethanes in drinking water and spontaneous abortion. *Epidemiology*. 1998;9:134-140.
26. Byrd RC. Positive therapeutic effects of intercessory prayer in coronary care unit population. *South Med J*. 1988;81:826-829.

27. Poole C. Induction does not exist in epidemiology, either. In: Rothman, KJ (ed.). *Causal Inference*. Chestnut Hill, MA: Epidemiology Resources Inc.; 1988.

28. Coffin JM. HIV viral dynamics. *AIDS*. 1996;10(3): S75-S84.

29. Duesberg PH, Mandrioli D, McCormack A, Nicholson JM, Rasnick D, Fiala C, et al. AIDS since 1984: no evidence for a new, viral epidemic—not even in Africa. *Ital J Anat Embryol*. 2011;116:73-92.

30. Cohen J. The Duesberg phenomenon. *Science*. 1994;266:1642-1649.

31. Gallo RC, Salahuddin SZ, Popovic M, Shearer GM, Kaplan M, Haynes BF, et al. Frequent detection and isolation of cytopathic retroviruses (HTLV-III) from patients with AIDS and at risk for AIDS. *Science*. 1984;224:500-503.

32. Cohen J. Fulfilling Koch's postulates. *Science*. 1994; 266:1647.

33. Schechter MT, Craib KJP, Montaner JSG, Le TN, O'Shaughnessy MV, Gelmon KA, et al. HIV-1 and the aetiology of AIDS. *Lancet*. 1993;341:658-659.

34. Ascher MS, Sheppard HW, Winkelstein W Jr, Vittinghoff E. Does drug use cause AIDS? *Nature*. 1993;362:103-104.

35. Mellors JW, Munoz A, Giorgi JV, Margolick JB, Tassoni CJ, Gupta P, et al. Plasma viral load and CD4+ lymphocytes as prognostic markers of HIV-1 infection. *Ann Intern Med*. 1997;126:983-985.

36. Engels EA, Rosenberg PS, O'Brien TR, Goedert JJ. Plasma HIV viral load in patients with hemophilia and late-stage HIV disease: a measure of current immune suppression. *Ann Intern Med*. 1999;131:256-264.

37. Goedert JJ, Kessler CM, Aledort LM, Biggar RJ, Andes WA, White GC II, et al. A prospective study of human immunodeficiency virus type 1 infection and the development of AIDS in subjects with hemophilia. *New Engl J Med*. 1989;321:1141-1148.

38. McNaghten AD, Hanson DL, Jones JL, Dworkin MS, Ward JW, Thompson M, et al. Effects of antiretroviral therapy and opportunistic illness primary chemoprophylaxis on survival after AIDS. *AIDS*. 1999;13(13):1687-1695.

39. *HIV/AIDS Surveillance Report: U.S. HIV and AIDS Cases Reported Through December 2001*. cdc.gov. https://www.cdc.gov/hiv/pdf/statistics_2001_HIV _Surveillance_Report_vol_13_no2.pdf. Accessed April 15, 2018.

40. *HIV Surveillance Report: Diagnoses of HIV Infection in the United States and Dependent Areas, 2016*. cdc .gov. https://www.cdc.gov/hiv/pdf/library/reports /surveillance/cdc-hiv-surveillance-report-2016 -vol-28.pdf. Published November 2017. Accessed December 2017.

41. *Results from the 2002 National Survey on Drug Use and Health: National Findings*. 2003. files.eric .ed.gov. https://files.eric.ed.gov/fulltext/ED479833 .pdf. Accessed April 15, 2018.

42. *Results from the 2013 National Survey on Drug Use and Health: Summary of Findings*. samhsa. gov. https://www.samhsa.gov/data/sites/default /files/NSDUHresultsPDFWHTML2013/Web /NSDUHresults2013.pdf. Published November 2014. Accessed June 26, 2018.

Chapter Questions

1. Define each of the following terms:
   a. Cause of disease
   b. Risk factor
   c. Component cause (as used in Rothman's sufficient-component cause model)
   d. Sufficient cause
   e. Necessary cause

2. Describe the temporal relationship between the induction period and latent period.

3. Indicate whether the following statements are true or false:
   a. Hill's guideline of temporality is more easily established in a prospective than a retrospective study.
   b. Strong associations are more likely to be causal than weak ones because they are less likely to be attributable to alternative explanations.
   c. A causal relationship between an exposure and a disease cannot be established unless all of Hill's guidelines are met.
   d. Hill's guideline of specificity means that an exposure can cause only one disease.

e. Prenatal exposure to the Zika virus is a necessary cause of Zika infection in newborns.

f. Prenatal exposure to the Zika virus is a sufficient cause of Zika infection in newborns.

g. Prenatal exposure to cigarette smoke is a necessary cause of low birth weight in newborns.

h. Prenatal exposure to cigarette smoke is a sufficient cause of low birth weight in newborns.

4. Suppose that an article was published on the relationship between caffeine consumption during pregnancy and the risk of low birth weight. Caffeine is in a wide variety of beverages, foods, and drugs, including coffee, tea, and colas. Suppose that the following statements were taken from the introduction and results section of this article. State which of Hill's guidelines is supported by each of the statements. For example, statement A supports Hill's guideline on analogy.

a. Caffeine has a similar molecular structure to that of other chemicals that are known to affect human cell division and growth.

b. Caffeine exposure during pregnancy could have a harmful effect because caffeine may interfere with cell division, metabolism, and growth.

c. Several animal studies have shown an association between caffeine and lower fetal weight.

d. Seven previously published epidemiological studies of caffeine intake during pregnancy have shown an increased risk of offspring with low birth weight among women who consumed high levels of caffeine.

e. In the current study, the risk of low birth weight increased as caffeine consumption increased. Compared with women who did not consume any caffeine during pregnancy, women who had low caffeine consumption had a 40% increased risk of giving birth to an infant with low birth weight, women who had moderate caffeine consumption had a 90% increased risk, and women who had high caffeine consumption had a 150% increased risk.

5. Indicate whether the following statements are true or false:

a. The presence of an association is indicative of a causal relationship.

b. Time order is an essential attribute of a cause.

c. Direction (X leads to Y but not vice versa) is an essential attribute of a cause.

d. If we have ruled out chance, bias, and confounding as explanations for an association, we may conclude that the association is causal.

e. Sir Bradford Hill's nine causal guidelines should be used as rigid criteria to establish causation.

f. According to the sufficient-component cause model, blocking the action of a necessary cause will prevent all cases of a disease by all of its causal mechanisms.

CHAPTER 16

Screening in Public Health Practice

LEARNING OBJECTIVES

By the end of this chapter the reader will be able to:

- Describe the general features of the natural history of disease.
- Distinguish between primary, secondary, and tertiary prevention.
- List the key characteristics of diseases appropriate for screening.
- Describe the important features of a screening test.
- Define and calculate sensitivity, specificity, predictive value positive, and predictive value negative.
- Discuss the outcome measures and study designs for evaluating the effectiveness of a screening program.
- Define lead-time bias, length-biased sampling, and volunteer bias.
- Describe the effect of screening on prostate cancer incidence and breast cancer mortality.

▶ Introduction

Screening is defined as follows:

> The presumptive identification of an unrecognized disease or defect by the application of tests, examinations or other procedures which can be applied rapidly. Screening tests sort out apparently well persons who probably have a disease from those who probably do not. A screening test is not intended to be diagnostic. Persons with positive or suspicious findings must be referred to their physicians for diagnosis and necessary treatment.[1(p257)]

A diagnostic test typically carries more risk and is more expensive than a screening test. People who are found to have the disease are then

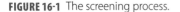

FIGURE 16-1 The screening process.

treated. Screening is used mainly to identify asymptomatic individuals at an earlier stage than if they waited for symptoms to arise. An important assumption is that earlier diagnosis will lead to earlier, more effective treatment that in turn will decrease the adverse effects of a disease and improve survival. The screening process is described in **FIGURE 16-1**.

Screening programs are currently popular in medicine and public health and will continue to grow as new technologies are developed to identify biological markers of early disease. In fact, policymakers have often responded too quickly to emerging public health problems by prematurely instituting screening programs. For example, mandatory screening for the human immunodeficiency virus (HIV) was instituted among immigrants and premarital couples to stop the spread of HIV long before effective treatments were available.[2]

Many new students of public health and even seasoned policymakers think that it is appropriate to screen for most diseases. However, screening is a complex activity with both beneficial and detrimental effects. Consequently, it is important for all public health practitioners to have a thorough understanding of screening principles. These concepts, which are described in this chapter, include the natural history of a disease; primary, secondary, and tertiary prevention; the hallmarks of a disease that make it appropriate for screening; the performance characteristics of screening tests and programs; and the methods and biases involved in evaluating the effectiveness of screening programs.

▶ Natural History of Disease

The **natural history** of a disease is defined as the course of a disease from its inception to its resolution.[1(p163)] It begins with the pathological onset of disease (point A in **FIGURE 16-2**), such as the transformation of a normal breast epithelial cell into a cancerous one or the infection of CD4 T lymphocytes with HIV. It continues with the preclinical stage, which lasts from the pathological onset to the first appearance of signs and symptoms (point A to point B). Thus, the person is unaware that he or she has a disease during the preclinical stage. The clinical stage lasts from the first appearance of symptoms to the end of the disease (point B to point E). Although the person usually seeks medical attention when symptoms develop, the actual time of diagnosis is a function of the availability of

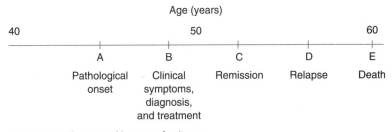

Age (years)

40   50   60
          A   B   C   D   E
    Pathological   Clinical   Remission   Relapse   Death
       onset   symptoms,
                  diagnosis,
                  and treatment

FIGURE 16-2 The natural history of a disease.

medical care and the individual's level of awareness. Once the diagnosis is made, treatment usually begins. Depending on the disease, the clinical stage may progress to death (point E), include remissions and relapses (points C and D, respectively), or regress either spontaneously or from successful treatment and cure (not shown in Figure 16-2). There is substantial variation in the length of each phase. Some individuals progress rapidly, and others progress slowly.

▶ Definition of Primary, Secondary, and Tertiary Prevention

The central goal of public health is to protect and promote health, in other words, to prevent disease, disability, and premature death. Prevention activities are customarily divided into three levels: primary, secondary, and tertiary. As described in the following sections, the main distinction between the levels is the stage at which they are implemented.

Primary Prevention

Primary prevention is defined as the maintenance of health through individual or community efforts so that the disease process never starts. Thus, primary prevention activities occur before pathological onset (point A in **FIGURE 16-3**) and reduce the incidence of disease. Examples of primary prevention activities include a healthy diet; regular exercise; avoidance of smoking; sunscreen use; seat belt and helmet use; immunizations against infectious diseases; policies to maintain a clean supply of water, air, and food; and safe home and work environments. Public and medical education campaigns at the individual and community levels and governmental legislation are among the many ways the general public becomes aware of and adopts behaviors and policies to prevent disease.

Although most primary prevention efforts target the general population, some efforts focus on special subgroups within the population. For example, women with a family history of or other breast cancer risk

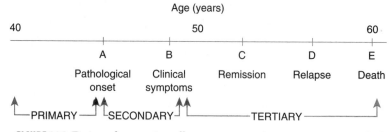

FIGURE 16-3 Timing of prevention efforts.

factors are being targeted to take drugs such as raloxifene to prevent the occurrence of breast cancer,[3] and groups at high risk of HIV infection have been targeted for intervention programs that reduce risky behaviors such as needle sharing[4] and unsafe sexual practices.[5]

All primary prevention activities assume that the action taken will reduce the occurrence of disease and its aftereffects. For example, behavioral interventions for men who have sex with men assume that reducing the frequency of unsafe sex will in turn reduce the incidence of HIV infection and disease progression.

Secondary Prevention

Secondary prevention is defined as the reduction in the expression and severity of clinical disease. Secondary prevention efforts do not prevent disease occurrence but instead identify asymptomatic individuals during the window between the pathological onset and the occurrence of clinical symptoms (between points A and B in Figure 16-3). Secondary prevention activities assume that early detection will lead to prompt and effective interventions that will ultimately improve survival. For many diseases, secondary prevention reduces disease prevalence by delaying the onset of clinical disease (point B) and by decreasing disease duration (points B to E). For example, screening for HIV infection, combined with the early use of several highly active antiretroviral drugs, substantially delays the onset of clinical symptoms, immune dysfunction, and mortality.[6]

For some diseases, secondary prevention may increase the disease incidence and prevalence (at least temporarily) because asymptomatic cases are identified at an earlier stage. For example, a portion of the increased incidence of prostate cancer in the late 1980s has been attributed to widespread use of screening in the U.S. population. This phenomenon is described in greater detail at the end of this chapter.

Secondary prevention of infectious diseases may have the added benefit of reducing or halting the spread of disease. For example, early screening, accompanied by counseling and drug therapy, reduces the spread of HIV by reducing risky behaviors and virus levels in semen.

TABLE 16-1 Levels of Prevention	
Prevention level	**Effect on disease**
Primary	Prevents disease from occurring. Goal is to reduce incidence.
Secondary	Delays onset and duration of clinical disease. Goal is to improve survival.
Tertiary	Slows disease progression; reduces disease sequelae. Goal is to improve survival.

Tertiary Prevention

The goal of **tertiary prevention** is to slow or block the progression of a disease, thereby reducing impairments and disabilities and improving the quality of life and survival among diseased individuals. It is implemented after a clinical diagnosis has been made (any time after point B in Figure 16-3) and may include prompt treatment, proper follow-up and rehabilitation, and patient education. A typical example of tertiary prevention is the use of drugs to prevent opportunistic infections among individuals with HIV infection. Fewer life-threatening infections and fewer difficult-to-follow treatment regimens and hospitalizations substantially improve the quality of life and survival among HIV-infected people. Another example of tertiary prevention is careful control of insulin levels and patient education to prevent retinopathy and other complications among patients with diabetes. The three levels of prevention and their effect on disease are summarized in **TABLE 16-1**.

▶ Appropriate Diseases for Screening

A disease must have certain characteristics to be appropriate for screening (see **TABLE 16-2**). First, the disease must be serious and have important consequences. Given the high cost and possible adverse consequences of screening, it is justifiable to screen for only major diseases, such as cancer of the cervix, breast, colon–rectum, prostate, and skin; noncancerous diseases, such as diabetes, hypertension, and glaucoma; and infectious diseases, such as HIV infection and tuberculosis.

Second, the disease must be progressive, and early treatment must be more effective than later treatment. This is because screening is carried out in the belief that the natural history of the disease can be altered by earlier treatment. Thus, breast cancer is a suitable disease for screening because its treatment is more effective when the cancer is discovered at an earlier stage than at a later stage.[7] On the other hand, pancreatic cancer is a serious disease that is not suitable for screening because mortality is high even with early diagnosis.[7]

TABLE 16-2 Characteristics of Diseases Appropriate for Screening

Disease is serious, with severe consequences.

Treatment is more effective at an earlier stage.

Disease has a detectable preclinical phase (DPCP).

DPCP is fairly long and prevalent in the target population.

Third, an appropriate disease must have a preclinical phase (from point A to B in Figure 16-2) that can be identified by a screening test. This phase is known as the detectable preclinical phase, or DPCP. The DPCP is a function of both the natural history of the disease and the technical capabilities of the screening test. When a disease process begins, abnormalities occur in the body, such as the division and shedding of abnormal cells, abnormal bleeding, or the production of compounds such as antigens and antibodies. A screening test is designed to identify these initial biological abnormalities so the affected individual comes to medical attention earlier. For example, breast cancer starts with the transformation of a single normal breast cell into a cancerous one. Over the next decade or so, the cancer cell and its progeny divide enough times to form a tumor large enough to be detectable by currently available screening methods. Presently, the smallest tumor detectable by screening mammography is a few millimeters.

Finally, an appropriate disease must have a DPCP that is fairly prevalent and has a long duration in the screened population. The prevalence of the DPCP in a population depends on three factors: the incidence of the disease, the average length of the preclinical phase, and any prior screening activities. Higher incidence and longer preclinical phases lead to a higher DPCP prevalence. Any prior screening activities will reduce the prevalence during the DPCP, particularly if the screening was recently conducted.

If the prevalence of the DPCP is high enough in the general population, mass screening—that is, screening of the entire population—is both feasible and cost effective. If the prevalence is not sufficiently high in the general population, screening efforts are targeted to high-risk groups, such as individuals over a certain age or with a family history of the disease. Screening at frequent intervals is recommended in very high-risk populations.

It is not efficient or cost effective to screen for diseases with a low DPCP prevalence because thousands of people would need to be screened to detect only a few cases. For the same reason, it is inefficient to screen for acute infectious diseases with a short DPCP (lasting hours to weeks).

HIV infection is an example of an appropriate disease that meets all the criteria for screening. It is a severe disease with dire consequences: the case-fatality rate among all reported adult AIDS cases during the period 1981 to 2015 was 56%.[8] It has a long and highly prevalent DPCP in the population, particularly subgroups such as men who have sex with men. In fact, the seroprevalence of HIV among Black men who have sex with men has been estimated to be as high as 41.5% in some communities.[9] Finally, there are many treatments that are effective at reducing the sequelae of HIV infection when given at an early stage.

FIGURE 16-4 illustrates the natural history of an HIV infection without treatment. Transmission occurs when viruses from one person's infected cells enter another person and infect some of that person's cells. In about half of the cases, the primary HIV infection is asymptomatic. However, for some cases, nonspecific symptoms of the acute HIV syndrome occur within a few days or weeks. (These symptoms are often attributed to a severe cold or influenza.) During the first few weeks after infection, HIV can be detected only by using a sophisticated and expensive test called polymerase chain reaction, or PCR test. This test is not used for screening because it is costly and difficult to perform.

By 6 weeks, most immune systems produce HIV antibodies in response to the infection, which is now detectable by the HIV antibody screening test.[10] (Note that recently developed antibody/antigen tests can detect HIV infection sooner.) Once infection is detectable by the screening test, the person has entered the DPCP. This phase is often quite long— its median length is 10 years without treatment. Even though the person has no symptoms during the DPCP, the virus is invading and destroying CD4 T lymphocytes and damaging the immune system. When CD4 T lymphocyte levels fall to 200 per microliter, the person meets the

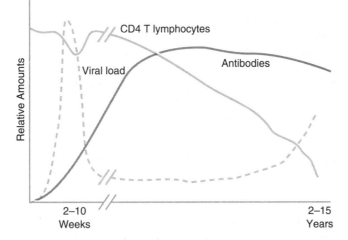

FIGURE 16-4 Natural history of HIV infection without treatment.

official case definition of AIDS. By this time, the individual's immune system is unable to respond to pathogens, and severe symptoms and life-threatening infections and malignancies may occur. The first occurrence of any symptoms marks the end of the preclinical phase.

The time course and clinical manifestations of HIV infection vary widely without treatment. Some individuals progress rapidly, and others move slowly. Thus, the first time a population is screened for HIV, the individuals identified are at varying stages of preclinical illness. The effectiveness of screening varies from one population to another because effectiveness depends on the relative proportions of individuals identified at the early, middle, and late stages of the preclinical phase. The AIDS diagnosis is delayed, and survival is dramatically improved when combination antiretroviral therapy is started in adults with HIV infection who have detectable virus in their plasma regardless of their CD4 T lymphocyte level.[6]

The only way to treat HIV infection as early as possible is to screen as early as possible. But who should be screened for HIV? In 2006 the Centers for Disease Control and Prevention (CDC) greatly expanded its HIV screening recommendations.[11] The CDC now advises that screening for HIV infection be routinely performed in *all* healthcare settings for *all* pregnant women and *all* adult and adolescent patients aged 13 to 64 years as part of their routine care. In addition, the new guidelines recommend repeat screening at least annually for persons at high risk for HIV infection, including injection drug users and their sex partners, persons who exchange sex for drugs or money, men who have sex with men, and sex partners of infected individuals.

Why did the CDC expand the target populations for screening? The answer lies in the epidemiological trends over the past decades. Although substantial decreases in HIV infection incidence and mortality have occurred since the 1990s, progress has been uneven, and diagnoses have increased in certain groups. For example, diagnoses have risen in Hispanic and Latino gay and bisexual men.[12] Cases in these minority groups are often identified late in the course of their infection, and therefore they may unknowingly transmit HIV to others and are less likely to benefit from treatment.[13] Thus, the new recommendations were designed "to foster earlier detection of HIV infection; identify and counsel persons with unrecognized HIV infection and link them to clinical and preventive services; and further reduce perinatal transmission of HIV in the United States."[11]

▶ Characteristics of a Screening Test

For screening to be successful, the screening test must be economical, convenient, relatively free of risk and discomfort, acceptable to a large number of individuals, and highly valid and reliable. Currently, screening tests that meet these criteria include serology tests for markers for

HIV, hepatitis B, and tuberculosis; mammograms for the detection of breast cancer; Pap smears for cervical cancer; blood pressure monitoring and cholesterol screening for heart disease; fecal occult blood tests for colorectal cancer; and vision tests for glaucoma. The following sections describe in more detail the characteristics of a suitable screening test.

Validity

The purpose of a screening test is to correctly identify individuals who do and do not have preclinical disease. Those who have preclinical disease should test positive, and those who do not have it should test negative. The ability of a screening test to successfully separate these two groups is a measure of its validity, which is expressed by its sensitivity and specificity. These two measures are described in more detail later in this chapter.

Reliability

The **reliability** of a test is its ability to give the same result on repeated testing. Reliability is influenced by the stability of the physiological state being measured (e.g., blood pressure varies by time of day and recent activities), the technical characteristics of the test method (such as the instrument being used), and interobserver and intraobserver agreement among the technicians conducting the test. Interobserver agreement refers to reliability between different technicians, and intraobserver agreement refers to reliability for the same technician over time. Although a valid test is always reliable, a reliable test is not always valid. A reliable test can incorrectly classify individuals as diseased or disease free with great consistency.

Source of Test Errors

All screening tests currently in use are affected by measurement errors. Mismeasurement may occur through sloppiness, such as mislabeling specimens, poor training of screening technicians, or poor equipment. Whatever the source, the outcome of mismeasurement is usually an incorrect test result. Although errors can often be corrected by performing a second test, a false-positive result and subsequent retesting can cause great distress for the patient. In addition, when a more invasive procedure is needed to follow-up a false-positive result, there may be morbidity from the procedure. For example, maternal serum alpha-fetoprotein is a prenatal blood test that is used to screen for birth defects known as neural tube defects (such as spina bifida). A positive result may be followed up with an amniocentesis that carries a small but real risk of miscarriage. In addition, false-negative results are harmful because the undetected disease continues to progress.

Criterion of Positivity

Even when test errors are minimized, the decision to term certain test results *positive* and others *negative* is somewhat arbitrary. The **criterion of positivity** is a point on a continuum that extends from clearly normal results (for healthy people) to clearly abnormal results (for people who have preclinical disease) (see **FIGURE 16-5**). Questionable results that may occur for some people with and without preclinical illness fall into a gray zone in the middle of the continuum. For example, the criterion of positivity may be the presence of dysplastic cells on a Pap smear test for cervical cancer, the presence of calcifications on a mammogram for breast cancer, or systolic and diastolic blood pressure readings greater than 130 and 80 mm Hg for hypertension. A particular criterion of positivity is selected to maximize the validity of the screening test. If the criterion is set high (point B in Figure 16-5), then only very abnormal results will be considered positive and slight abnormalities will be missed. Thus, there will be more false-negative results. If the criterion is set low (point A), then any slight abnormality will be considered positive and there will be more false-positive results.

FIGURE 16-6 illustrates the use of the criterion of positivity for the enzyme immunoassay (EIA)—the first screening test developed for detecting antibodies to HIV antigen—in a population with HIV infection and a population without HIV infection. The EIA is performed by incubating a person's serum with recombinant HIV antigens. If HIV antibodies are present in the serum, they will bind to the antigen-covered walls and turn yellow. The degree of the yellow color is measured by a laboratory instrument called a spectrophotometer. The amount of color in a sample is compared with the colors in the control samples.

Clearly negative   Gray zone   Clearly positive

– – – – – – – – – – – – – ??????????????????????????+++++++++++++++++++++

                  A   B

              LOW   HIGH

FIGURE 16-5 Criterion of positivity.

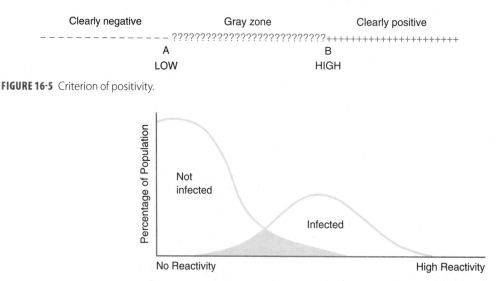

FIGURE 16-6 Schematic representation of HIV EIA result in two populations.

Note from Figure 16-6 that there is overlap between the two populations in the way they react to the EIA. Although most uninfected people have no reactivity, some uninfected individuals have a low degree of reactivity. Likewise, although most infected people have a high degree of reactivity, some infected individuals have a low degree of reactivity. (The area of overlap in Figure 16-6 is analogous to the gray zone in Figure 16-5.) The criterion of positivity for this screening test is generally set at a low level (see point A in Figure 16-5) because of the severe consequences of a false-negative result. The EIA was first used to screen donated blood. Any donated blood that tested positive was discarded, and the individual who donated this blood was retested with a second EIA and another test called a Western blot, which does a better job of weeding out false-positive results. The individual was notified only if both follow-up tests were also positive.

Sensitivity and Specificity

Sensitivity and **specificity** are measures of the validity of a screening test, that is, its ability to determine the "truth" about the presence or absence of preclinical disease. Sensitivity is the probability that a test correctly classifies positive individuals who have preclinical disease. Sensitivity is expressed as a percentage: the number of individuals with preclinical disease who test positive is in the numerator, and the total number of individuals with preclinical disease is in the denominator.

$$\frac{\text{Number of individuals with preclinical disease who test positive}}{\text{Number of individuals with preclinical disease}} \times 100$$

Specificity is the probability that a test correctly classifies individuals without preclinical disease as negative. Specificity is also expressed as a percentage: the number of individuals without preclinical disease who test negative is in the numerator, and the total number of individuals without preclinical disease is in the denominator.

$$\frac{\text{Number of individuals without preclinical disease who test negative}}{\text{Number of individuals without preclinical disease}} \times 100$$

TABLE 16-3 presents the results of a screening test in a population in the form of a two-by-two table. The sensitivity is equal to $a/(a + c)$, and the specificity is equal to $d/(b + d)$.

Denominator data for determining the sensitivity $(a + c)$ and specificity $(b + d)$ are usually determined in one of two ways. First, a gold-standard diagnostic procedure (i.e., a very accurate and commonly used procedure) can be used to make a definitive diagnosis and to determine the total number of individuals with and without the disease. Second, when the gold-standard procedure is too invasive or expensive, the population is followed for a period of time to determine who develops the disease.

TABLE 16-3 Calculating Sensitivity, Specificity, and Predictive Value Using a Two-by-Two Table

Screening test result	Disease present		
	Yes	No	Total
Positive	a	b	a + b
Negative	c	d	c + d
Total	a + c	b + d	a + b + c + d

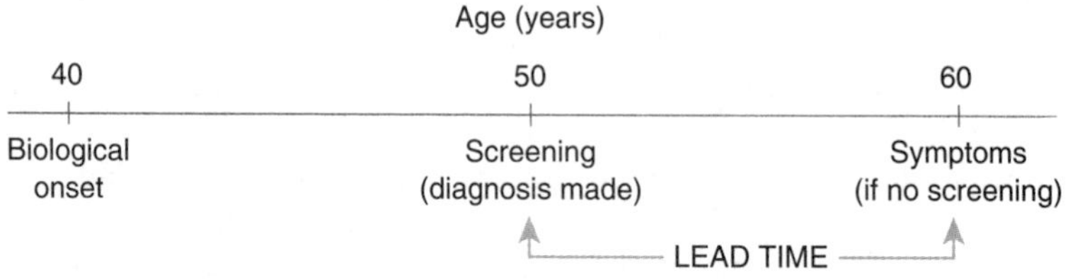

Age (years)

40   50   60

Biological onset   Screening (diagnosis made)   Symptoms (if no screening)

————— LEAD TIME —————

FIGURE 16-7 Lead time in a hypothetical individual.

For example, the sensitivity and specificity of physical examination and mammography for the detection of breast cancer were originally determined by following a group of study participants for about 10 years.[14(pp74-80)] Any woman who developed clinical symptoms of breast cancer within a year of a negative screening test was considered a false negative.

▶ Lead Time

Lead time is the amount of time that the disease diagnosis is advanced by screening. In other words, it is the length of time from disease detection by screening to the time that the diagnosis would have been made on the basis of symptoms.[15] For example, suppose that a person's disease is detected by screening at age 50 and that this person would have been diagnosed at age 60 when symptoms developed (see **FIGURE 16-7**). The lead time for this individual is 10 years. Note that lead time varies from one person to another, depending on the stage of preclinical disease at screening and the duration of preclinical disease in the individual.[14(pp11-12)] The lead time will be longer if detection by screening occurs in the early part of the preclinical phase and shorter if detection occurs close to the onset of symptoms.

Because we can never know when the disease would have been diagnosed as a result of symptoms, it is impossible to determine the actual lead time in a screened individual. However, it is possible to estimate the distribution of lead times in a screening program by comparing the rate of clinical disease over time in the screened group and comparable unscreened group.[14(p12)]

▶ Predictive Value: A Measure of Screening Program Feasibility

A screening program is defined as "a set of procedures for early detection and treatment of a disease that is available to a population."[14(p2)] It contains both diagnostic and therapeutic components and includes the screening test and the follow-up evaluations for people with positive test results.[14(pp5-6)] The therapeutic component consists of treatment of confirmed cases of disease. Thus, a screening program is much more than just a screening test. Furthermore, the feasibility and success of a screening program depend a great deal on the population in which it is applied.

The **predictive value** is the main way to measure a screening program's feasibility. Predictive value has two components: predictive value positive (PVP) and predictive value negative (PVN). The PVP is the proportion of individuals with a positive test who have preclinical disease. It is calculated as a percentage: the number of individuals with preclinical disease who test positive is in the numerator, and the total number of individuals who test positive is in the denominator.

$$\frac{\text{Number of individuals who test positive and have preclinical disease}}{\text{Number of individuals who test positive}} \times 100$$

The PVN is defined as the proportion of individuals without preclinical disease who test negative. It is calculated as a percentage: the number of individuals without the disease who test negative is in the numerator, and the total number of individuals who test negative is in the denominator.

$$\frac{\text{Number of individuals who test negative and do not have preclinical disease}}{\text{Number of individuals who test negative}} \times 100$$

Note from the two-by-two table presented in Table 16-3 that the PVP equals $a/(a+b)$ and the PVN equals $d/(c+d)$. The key components of PVP are the number of true positive cases detected (a) and the number of false positives (b), and the key components of PVN are the number of true negatives (d) and the number of false negatives (c).

A high PVP is essential for a successful screening program. It implies that the screening program is effective because the program detects a large proportion of actual cases among individuals with positive results.

A low PVP implies that resources are being wasted on diagnostic follow-ups of false-positive results. A low PVP can have additional consequences if a positive screening test is followed by a potentially harmful diagnostic evaluation, as was described earlier for the maternal serum alpha-fetoprotein test.

PVP is influenced by the sensitivity and specificity of the screening test and by the prevalence of the DPCP in the screened population. PVP is influenced more by specificity than sensitivity because the specificity determines the number of false-positive results.

The following paragraphs describe two hypothetical breast cancer screening programs to illustrate the validity and feasibility measures described. Suppose that a newly developed blood test to detect breast cancer is being evaluated by a private company that hopes to market the test for use in the population. The company tries out the test on 1,000 women with known breast cancer. Of these, 950 have a positive finding, establishing the sensitivity at 95% $[a/(a + c) = 950/1,000]$. The company uses the same blood test to test 1,000 women who are considered free of breast cancer on the basis of a mammogram and physical examination. Of these women, 980 are negative and 20 are positive. Thus, the specificity of the test is established at 98% $[d/(b + d) = 980/1,000]$. The new blood test is licensed for commercial and research use on the basis of this information.

Two Massachusetts public health officials decide to institute a breast cancer screening program using the blood test just described, with the intention of identifying breast cancer very early in the DPCP. They plan to follow up all positive blood tests with a biopsy, which will separate truly positive screening test results from false-positive ones. One public health official decides to screen a low-risk population, and the other decides to screen a high-risk population. They both decide to use the same laboratory to conduct the new blood test so that the results of the two programs can be compared.

The public health official interested in screening a low-risk population sets up a program among women from the general population who are older than 50 years of age, where the estimated prevalence of preclinical breast cancer is 5 per 1,000, or 0.5%. He screens 40,000 randomly selected Massachusetts women in this age group. The results of his efforts are described in **TABLE 16-4**.

Among the 200 individuals in the DPCP (200/40,000 = 0.5% prevalence), 190 are identified as positive and 10 are missed. This result reflects that the sensitivity of the blood test is 95% (190/200 = 95%). The 10 who are missed show evidence of breast cancer on a traditional mammogram within a year after testing and are therefore considered false negatives. Among the 39,800 disease-free individuals, 39,004 test negative and 796 test positive. This result reflects that the specificity of the blood test is 98% (39,004/39,800 = 98%). Of the 39,014 individuals who test negative, 39,004 truly do not have breast cancer, and therefore the PVN is nearly 100% (39,004/39,014 = 99.97%). Of the 986

TABLE 16-4 Results of a Hypothetical Breast Cancer Screening Program in a Low-Prevalence Population

	Breast cancer		
Blood test	**Yes**	**No**	**Total**
Positive	190	796	986
Negative	10	39,004	39,014
Total	200	39,800	40,000

TABLE 16-5 Results of a Hypothetical Breast Cancer Screening Program in a High-Prevalence Population

	Breast cancer		
Blood test	**Yes**	**No**	**Total**
Positive	380	792	1,172
Negative	20	38,808	38,828
Total	400	39,600	40,000

individuals who test positive, 190 have breast cancer as confirmed by a biopsy, and therefore the PVP is 19.3% (190/986 = 19.3%). Thus, the net result of screening this low-risk population is that 190 women with breast cancer in the DPCP are identified. On the other hand, 796 women have a false-positive result upon follow-up with a biopsy.

The second public health official is concerned about the low PVP associated with screening a low-risk population, and therefore she sets up her screening program among Massachusetts women at high risk for developing breast cancer. High-risk women are identified from an outreach program for women older than 50 years of age with a family history of breast cancer. The estimated prevalence of breast cancer in this high-risk population is 10 per 1,000, or 1.0%. She proceeds to screen 40,000 randomly selected high-risk individuals using the new screening blood test. The results of her efforts are described in **TABLE 16-5**.

Among the 400 women in DPCP (400/40,000 = 1.0% prevalence), 380 are identified as positive and 20 are missed given that the sensitivity of the test is 95% (380/400 = 95%). The 20 who are missed show evidence of breast cancer within a year after testing and so are considered false negatives. Among the 39,600 disease-free individuals, 38,808 test negative and 792 test positive given that the specificity of the test is 98% (38,808/39,600 = 98%). Of the 38,828 individuals who test negative, 38,808 truly do not have breast cancer, and therefore the PVN is again nearly 100% (38,808/38,828) = (99.95%). Of the 1,172 individuals who test positive, 380 have breast cancer, and therefore the PVP is 32.4% (380/1,172 = 32.4%). Thus, the net result of screening this high-risk population is that 380 women with breast cancer in the DPCP are identified. Note that there is a much higher yield from screening the high-risk population, even with identical tests. This is because a high-risk woman with a positive test result is much more likely to have breast cancer than a low-risk woman with a positive test result.

▶ Evaluating a Screening Program

Formal evaluation of a screening program may be unnecessary in certain circumstances, such as when the intervention is simple and highly effective.[14(pp12-13)] For example, it is not necessary to evaluate screening for vision and hearing problems among children, but failure to screen would be considered unethical.

Formal evaluations are not conducted when policymakers believe, often without objective evidence, that early detection and treatment are beneficial and prematurely institute mandatory screening programs. For example, compulsory HIV screening was instituted among blood donors, immigrants, and premarital couples before effective treatments were available and evaluation programs were in place.[2] These programs quickly became the standard of care, and formal evaluations were never conducted.

When public health officials conduct a formal evaluation of screening programs, they look at several features of the program, including the potential for bias and outcome measures.

▶ Bias

Lead-Time Bias

The customary way to evaluate the success of a screening program is to compare the survival experience of a screened population with that of a similar unscreened population. Survival is assessed either as the percentage of patients alive as of a certain time after diagnosis (e.g., the percentage surviving 5 years after diagnosis) or by the average number of years that a patient lives after diagnosis. Note that survival is measured from the time of diagnosis to the time of death and that the diagnosis time is, by definition, different for screened individuals (shortly after screening) and unscreened individuals (at the onset of symptoms) (see Figure 16-7). Thus, survival may appear longer among screened individuals simply because their diagnoses were made earlier, not because they actually lived longer. This phenomenon, which is known as **lead-time bias**, overestimates the benefit of screening and needs to be taken into account when evaluating a screening program.

FIGURE 16-8 illustrates lead-time bias using three hypothetical men with prostate cancer. The first man was an unscreened case of prostate cancer. Biological onset of disease began at age 40 years (A), but the man underwent no screening during the detectable preclinical phase (B to C). He was diagnosed with cancer only when symptoms occurred at age 65 (C), and although he was treated, he died from prostate cancer at age 80 (D). There was no lead time in his case because there was no screening. This man's survival time was 15 years, from diagnosis at age 65 to death at age 80.

The second man was a screen-detected case who was diagnosed at age 50 years (B). He would have been diagnosed at age 65 (C) if he had waited for symptoms to occur, and therefore his lead time was 15 years (B to C). He died at age 80 (D), and therefore his survival time was 30 years (B to D). Screening appears to be effective because survival was longer for case 2 than case 1 (30 vs. 15 years). However, early treatment was not effective in postponing his mortality. Both case 1 and 2 died at exactly the same age. The apparent survival benefit for case 2 results from lead-time bias.

Case 1

Age (years)

40	50	65	80
A	B	C	D
Biological onset	Becomes detectable (but not screened)	Symptoms (diagnosis made)	Death

Case 2

Age (years)

40	50	65	80
A	B	C	D
Biological onset	Becomes detectable (found at screen)	Symptoms (if not screened)	Death

Case 3

Age (years)

40	50		78	83
A	B		C	D
Biological onset	Becomes detectable (found at screen)		Symptoms	Death

FIGURE 16-8 The natural history of three men with prostate cancer: an illustration of lead-time bias.

The third man was also a screen-detected case. He was diagnosed by screening at age 50 years (B), and early treatment was somewhat effective. Therefore, it delayed the onset of symptoms to age 78 (C) and death to age 83 (D). His survival time is 33 years from age 50 to age 83. Case 3 lived 3 years longer than the first two men, and therefore he illustrates the benefit of screening—the postponement of morbidity and mortality.

Length-Bias Sampling

Length-bias sampling is another bias that should be considered when evaluating a screening program. This bias occurs because screening tends to identify cases with less aggressive forms of the disease.[15(p14)] Screening tends to detect cases with a long preclinical course, which in turn should have a long clinical course and better survival.

FIGURE 16-9 illustrates length-bias sampling using two hypothetical men with prostate cancer. The first man experiences biological onset of disease at age 40 years. He is identified by screening at age 50 years when his DPCP begins. He undergoes treatment, but symptoms develop at age 60. Death from prostate cancer occurs at age 70 because the treatment is ineffective. Thus, his DPCP is 10 years and his survival time is 20 years. This man is considered a slow progressor because his entire disease course lasts 30 years (A to D) and his DPCP (B to C) and clinical phase (C to D) last 10 years each.

Case 2 has a very different natural history because his disease course is quite rapid. Like case 1, his biological onset is at age 40 years. However, his DPCP starts at age 45, his symptoms appear and he is diagnosed at age 50 (C), and death occurs at age 55 (D). The entire disease course lasts 15 years—half of that of case 1.

Case 1

Age (years)

40	50	60	70
A	B	C	D
Biological onset	Becomes detectable, diagnosed by screening	Symptoms	Death

Case 2

Age (years)

40	45	50	55
A	B	C	D
Biological onset	Becomes detectable, but not screened	Symptoms (diagnosed)	Death

FIGURE 16-9 The natural history of two men with prostate cancer: an illustration of length-bias sampling.

Which type of case is a typical screening program more likely to identify? The answer is case 1 simply because his DPCP is twice as long as that of case 2. Thus, length-bias sampling makes a screening program appear to have a beneficial effect on survival because people who are destined to have a favorable course are selectively identified.

Volunteer Bias

The third type of bias to consider when evaluating a screening program is called **volunteer bias**. This type of bias occurs in only observational studies of screening efficacy. It means that the decision to be screened is influenced by a person's health awareness, which in turn may be related to his or her subsequent morbidity and mortality.[14(p17)] One could argue that either healthy people are more likely to volunteer for screening than sick people or sick people are more likely to be screened than healthy people. The former would overestimate the benefit of the screening program, and the latter would underestimate it. In either case, the results are confounded by patient characteristics that are difficult to assess and control.

▶ Selecting an Outcome

Epidemiologists use several outcome measures to evaluate the success of a screening program, including (1) process measures, (2) survival, (3) shift in stage distribution, (4) overall mortality, and (5) cause-specific mortality. Process measures include the number of people who have been screened and the number of cases of disease that have been detected by screening. These measures are simple to obtain, but they do not gauge screening effectiveness; that is, they do not indicate whether the screening program has decreased the adverse effects of disease and improved survival.

A more direct way of assessing screening effectiveness is to compare the survival of screen-detected cases with that of unscreened cases. Survival is commonly assessed in terms of the percentage of individuals alive as of a certain time after diagnosis. Screen-detected cases may appear to survive longer than unscreened cases as a result of lead-time bias, length-bias sampling, or volunteer bias. Thus, using survival as an outcome measure may give a false impression of the benefit of screening.

An alternative assessment measure is the comparison of disease-stage distribution among individuals identified by screening versus those identified by other methods. If screening is effective, the stage distribution should shift toward earlier cases of disease. For example, following the introduction of prostate cancer screening in Norway, there was a 64% increase in the incidence of localized disease and a 36% decrease in the incidence of distant disease among men aged 66 to 74 years.[16] Nevertheless, it is difficult to determine whether such shifts result from a real screening benefit or from confounding caused by volunteer bias or length-bias sampling.

Another way to assess the effectiveness of screening is to compare the overall mortality rate among screened and unscreened populations. If the overall mortality rate is lower in the screened population, then one may conclude that the combination of screening and early treatment has been effective in postponing death. Although the total mortality rate is not influenced by lead-time bias or length-bias sampling, it may be an insensitive endpoint if the disease of interest accounts for only a small proportion of deaths. For example, even though prostate cancer is the most common cancer among U.S. men, it accounts for only about 8% of cancer deaths among males.[17] Thus, disease-specific mortality rate is considered the best outcome measure for evaluating a screening program. However, even disease-specific mortality is not appropriate for outcomes that do not lead to death. For example, the occurrence of blindness is the best outcome for assessing the effectiveness of glaucoma screening. It does not make sense to use glaucoma mortality to measure the effectiveness of screening because blindness does not usually cause death.

▶ Study Designs to Evaluate Screening Programs

The effectiveness of a screening program can be evaluated using a variety of study designs. These designs are briefly covered here in the context of screening. The designs fall into two major categories: experimental and observational. The experimental approach for evaluating screening programs consists mainly of randomized, controlled clinical trials. Observational studies include cohort, case–control, and ecological studies.

Experimental Studies

In an experimental study, the investigator randomly assigns individuals to be screened or not screened and then follows the two groups for the outcomes of interest (such as mortality, survival, and morbidity). Experimental studies can be performed only when there is a state of **equipoise** regarding screening effectiveness within the medical community. There must be genuine confidence that screening is worthwhile to administer it to some individuals and genuine reservations to withhold it from others.

The main advantage of experimental studies is that if the study size is sufficiently large, both known and unknown confounders will be balanced between compared groups. A second advantage is the elimination of confounding from volunteer bias. Thus, an experimental evaluation will provide the most rigorous data on the effectiveness of screening. In addition, it can give estimates of lead time and evaluate the effect of length-bias sampling.

Although experimental designs have strong methodological appeal, they also have some important drawbacks. First, several thousand participants are typically needed to demonstrate a relatively modest level of efficacy. Second, follow-up may take many years, and much time and effort must be expended to keep losses to a minimum. These issues make experimental evaluations of screening programs very expensive and reduce their feasibility and relevance, particularly when advances in screening technology and treatment are occurring rapidly. Swift advances in medical knowledge also reduce the acceptability of participating in long-term, randomized trials among physicians and patients and may raise ethical concerns for the unscreened patients. Consequentially, epidemiologists usually employ observational designs to evaluate screening programs.

Cohort Studies

In cohort studies, participants decide themselves whether to be screened. Participants are followed to ascertain the outcomes of interest. Thus, they are more susceptible to confounding than experimental studies. If the confounder is known, the investigator can measure and adjust for its effect in the design or analysis, but if the confounder is unknown, adjustment is not possible. Cohort studies also suffer from one of the same problems as experimental studies; namely, a large number of subjects must be followed for a long period of time.

On the other hand, because participants choose to be screened, the ethical dilemmas present in experimental studies are avoided. Also, although experimental studies must always be prospective, cohort studies can be either prospective or retrospective. Retrospective cohort studies of screening efficacy, which are more efficient than prospective ones, are quite feasible if detailed data on screening and confounding characteristics are documented in existing data sources, such as medical records.

Case–Control Studies

In a case–control study, the investigator selects cases who are individuals either with a recent diagnosis or who have died from the disease targeted by screening. Controls are selected from the population that gave rise to the cases. For example, if cases include newly diagnosed patients, controls are selected from the same geographic area or hospital from which the cases were identified. The investigator obtains information on screening status (e.g., if participants were ever screened or date of last screening) and potential confounders either by interview or medical record review. The usual challenges associated with obtaining accurate exposure information and controlling for confounding apply. The main advantage of the case–control approach is efficiency; nevertheless, the study must be carefully designed to minimize information and selection bias.

Ecological Studies

An ecological, or correlational, study can be used to evaluate the effect of a screening program. This type of study describes the relationship between screening frequency and an outcome measure among many populations at the same time or the same population at different times. Ecological studies are efficient because they are based solely on easy-to-obtain group-level data about the screening program (such as the proportion of the population screened) and group-level outcome data (such as disease-specific mortality rates in screened and unscreened areas).

The limitations of ecological studies include the lack of individual-level data and the resulting difficulty with making inferences from the group to the individual. In addition, data on confounding variables are usually missing. Ecological studies are most informative when a new screening program is introduced into an isolated, well-defined population.[14(pp97-100)] For example, in 1964, a cervical cancer screening program targeting women aged 25 to 59 years was initiated in Iceland.[18,19] By 1977, more than 85% of the population had been screened. The cervical cancer mortality rate among women in the targeted age group rose until 1970 but then dropped by 60%. No change in cervical cancer mortality rate was observed in older women who were not specifically targeted for screening. These data strongly suggest that the introduction of the screening program in Iceland had a beneficial effect on cervical cancer mortality rates.

▶ Examples of the Effect of Screening on Public Health

The Effect of Screening on Disease Incidence: The Case of Prostate Cancer

Prostate cancer is the most common cancer among men, accounting for about 19% of newly diagnosed cancers in 2017.[17] This form of cancer has received a great deal of attention because many famous men have publicly acknowledged that they have been affected.[20] Currently known risk factors include African American race, increased age, and family history of prostate cancer.[21] Most prostate cancer cases appear to progress slowly; that is, they have long preclinical and clinical phases. In fact, prostate cancer is usually not life threatening and is most commonly diagnosed at autopsy among elderly men who never had any symptoms and died of other causes.[22]

Currently available screening methods include the prostate-specific antigen (PSA) blood test and digital rectal examination. Although the decrease in prostate cancer mortality over time suggests that prostate cancer screening is beneficial, the U.S. Preventive Services Task Force recently recommended against using PSA-based screening for prostate cancer because the reduction in mortality following screening is very small compared to the harms of treating this typically benign disease.[23]

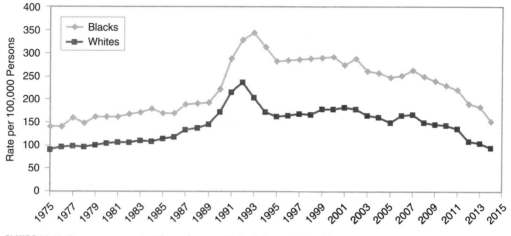

FIGURE 16-10 Prostate cancer incidence by race, United States, 1975–2014.

Data from Howlader N, Noone AM, Krapcho M, Miller D, Bishop K, Kosary CL, et al. (eds). *SEER Cancer Statistics Review, 1975–2014*. cancer.gov. https://seer.cancer.gov/csr/1975_2014/.
Published April 2017. Accessed April 2017.

In fact, significant harms, such as erectile dysfunction and urinary incontinence, can result from surgical treatment.

Prostate cancer trends in the United States provide a real-life example of changes in incidence that occur following the widespread use of a screening program. Note from **FIGURE 16-10** that prostate cancer incidence increased slowly until the late 1980s, when incidence rose sharply.[7] An abrupt decline in incidence began in 1992 for Whites and in 1993 for Blacks. These changes are likely attributable in part to the effects of screening. When a screening test becomes widely used in a population, the incidence rate of the target disease increases at first and then declines as a result of the earlier diagnosis of cases. Further evidence of the effect of prostate cancer screening on disease incidence is that by the late 1980s, a higher proportion of those diagnosed were at early stages.[7] Randomized trials have been conducted in the United States and Europe to determine whether this trend translated into lower mortality rates.[24,25] Results from the Prostate, Lung, Colorectal, and Ovarian Cancer Screening Trial, a large randomized study, showed that there was no evidence of a mortality benefit for annual screening after 15 years of follow-up.[24]

The Effect of Screening on Mortality: The Case of Breast Cancer

Since the 1960s, investigators have conducted numerous randomized, controlled clinical trials of the effectiveness of breast cancer screening, including mammography and breast self-examination.[26] These studies have been conducted in Europe, Canada, and the United States and have collectively enrolled and followed nearly 500,000 women for up to 18 years. In these trials, a group of women offered screening was compared with a group of women not offered screening. (The latter group received "usual care.") Women were assigned to each group using a variety of randomization methods. In some studies, population-based lists of women were compiled, and individual women were randomly assigned to the study and control groups. In other studies, clusters of women (e.g., all women registered in a certain medical practice) were randomly assigned to the groups.

Through the 1990s, the studies indicated that the use of screening mammography (either alone or in combination with a clinical examination) reduced the risk of dying by about 30% among women 50 to 69 years of age after 10 to 12 years of follow-up.[27] Even though the risk of a false-positive result in this age group was 47.3% after 10 years of mammograms, there was a widespread consensus that all women in this age group should be screened.[27] During this period, the balance of risks and benefits appeared to be less clear for women aged 40 to 49 years. In randomized trials of mammographic screening, there was no meaningful decrease in mortality after 5 to 7 years of follow-up and only a marginal benefit after 12 to 14 years of follow-up.[27] Furthermore, the risk of a false-positive result in this age group was 56.2% after 10 years of screening.[28] False-positive mammography results are not trivial because they lead to more outpatient appointments, mammograms, biopsies, and great emotional stress. As a result, the 1997 National Institutes of Health Consensus Development Conference concluded that a universal recommendation for mammography for all women in their 40s was not warranted.[29]

In 2009 and again in 2016, the U.S. Preventive Services Task Force assessed the available evidence related to screening practice recommendations issued in agreement with the Consensus Development Conference.[30,31] In particular, the 2016 recommendations for mammography screening among asymptomatic women who are not high risks for breast cancer stated that "the decision to start screening should be an individual one" for women aged 40 to 49 years and that screening should be conducted every 2 years for women aged 50 to 75 years. They also stated that there is insufficient evidence regarding benefits of screening mammography for women aged 75 years and older.[31] These recommendations are supported by numerous analyses that show this screening strategy achieves the most benefit in terms of mortality reduction with the least amount of harm from false-positive results, unnecessary biopsies, and overdiagnosis (e.g., the diagnosis of small tumors that never would have become large).[32]

Summary

Screening is defined as "the presumptive identification of unrecognized disease or defect by the application of tests, examinations or other procedures which can be rapidly applied."[1(p165)] It is used mainly to identify asymptomatic individuals at an earlier stage than if they waited for symptoms to develop, under the assumption that earlier diagnosis will lead to more effective treatment and improve the consequences of disease. Lead time is defined as the amount of time that the disease is advanced by screening. It spans the length of time from disease detection by screening to the time that the diagnosis would have been made on the basis of symptoms. The actual lead time in a screened individual cannot be determined because we can never know when the disease would have been diagnosed as a result of symptoms. However, lead-time distributions can be estimated in certain settings. Screening is part of prevention activities that may deter the initial occurrence of disease (primary prevention), delay the onset and duration of clinical disease (secondary prevention), slow disease progression, and reduce disease sequelae (tertiary prevention).

To be suitable for screening, a disease must be serious with important consequences and must be progressive with an effective early stage treatment. In addition, suitable diseases must have a detectable preclinical stage that is fairly long and prevalent in the targeted population. Examples of appropriate diseases include breast and prostate cancer, HIV infection, hypertension, and glaucoma.

The characteristics of a successful screening test, examination, or procedure include low cost, minimal risk, convenience, acceptability, and reliability. The test must also have a high degree of validity, as measured by sensitivity and specificity. Sensitivity is the probability that a test correctly classifies individuals with preclinical disease as positive; specificity is the probability that a test correctly classifies individuals without preclinical disease as negative. These two measures are influenced in part by the criterion of positivity—the point at which a test result is deemed positive.

A screening program is defined as "a set of procedures for early detection and treatment of a disease that is available to a population" and includes both diagnostic and therapeutic components.[14(pp5-6)] The predictive value is the principal way to assess a screening program's feasibility. Predictive value positive is the proportion of individuals with a positive test who have preclinical disease; predictive value negative is the proportion of individuals with a negative test who do not have preclinical disease. A high predictive value positive, which is crucial to the success of a screening program, is attained by increasing the sensitivity and specificity of the screening test and by targeting a population whose detectable preclinical phase is fairly prevalent.

Outcome measures that can be used to evaluate the success of a screening program include process measures such as the number of people screened, the stage distribution of screened versus unscreened cases, and overall mortality and cause-specific mortality among screened and unscreened cases. Cause-specific mortality is the best outcome measure for diseases that are generally fatal. Study designs that are used to evaluate the effectiveness of screening programs include experimental, case–control, cohort, and ecological studies.

When evaluating a screening program, one must consider three sources of bias: lead-time bias, length-bias sampling, and volunteer bias. Lead-time bias can overestimate the benefit of screening when survival is used to evaluate a screening program. It occurs because survival is measured from the time of diagnosis until death and diagnoses occur earlier with screening even when death is not delayed. Length-bias sampling can exaggerate the benefit of a screening program because screening tends to detect less aggressive forms of disease that have a long preclinical phase. Volunteer bias occurs when observational studies are used to evaluate a screening program and stems from confounding between screened and unscreened populations.

References

1. Porta M. *A Dictionary of Epidemiology*. 6th ed. New York, NY: Oxford University Press; 2014.
2. Cleary PD, Barry MJ, Mayer KH, Brandt AM, Gostin L, Fineberg HV, et al. Compulsory premarital screening for the human immunodeficiency virus. *JAMA*. 1987;258:1757-1761.
3. Cuzick J, Sestak I, Bonanni B., Costantino JP, Cummings S, DeCensi A, et al. Selective oestrogen receptor modulators in prevention of breast cancer: an updated meta-analysis of individual participant data. *Lancet*. 2013;381:1827-1834.
4. Bertrand K, Roy E, Vaillancourt E, Vandermeerschen J, Berbiche D, Boivin J-F. Randomized controlled trial of motivational interviewing for reducing injection risk behaviors among people who inject drugs. *Addiction*. 2015;110:832-841.
5. Hidalgo MA, Kuhns LM, Hotton AL, Johnson AK, Mustanski B, Garofalo R. The MyPEEPS randomized controlled trial: a pilot of preliminary efficacy, feasibility, and acceptability of a group-level, HIV risk reduction intervention for young men who have sex with men. *Arch Sex Behav*. 2015;44:475-485.
6. Gunthard HF, Saag MS, Benson CA, del Rio C, Eron JJ, Gallant JE, et al. Antiretroviral drugs for treatment and prevention of HIV infection in adults: 2016 recommendations of the International Antiviral Society-USA Panel. *JAMA*. 2016;316:191-210.
7. Howlader N, Noone AM, Krapcho M, Miller D, Bishop K, Kosary CL, et al. (eds.). *SEER Cancer Statistics Review, 1975-2014*. cancer.gov. https://seer.cancer.gov/csr/1975_2014/. Published April 2017. Accessed April 2017.
8. *HIV Surveillance Report: Diagnoses of HIV Infection in the United States and Dependent Areas, 2016*. cdc.gov. https://www.cdc.gov/hiv/pdf/library/reports/surveillance/cdc-hiv-surveillance-report-2016-vol-28.pdf. Published November 2017. Accessed December 2017.
9. Lieb S, Prejean J, Thompson DR, et al. HIV prevalence rates among men who have sex with men in the southern United States: population-based estimates by race/ethnicity. *AIDS Behav*. 2011;15:596-606.
10. Horsburgh CR, Jason J, Longini IM Jr, Mayer KH, Schochetman G, Rutherford GW, et al. Duration of human immunodeficiency virus infection before detection of antibody. *Lancet*. 1989;334:637-640.
11. Branson BM, Handsfield HH, Lampe MA, Janssen RS, Taylor AW, Lyss, SB, et al. Revised recommendations for HIV testing of adults, adolescents, and pregnant women in health-care settings. *MMWR*. 2006;55(RR-14):1-17. https://www.cdc.gov/mmwr/preview/mmwrhtml/rr5514a1.htm. Accessed June 2017.
12. HIV in the United States: at a glance. cdc.gov. https://www.cdc.gov/hiv/statistics/overview/ataglance.html. Accessed June 2017.
13. Centers for Disease Control and Prevention. Late HIV testing—34 States, 1996-2005. *MMWR*. 2009; 58(24):661-665. https://www.cdc.gov/mmwr/preview/mmwrhtml/mm5824a2.htm. Accessed June 2017.
14. Morrison AS. *Screening in Chronic Disease*. 2nd ed. New York, NY: Oxford University Press; 1992.
15. Hutchison GB, Shapiro S. Lead time gained by diagnostic screening for breast cancer. *J Natl Cancer Inst*. 1968;41:665-681.
16. Møller MH, Kristiansen IS, Beisland C, Rørvik J, Støvring H. Trends in stage-specific incidence of prostate cancer in Norway, 1980-2010: a population-based study. *BJU Int*. 2016;118:547-555.
17. *Cancer Facts & Figures 2017*. Figure 3, page 10. cancer.org. https://www.cancer.org/content/dam/cancer-org/research/cancer-facts-and-statistics/annual-cancer-facts-and-figures/2017/cancer-facts-and-figures-2017.pdf. Accessed June 2017.
18. Johannesson G, Geirsson G, Day N. The effect of mass screening in Iceland, 1965-74, on the incidence

and mortality of cervical cancer. *Int J Cancer.* 1978;21:418-425.

19. Johannesson G, Geirsson G, Day N, Tulinius H. Screening for cancer of the uterine cervix in Iceland 1965-1978. *Acta Obstet Gynecol Scand.* 1982;61:199-203.

20. Takeda A. 16 famous men who have had prostate cancer. everydayhealth.com. http://www.everyday health.com/prostate-cancer-pictures/famous-men -who-battled-prostate-cancer.aspx. Accessed June 2017.

21. Prostate Cancer Risk Factors. cancer.org. https:// www.cancer.org/cancer/prostate-cancer/causes -risks-prevention/risk-factors.html. Accessed June 2017.

22. Gittes RF. Carcinoma of the prostate. *New Engl J Med.* 1991;324:236-245.

23. Moyer VA, LeFevre ML, Siu AL, Baumann LC, Bibbins-Domingo K, Curry SJ, et al., on behalf of the U.S. Preventive Services Task Force. Screening for prostate cancer: U.S. Preventive Services Task Force recommendation statement. *Annals Int Med.* 2102;157:120-134.

24. Pinsky PF, Prorok PC, Yu K, Kramer BS, Black A, Gohagan JK, et al. Extended mortality results for prostate cancer screening in the PLCO trial with median follow-up of 15 years. *Cancer.* 2017;123:592-599.

25. Schroder FH, Hugosson J, Roobol MJ, Tammela TLJ, Zappa M, Nelen V, et al. Screening and prostate cancer mortality: results of the European Randomised Study of Screening for Prostate Cancer (ERSPC) at 13 years of follow-up. *Lancet.* 2014;384:2027-2035.

26. Nelson HD, Tyne K, Naik A, Bougatsos C, Chan BK, Humphrey LL. Screening for breast cancer: an update for the U.S. Preventive Services Task Force. *Ann Intern Med.* 2009;151:727-737.

27. Fletcher SW, Black W, Harris R, Rimer BK, Shapiro S. Report of the International Workshop on Screening for Breast Cancer. *J Natl Cancer Inst.* 1993;85:1644-1656.

28. Elmore JG, Barton MB, Moceri VM, Polk S, Arena PJ, Fletcher SW. Ten-year risk of false positive screening mammograms and clinical breast examinations. *New Engl J Med.* 1998;338:1089-1096.

29. National Institutes of Health Consensus Development Panel. National Institutes of Health Consensus Development Conference Statement: breast cancer screening for women ages 40-49, January 21-23, 1997. *J Natl Cancer Inst.* 1997;89:1015-1020.

30. DeAngelis CD, Fontanarosa PB. U.S. Preventive Services Task Force and breast cancer screening. *JAMA.* 2010;303(2):172-173.

31. Siu AL on behalf of the U.S. Preventive Services Task Force. Screening for Breast Cancer: U.S. Preventive Services Task Force Recommendation Statement. *Ann Int Med.* 2016;164:279-297.

32. Mandelblatt JS, Cronin KA, Bailey S, et al. Effects of mammography screening under different screening schedules: model estimates of potential benefits and harms. *Ann Int Med.* 2009;151:738-747.

Chapter Questions

1. Define each of the following terms:
   a. Natural history of a disease
   b. Detectable preclinical phase
   c. Criterion of positivity
   d. Sensitivity
   e. Specificity
   f. Predictive value of a positive test
   g. Lead time

2. State the main differences between primary, secondary, and tertiary prevention.

3. What types of diseases are appropriate for screening?

4. Suppose that 100,000 men were screened for prostate cancer for the first time. Of these, 4,000 men had a positive result on the screening blood test; of those who tested positive, 800 had a biopsy indicating a diagnosis of prostate cancer. Among the remaining 96,000 men who screened negative, 100 developed prostate cancer within the following year and were assumed to be false negatives to the screen.
   a. Set up the two-by-two table for these data.
   b. What is the prevalence of prostate cancer in this population?

    c.   Calculate and interpret the sensitivity of this screening test.

    d.   Calculate and interpret the specificity of this screening test.

    e.   Calculate and interpret the predictive value positive of this screening test.

    f.   There is a widespread assumption that screening a population to detect the early stages of disease is always beneficial. However, there are risks and costs that must be weighed against the benefits of screening. Briefly describe two hidden costs of screening for prostate cancer in this example.

5.   Consider the following events in one woman's life. Note that some events are hypothetical and some are real.

Event	Age (years)
Birth	0
Cervical cancer begins	30
Cervical cancer is detectable by screening	40
Woman is screened, cancer is detected, treatment begins	45
If no screening, symptoms would have developed and cancer would have been detected	60
If no screening, death would have occurred	70
Death occurs	80

    a.   Compute the total preclinical phase of this woman's cervical cancer. Assume that she did not get screened.

    b.   Compute the detectable preclinical phase of this woman's cervical cancer. Assume that she did not get screened.

    c.   Compute the lead time for this patient.

    d.   Did screening increase the life span of this patient? Justify your answer.

6.   Describe the three types of bias that must be considered when evaluating the results of a screening program.

7.   Indicate whether the following statements are true or false:

    a.   The purpose of screening is to identify symptomatic cases of disease.

    b.   Screening is conducted to reduce morbidity and improve survival.

    c.   The predictive value positive is more influenced by the specificity than the sensitivity of the screening test.

    d.   The specificity of a screening test determines the number of false-positive results.

e. The incidence of the target disease will likely increase when a new screening test becomes widely used.

f. Unlike cohort studies, experimental studies of screening effectiveness avoid volunteer bias.

8. Some years ago, the International Olympic Committee wanted a screening test that would correctly identify a high proportion of athletes who used illegal performance-enhancing drugs. On the other hand, the athletes were concerned about a screening test that would incorrectly identify persons as using illegal performance-enhancing drugs when in fact they were not using them. Which of the following screening test characteristics were important to each group?

a. High sensitivity for Olympic officials and high specificity for athletes

b. High specificity for Olympic officials and high sensitivity for athletes

c. High positive predictive value for Olympic officials and high sensitivity for athletes

d. High specificity for Olympic officials and high predictive value negative for athletes

CHAPTER 17

Ethics in Research Involving Human Participants

Contributed by Molly Pretorius Holme

LEARNING OBJECTIVES

By the end of this chapter the reader will be able to:
- Describe historical events that have shaped current guidelines and regulations for the ethical conduct of epidemiological research with human subjects.
- Recognize ethical conflicts in historical and contemporary case examples.
- Identify key principles, guidelines, and regulations governing research with human subjects.
- Discuss the required elements of informed consent.
- Evaluate informed consent processes.

▶ Introduction

A number of guidelines have been developed to help researchers and reviewers of research ensure the ethical conduct of studies involving human subjects. This chapter describes the development of these guidelines and the application of the principles they promote: respect for individual autonomy, beneficence, nonmaleficence, and justice.

Many of the ethical guidelines, principles, and regulations that are currently applied to research involving human subjects were formalized in response to specific events that highlighted serious ethical offenses and breaches of public trust. Some of these events were deliberate, atrocious acts committed under the guise of research; others were a result of very unfortunate mistakes, ignorance, or carelessness. Many studies that are deemed unethical today were viewed at the time as acceptable. Understanding the history of these events and the legacy of those who were harmed helps us understand the context and importance of the rules and regulations with which we must comply today. This chapter provides historical and contemporary examples of ethical conflicts in research involving human subjects and the response of the public, the scientific community, and governments.

An institutional review board (IRB) should review research involving human subjects before research activities are initiated. This process, the role of the IRB, and investigators' responsibilities are also discussed.

Informed consent is a key component of the ethical conduct of research with human volunteers. This chapter concludes with an overview of the informed consent process and the essential elements to include in an informed consent form.

▶ Historical Perspective

Nazi War Crimes and the Nuremberg Code

Prior to and during World War II, Nazi physicians and scientists conducted experiments on concentration camp prisoners without their consent (see **TABLE 17-1**). Many of these experiments involved exposing subjects to extreme suffering for observational purposes, such as to determine the time to death for individuals submerged in freezing water or to determine the ability of subjects to withstand high altitude conditions by forcing them into low-pressure chambers. Other experiments involved deliberately inflicting wounds or burns, infecting subjects with diseases, or poisoning them to test various treatments or to perform autopsies afterward.

During the Nuremberg Military Tribunals at the end of World War II, the scientists who conducted these experiments were held accountable for their actions, and many issues in research ethics received public scrutiny. The 10 principles outlined in the Nuremberg Code,[1(pp181-182)] which was formulated during this process, were among the first rules for experimentation involving human subjects. The first and most famous principle from this historical code states, "The voluntary consent of the human subject is absolutely essential."[1(pp181-182)] The Nuremberg principles served to inform the development of subsequent professional and governmental codes that would guide the ethical conduct of research with human subjects.

The Tuskegee Syphilis Study

In 1932, the U.S. Public Health Service (PHS) began a study of the natural course of untreated syphilis among rural Black males in Macon County, Alabama (see Table 17-1). About 400 men with syphilis and 200 uninfected controls were enrolled in the study. Informed consent was not obtained from study participants. They were not told about the study's objective nor that they suffered from a contagious, sexually transmitted

TABLE 17-1 Examples of Ethical Problems Identified in Research Involving Human Subjects and the Development of Guidelines and Regulations: A Timeline

Event	Year	Document or regulation
Tuskegee Syphilis Study began	1932	
Nazi war crimes	1940s	
	1947	Nuremberg Code
Thalidomide disaster	1950s–1960s	
	1962	U.S. Kefauver–Harris Amendments to the Food, Drug, and Cosmetics Act
	1964	Declaration of Helsinki (I)
Beecher article published	1966	
	1966	U.S. PHS Directive (requirement for independent committee review)
Tuskegee Syphilis Study exposed and halted	1972	
	1974	U.S. National Research Act
	1975	Declaration of Helsinki (II), Tokyo
	1979	Belmont Report
	1982	CIOMS/WHO International Ethical Guidelines for Biomedical Research Involving Human Subjects
	1983	Declaration of Helsinki (III), Venice
	1989	Declaration of Helsinki (IV), Hong Kong
	1991	U.S. Federal Policy for the Protection of Human Subjects ("The Common Rule")

(continues)

TABLE 17-1 Examples of Ethical Problems Identified in Research Involving Human Subjects and the Development of Guidelines and Regulations: A Timeline *(continued)*

Event	Year	Document or regulation
	1993	CIOMS/WHO International Ethical Guidelines for Biomedical Research Involving Human Subjects (revised)
	1996	Declaration of Helsinki (V), South Africa
	1996	U.S. Health Insurance Portability and Accountability Act (HIPAA)
	1997	ICH Consolidated Guidance for Good Clinical Practice in Research
Jesse Gelsinger dies in gene therapy trial	1999	
	2000	Declaration of Helsinki (VI), Scotland
	2000	Indian Council of Medical Research (ICMR) Ethical Guidelines for Biomedical Research on Human Subjects
Ellen Roche dies in asthma study	2001	
	2002	CIOMS/WHO International Ethical Guidelines for Biomedical Research Involving Human Subjects (revised)
	2003	The Privacy Rule (U.S. DHHS)
	2008	Declaration of Helsinki (VII), South Korea
	2013	Declaration of Helsinki (VIII), Brazil
	2016	CIOMS/WHO International Ethical Guidelines for Health-related Research Involving Humans
	2017	Final Revisions to the Common Rule published ("The Final Rule")
	2018	Most provisions of "The Final Rule" go into effect

disease. Study procedures such as spinal taps were represented as "free treatment," and burial stipends motivated family members to allow autopsies on participants who reached the study's "end point."[2]

For many of these men, the study offered their first encounter with a doctor. Part of the physicians' initial justification for the study was therefore that participants were receiving general medical attention they would otherwise never access and that the treatment for syphilis available at the start of the study (an arsenic–mercury compound) was painful, toxic, and sometimes fatal.[2] Nonetheless, when penicillin became widely available by 1947 as a standard cure for syphilis, treatment was denied to Tuskegee subjects so as not to interfere with the scientific aims of the study.[2] Worse still, the PHS actively sought to prevent study subjects from obtaining treatment and information from other sources.[2] Arrangements were made for the World War II draft board to exclude any Tuskegee participants from a list of draftees requiring treatment for venereal disease. State and local health departments cooperated with the PHS, assisting with the retention of Tuskegee study subjects and referring them to Tuskegee researchers before prescribing antibiotics.[2]

The Tuskegee Syphilis Study was not a clandestine endeavor. Throughout the study, articles were published in prominent journals. In 1969, a review panel at the Centers for Disease Control and Prevention determined that the study should continue. Surprisingly, this decision was made 3 years after the PHS had developed its own ethical guidelines on human experimentation, 5 years after the release of the Declaration of Helsinki (discussed later), and long after the establishment of the Nuremberg principles.[3] The researchers and those who reviewed the study assessed that the participants' disease was too far advanced to benefit from penicillin and that therapy might actually cause severe complications.[2]

The Tuskegee Syphilis Study, which was halted in 1972 only when national press reports prompted public outrage, was the longest nontherapeutic experiment on human beings in medical history.[2] By the time the study was stopped, dozens of the participants had died of syphilis or related complications, many of their wives had been infected, and many of their children had been born with congenital syphilis.

This study, with its long-standing and intentional withholding of information and treatment, is a tragic example of research objectives being placed above the welfare of study participants and their families. The study has come to symbolize racism in medicine and science, ethical misconduct in research, and governmental exploitation of the vulnerable. The history of this study in the United States has contributed to persistent mistrust of public health authorities today, particularly among racial and ethnic minority groups.[4] President Clinton formally apologized for the study's injustices on behalf of the U.S. government in 1997.

Dr. Henry Beecher's Call for "Responsible Investigators"

The Tuskegee Syphilis Study was not the only biomedical experiment publishing results obtained under unethical conditions. In 1966, Henry K. Beecher 's article titled "Ethics and Clinical Research" was published in the *New England Journal of Medicine*[5] (see Table 17-1). In this landmark article, Beecher reported on 22 research studies with serious ethical problems, highlighting the ongoing regularity of ethical violations in research practice, despite the contemporaneous existence of numerous ethical codes and guidelines. He paid special attention to the inadequate information provided to subjects about the nature of research and a lack of truly informed consent. Foreshadowing current editorial policies for most peer-reviewed journals, he questioned whether results obtained from unethical practices should ever be published.

In the context of an enormous growth in resources for clinical research and academic pressures on investigators, Beecher advocated strongly for self-regulation among scientists and emphasized the importance of maintaining public trust: "It will certainly be charged that any mention of these matters does a disservice to medicine, but not one so great, I believe, as a continuation of the practices to be cited."[5] Prompted in part by this pivotal article, the National Institutes of Health (NIH) and the Food and Drug Administration (FDA) soon began peer review of human experimentation and required written documentation of informed consent, essentially an early form of IRB review.

The Thalidomide Disaster and Increased U.S. FDA Regulation

In addition to regulating research conduct, governments regulate the products that are tested on human beings. In the United States, Congress enacted the Kefauver–Harris bill in 1962, which mandated additional FDA regulations on the testing of investigational new drugs. This regulatory action was spurred by the European thalidomide disaster, in which safety tests failed to demonstrate the drug's teratogenicity, and it was prescribed to pregnant women for morning sickness (see Table 17-1). Even though the drug had not been approved for use in the United States, millions of samples were distributed to practicing physicians. In the early 1960s, approximately 12,000 children in 46 countries were born with severe birth defects stemming from thalidomide exposure. The 1962 drug amendments in the United States required drug manufacturers to demonstrate the effectiveness and safety of products prior to marketing, to report adverse events to the FDA, and to fully disclose the risks and benefits of their products in advertisements targeting physicians. The bill also required informed consent from clinical research participants.

The Declaration of Helsinki

In 1964, the World Medical Association held a conference in Helsinki, Finland, to formalize universally applicable ethical principles that would guide physicians in medical research involving human subjects.[6] The Declaration of Helsinki that resulted from this conference was revised several times at later conferences (see Table 17-1) and remains an international standard for biomedical research involving human subjects.[7] The Declaration of Helsinki includes "freely given informed consent" as a key requirement of ethical research. The first revision (Helsinki II, 1975) included a statement that human subjects research should be reviewed by an independent committee. The Declaration of Helsinki is also well known for its distinction between therapeutic and non-therapeutic research. Other important assertions in the Declaration of Helsinki include that research with human subjects should be based on the results of preclinical experiments in the laboratory and, as appropriate with animals, research should be conducted by scientifically qualified individuals and the risks of participating in research should not exceed the benefits.

In contrast to the Nuremberg Code, which was developed by a tribunal in the context of a trial for war crimes, the Declaration of Helsinki represents the first substantial effort by a professional body in medicine to self-regulate the ethical conduct of research.

U.S. Federal Requirements for Independent Committee Review

The PHS Directive of 1966 required U.S. federal grant recipients to confirm that their research would undergo independent committee review. This directive represented a major turning point in the regulation of human research because it dismissed the expectation that investigators use their discretion to put the interests of human subjects over the interests of science and society. Over time, it had become increasingly apparent that the potential for misconduct or confusion about the ethical appropriateness of research practices was a threat to the scientific community and to society. The scientific community's reputation was at stake, and society stood to lose the benefits of scientific progress gained by conducting research. This directive was the beginning of the creation of a complex system of external regulatory oversight for human subjects research conducted in the United States.

The U.S. National Research Act of 1974, galvanized in part by publicity from the Tuskegee Syphilis Study, specifically required institutions to establish review boards with at least five members from diverse backgrounds, including one nonscientist. These IRBs, discussed later in this chapter, would look out for the rights and welfare of human research volunteers in federally funded studies.

The Belmont Report

The U.S. National Research Act of 1974 established the National Commission for the Protection of Human Subjects of Biomedical and Behavioral Research. The Belmont Report,[8] published in 1979, is a summary of the basic ethical principles identified by the Commission over 4 years of deliberations (see Table 17-1). Three major principles that apply to research with human subjects are identified in the Belmont Report: respect for persons, beneficence, and justice. These remain fundamental principles in current U.S. regulations for human subjects research.

Respect for persons is based on the conviction that "individuals should be treated as autonomous agents" and that "persons with diminished autonomy are entitled to protection."[8] A requirement of respect for persons is that people, to the extent that they are able, must be allowed to decide what will or will not happen to them. The decision to participate in research must be voluntary and informed. The essential elements of informed consent are discussed later in this chapter.

Through the principle of beneficence, researchers are obligated to maximize possible benefits and minimize possible harms. Possible risks to study participants should be systematically weighed against possible benefits. External information, such as safety reports or results from other studies, should inform the assessment of risks and benefits on an ongoing basis.

In addition to physical risks and benefits, social, psychological, legal, and financial risks and benefits must be considered. For example, will volunteers in an HIV vaccine trial face discrimination or have problems obtaining health insurance if the experimental vaccine causes them to produce HIV antibodies that result in a false-positive HIV test? Researchers are responsible for considering such possibilities in advance and implementing appropriate safeguards. In the example given, this might include ensuring that HIV vaccine trial volunteers receive identification cards with a contact they can call anytime to resolve questions about their HIV status. Regardless of the investigators' efforts to minimize risks or inconveniences, potential difficulties such as these must be discussed with each volunteer during the informed consent process.

The principle of beneficence also applies to information obtained through research. Data must be collected, stored, and analyzed in ways that minimize risk to participants. This includes protecting participant confidentiality by storing personal identifiers in secure locations and preventing opportunities for identifiable information about research participants to be released.

The principle of justice helps determine whether the burdens and benefits of research are fairly distributed. In the United States during the 19th and early 20th centuries, the poor bore a disproportionate burden of the risks associated with serving as research subjects while the new findings and procedures resulting from scientific research largely benefited wealthy people receiving private health care. Cases such as the

Nazi concentration camp experiments or the Tuskegee Syphilis Study are examples of injustices. The subjects included in those experiments bore the burdens of participation but stood to gain nothing from the outcomes of the research. The selection of research subjects must therefore be carefully considered: Are certain groups being singled out simply because they are easily available, or are there valid reasons to include them that are directly related to the problem being studied? Do the groups represented by the subjects stand to benefit from the findings that may result from the research?

▶ International Ethical and Research Practice Guidelines

In addition to the Declaration of Helsinki, there are a number of ethical research and practice guidelines that are internationally oriented. A few are discussed in the following sections or listed in Table 17-1.

WHO/CIOMS Guidelines

In 1982, the World Health Organization (WHO) and the Council for International Organizations of Medical Sciences (CIOMS) published International Ethical Guidelines for Biomedical Research Involving Human Subjects. This document built on Helsinki II and addressed issues of informed consent; standards for external review; and protections for vulnerable persons participating in medical research. These guidelines have been revised to provide further commentary on issues such as fair research benefits in low-resource settings, community engagement in research, and the storage and use of biological material and health-related data. The 2016 guidelines also revisited the blanket classification of certain populations as "vulnerable" to emphasize that with appropriate protections these groups should not be excluded from research. The CIOMS guidelines pay special attention to the needs of resource-limited countries and multinational research partnerships.[9]

International Conference on Harmonization Guidelines for Good Clinical Practice

The International Conference on Harmonization (ICH) guidelines provide a unified standard for conducting human clinical trials in the European Union, Japan, and the United States to facilitate mutual acceptance of resulting data, reduce the need for duplicative studies, and reduce delays in international access to beneficial products and procedures. The ICH guidelines for Good Clinical Practice (GCP)[10] offer an international ethical and scientific quality standard for the design, conduct, recording, and reporting of trials involving human subjects. Detailed guidance is provided for IRBs, trial sponsors, and investigators, and training in GCP is recommended for individuals involved in clinical research.

▶ The U.S. Regulatory Framework for Human Subjects Research

U.S. Federal Policy for the Protection of Human Subjects

The U.S. Food and Drug Administration (FDA) and the Department of Health and Human Services (DHHS) codified human subjects regulations based on the Belmont Report in 1981.

The FDA regulations provide protections for human subjects when products such as drugs, devices, biologics, and food additives are tested. These include Title 21 Code of Federal Regulations (CFR) Parts 50 (protection of human subjects), 54 (financial disclosure by investigators), 56 (IRBs), 312 (investigational new drug application), and 314 (applications for FDA approval to market a new drug).

The U.S. Federal Policy for the Protection of Human Subjects, referred to as the "Common Rule" was adopted by several federal agencies and published in 1991; the DHHS outlines these regulations in Title 45 CFR 46 Subpart A. Additional protections for vulnerable subjects— pregnant women, prisoners, and children—are outlined in Subparts B–D.[11] Final revisions to the Common Rule (called "the Final Rule") were issued in January 2017[12] and went into effect in July 2018.

The U.S. Federal Policy provides definitions of *research*, *human subject*, and other relevant terms for the activities to be covered by the policy. Researchers should familiarize themselves with these definitions because their applicability to a given project will determine some aspects of the required review process. An IRB can also advise if there is any doubt about whether a project involves human subjects research by the federal definitions.

The Federal Policy includes three major components of protections for human research subjects: (1) institutional assurances, (2) IRB review, and (3) informed consent (discussed later in this chapter).

Institutional Assurances

The U.S. Office for Human Research Protections (OHRP) monitors compliance with 45 CFR 46.[11] One way that OHRP monitors compliance with these regulations is to issue a type of permit, termed an *assurance*, to institutions that receive federal funds to conduct research with human participants. This assurance (called a federal-wide assurance, or FWA) obligates an institution to comply with the Federal Policy. The terms of the assurance include important responsibilities such as reporting unanticipated problems or noncompliance, ensuring appropriate IRB review, and ensuring a suitable informed consent process.

The Institutional Review Board (IRB)

When research involving human subjects is supported by U.S. federal funds, it is subject to the Federal Policy for the Protection of Human Subjects, which mandates IRB review. Although investigators may not be legally required to obtain IRB approval for research that is not federally funded, major research institutions require it regardless of funding source, and it is a generally accepted aspect of ensuring ethical research practice.

Researchers must obtain approval from an IRB before initiating any research with human volunteers. To obtain approval, investigators submit to the IRB a study application or protocol, consent and recruitment materials, and detailed information about the planned conduct of the research. The investigator should demonstrate provisions for human subjects protections such as the following: (1) appropriate procedures for informed consent, (2) adequate protections for subjects' privacy and confidentiality of the information collected, (3) minimization of risks to subjects, (4) reasonable risks relative to the possible benefits, (5) special protections if vulnerable subjects are to be included, and (6) fairness in the selection of subjects. Researchers are also responsible for following the IRB-approved research protocol, obtaining IRB approval for any changes to the protocol, obtaining IRB reapproval for research activities on an annual basis, using only the approved and current version of the informed consent form (when informed consent is to be documented in writing), and informing the IRB and other appropriate authorities about any adverse or unexpected events involving risk to human subjects. Investigators must never initiate changes to a research protocol without IRB review and approval, unless such changes are necessary for the immediate safety of the research participants.

The Health Insurance Portability and Accountability Act (HIPAA)

The Health Insurance Portability and Accountability Act (HIPAA) was passed in 1996 to facilitate the processing of electronic healthcare information. The Act also addresses the security and privacy of health data. In response, the DHHS issued Standards for Privacy of Individually Identifiable Health Information—the Privacy Rule—which went into effect in 2003. This rule applies to individually identifiable health information obtained or kept by a covered entity (health plans and care providers that transmit electronically available information, for example, to process claims). Researchers may access protected health information by obtaining either consent from each patient of interest or a waiver from an IRB or Privacy Board. There are also five other modes by which a researcher may be allowed to access protected health information for research purposes. Researchers must work with the privacy officer at the data source to identify the appropriate mode of access and to comply with its requirements.

▶ Limitations Posed by Ethical Requirements

Although oversight is an essential aspect of protecting human research volunteers, stringent regulatory requirements and the restrictions that some ethical review committees may place on researchers can hinder the conduct of certain types of research. In addition, the costs of maintaining an IRB are not trivial nor are the administrative burdens associated with regulatory requirements.

Certain ethical restrictions may even compromise the quality of scientific research. For example, biased samples can result when researchers are not permitted to contact potential study volunteers and volunteers must instead opt in to participate in research based only on preliminary information from advertisements or provider letters. Research in some settings has shown that a patient's decision not to opt in is often based on a perception that his or her case is not interesting enough and not because of a lack of willingness to volunteer for research.[13] A requirement to opt in can mean that some participants, such as those who are more severely ill or underprivileged, may be more likely to be excluded, the incidence or prevalence of the condition under study may be under- or overestimated, or the estimated association between an exposure or a risk factor and the outcome may be biased.[14] Paradoxically, it may be unethical to conduct a study that has a diminished capacity to provide valid results. The negative effect of potentially biased study results thus warrants consideration in relation to the potential confidentiality costs of various recruitment methods.[14] Fortunately, there is usually room for dialogue about study-specific risk–benefit ratios, and researchers should be prepared to work together with ethical review committees to reach compromises that protect both the research subjects and the quality of the expected results.

▶ Contemporary Examples

In 1999, while participating in a gene therapy trial at the University of Pennsylvania that was subsequently found to be ethically problematic, 18-year-old Jesse Gelsinger died. Problems with the trial included undisclosed risks and conflicts of interest. Both the lead researcher for the trial and the university held stock in a company for gene therapy development, and this financial conflict was not disclosed to trial participants. A conflict of interest can cloud the entire conduct of a study, particularly in hindsight when problems are identified. For example, would the risks have been disclosed more thoroughly had the researchers not had a financial interest in completing the study? An investigation also exposed flaws in the system of patient safety oversight. After Gelsinger's death, the NIH was notified of 652 previously unreported serious adverse events from gene therapy studies.

In 2001, Ellen Roche, a healthy 24-year-old, died from the effects of inhaling hexamethonium for an asthma study at the research institution where she was employed. The study had been designed and approved without proper reference to existing literature on the risks associated with the intervention. Considering the principle of beneficence, these investigators were responsible for pursuing all the information available to fully consider the risk–benefit ratio associated with participation in their research, both before and during the conduct of the study. Failure to do so can have disastrous effects, as exemplified by the death of this volunteer.

Fortunately, research participant deaths are rare. However, these examples underscore the critical importance of following ethical guidelines and upholding scientific integrity. As Jesse Gelsinger's father reminds us of his son's altruism, "If researchers, industry, and those in government apply Jesse's intent—not for recognition or for money, but only to help—then they will get all they want and more. They'll get it right."[15]

▶ The Informed Consent Process

Information, Comprehension, and Voluntariness

The informed consent process includes three basic elements: information, comprehension, and voluntariness.[8] Informed consent is an educational and decision-making process in which potential volunteers must be effectively informed of the purpose, procedures, and possible risks and benefits associated with participation in a study. The process of obtaining informed consent is expected to go beyond signing a form, by prompting a meaningful discussion between volunteers and researchers in which volunteers are able to ask any questions they may have. Potential volunteers should be given adequate time to consider their choice to participate and to consult with others if they wish.

It is the investigator's responsibility not only to provide the information required for potential subjects to make a decision about participation but also to ensure that research subjects comprehend this information. This responsibility involves consideration of maturity, education levels, and literacy, among other factors, when designing consent materials for different populations. Sometimes, an assessment of understanding is appropriate.

The researcher could also pose hypothetical or open-ended questions about the study to probe volunteers' reasons for participation and to identify their concerns. Such measures can help to uncover and correct volunteers' misperceptions about what is involved before they are enrolled.

It must be clear to participants that they are being invited to participate in research and that the objectives therein are not necessarily based on their individual best interests or preferences. Consider, for example, an HIV vaccine trial in which participants are randomized to receive either an experimental vaccine or a placebo. Neither will necessarily benefit the volunteers. Potential volunteers must not participate in the trial with the misperception that they will be protected against HIV. The vaccine is experimental and may not be efficacious, and volunteers could receive the placebo, which confers no protection. The education of potential volunteers about vaccine trial concepts prior to enrollment is critical in obtaining informed consent under these circumstances.

The decision to participate in research must be truly voluntary—free of coercion or undue influence. Participants must understand that their medical care and access to other services will not be affected by their decision to enroll or not enroll or to withdraw from a study. Researchers should be particularly cautious about enrolling subjects who may be unduly influenced by the compensation provided for participating in a trial, especially one that involves more than minimal risk. The amount of compensation to be offered for trial participation should be given thoughtful consideration by study staff and review boards familiar with the community selected to participate in the research.

Documentation of Informed Consent

Informed consent should usually be documented with a written consent form. The form must be preapproved by an IRB and signed by research participants or their legally authorized representative. The researcher obtaining the consent often also signs the form. Participants are given a copy of the form to keep, and the original is filed in a secure location at the study site. Complete and accurate documentation is essential to demonstrate that appropriate informed consent was obtained prior to initiating any study procedures. Investigators should regularly review all informed consent documentation throughout the study to ensure it is properly maintained.

Special consideration should be given to methods for obtaining consent from participants with low literacy, including the use of visual aids. It is good practice to read informed consent forms aloud to potential participants to be sure they receive all the information therein. When consent is to be obtained orally, an impartial witness should observe the process. An IRB must approve in advance a written summary of what is to be said to the research participant. The witness and the researcher obtaining consent should sign a copy of this summary. Both the participant and the witness should sign a short form stating that the required elements of informed consent have been presented orally to the subject.

In some instances, the requirement for written informed consent may be waived. For example, when conducting an otherwise anonymous survey, the consent form becomes the only record identifying the research participant. In such cases, if the primary risk associated with participating in the survey is a potential breach of confidentiality, the required information about study participation can be presented to the participants in a written statement that they need not sign. However, an IRB must ascertain whether the appropriate criteria have been met for a waiver of written informed consent. The investigator does not makes this assessment alone.

There are a number of items that should be included in an informed consent form. **TABLE 17-2** includes a list of general requirements for informed consent based on the U.S. Federal Policy for the Protection of Human Subjects.

TABLE 17-2 Informed Consent Form Checklist
Basic elements

- A statement that the study involves research

- An explanation of the purposes of the research

- The expected duration of the subject's participation

- A description of the procedures to be followed

- Identification of any procedures that are experimental

- A description of any reasonably foreseeable risks or discomforts to the subject

- A description of any benefits to the subject or to others that may reasonably be expected from the research

- A disclosure of appropriate alternative procedures or courses of treatment, if any, that might be advantageous to the subject

- A statement describing the extent, if any, to which confidentiality of records identifying the subject will be maintained

- For research involving more than minimal risk, an explanation as to whether any compensation, and/or medical treatments are available if injury occurs and, if so, what they consist of, or where further information may be obtained

(continues)

TABLE 17-2 Informed Consent Form Checklist *(continued)*

Basic elements

- An explanation of who to contact for answers to questions about the research and research subjects' rights, and who to contact in the event of a research-related injury to the subject

- A statement that participation is voluntary, refusal to participate will involve no penalty or loss of benefits to which the subject is otherwise entitled, and the subject may discontinue participation at any time without penalty or loss of benefits to which the subject is otherwise entitled

Additional items that may be appropriate

- A statement that the particular treatment or procedure may involve risks to the subject (or to the embryo or fetus if the subject is or may become pregnant) that are currently unforeseeable

- Anticipated circumstances under which the subject's participation may be terminated by the investigator without regard to the subject's consent

- Any additional costs to the subject that may result from participation in the research

- The consequences of a subject's decision to withdraw from the research and procedures for orderly termination of participation by the subject

- A statement that significant new findings developed during the course of the research that may relate to the subject's willingness to continue participation, will be provided to the subject

- The approximate number of subjects involved in the study

Reproduced from the Code of Federal Regulations, Department of Health and Human Services. *Title 45: Public Welfare; Part 46: Protection of Human Subjects*. http://www.hhs.gov/ohrp/policy/ohrpregulations.pdf. Accessed August 11, 2017.

Methods for Improving and Evaluating Informed Consent

Obtaining truly informed consent is not easy. Many participants do not wish to be bothered with a lengthy form that they perceive to be legalistic. Many investigators are challenged by the task of explaining complex scientific objectives to laypeople. Study participants may provide consent without fully comprehending the implications of participating in the research or because they are overly optimistic about the intervention under study.

Consider again the example of an HIV vaccine trial. Phases II and III HIV vaccine trials recruit people at high-risk for HIV infection. Because of the HIV risk inclusion criteria, potential volunteers for these trials in the United States may be involved with injection drug use or other illegal activities, commercial sex work, or other risky sexual behaviors and may be drawn from marginalized populations. These potential volunteers are thus particularly vulnerable to social harms, and special protections for their rights and welfare throughout the trial must be carefully considered and implemented. Some volunteers may have low levels of education, may be unfamiliar with scientific research concepts, and may be unduly influenced to participate by the hope that the vaccine will protect them from HIV infection. These factors challenge the informed consent process.

Policy revisions have been proposed in response to concerns that consent forms are often too lengthy and complicated or more focused on protecting investigators or institutions from liability than on informing research volunteers. Final revisions to the Common Rule require that informed consent forms begin with a concise and focused presentation of the key information that is most likely to assist a potential volunteer in understanding the reasons one might or might not want to participate in the research. The information that is key to the decision-making process should be presented clearly and up front.

Community input can be invaluable when designing an informed consent process. Many research initiatives partner with a Community Advisory Board (CAB), which can advise on the needs and expectations of the community from which research participants are drawn and on the cultural appropriateness of the planned research and consent methods.

A randomized experimental study of a prototype informed consent process for HIV vaccine efficacy trials tested the hypothesis that informed consent is enhanced by presenting study information in both written and verbal formats; minimizing the reading level and enhancing the visual display of written documents; involving educators who are not physicians or investigators in discussions with potential participants; and providing ample time and opportunity for participants to review, consider, inquire about, and discuss the research.[16] This study found that despite low baseline knowledge of HIV vaccine trial concepts, participation in an enhanced informed consent process was associated with substantial and sustained increases in knowledge among persons targeted for participation in HIV vaccine efficacy trials in multiple U.S. cities.[16] Another study compared the use of a standard consent form to a concise version within a large international trial of the timing of antiretroviral therapy initiation in HIV-positive adults (START).[17] Investigators found that the easier to read, more concise consent form was not inferior to the standard longer form, supporting ongoing efforts to simplify informed consent documents. Such efforts to identify and implement effective improvements to the informed consent process in varying types of studies and social contexts represent important and meaningful ways to apply the principle of respect for persons.

Summary

Scientific research cannot be effectively conducted without safeguards and public trust. Historical and contemporary events have drawn attention to the importance of developing and enforcing guidelines for research involving human subjects. Numerous guidelines exist to help researchers protect the rights and welfare of human research participants. Researchers are responsible for understanding and following the applicable ethical and practice guidelines. Failure to do so can have broad and serious repercussions.

Researchers are also responsible for justifying their study designs, working with the appropriate authorities for oversight of their research, maintaining precise records, protecting subject confidentiality, and ensuring that information about a study is presented to subjects in a way that they can understand. Informed consent based on information, comprehension, and voluntariness is a cornerstone of the ethical conduct of research with human volunteers.

References

1. *Trials of War Criminals Before the Nuernberg Military Tribunals Under Control Council Law No. 10*. Vol. 2. Washington, DC: U.S. Government Printing Office; 1949. https://www.loc.gov/rr/frd/Military_Law/pdf/NT_war-criminals_Vol-II.pdf.

2. Jones JH. *Bad Blood*. New York, NY: Free Press; 1993.

3. Fourtner AW, Fourtner CR, Herreid CR. Bad blood: a case study of the Tuskegee syphilis project. http://sciencecases.lib.buffalo.edu/cs/files/2-bad_blood.pdf. Accessed August 11, 2017.

4. Thomas SB, Quinn SC. The Tuskegee Syphilis Study, 1932 to 1972: implications for HIV education and AIDS risk education programs in the Black community. *Am J Public Health*. 1991;81:1498-1504.

5. Beecher HK. Ethics and clinical research. *New Engl J Med*. 1966;274:1354-1360.

6. Declaration of Helsinki: recommendations guiding medical doctors in biomedical research involving human subjects. Adopted by the 18th World Medical Assembly, Helsinki, Finland, 1964. *New Engl J Med*. 1964;271:473.

7. World Medical Association. Declaration of Helsinki. wma.net. https://www.wma.net/policies-post/wma-declaration-of-helsinki-ethical-principles-for-medical-research-involving-human-subjects/. Accessed July 11, 2017.

8. National Commission for the Protection of Human Subjects of Biomedical and Behavioral Research. *The Belmont Report: Ethical Principles and Guidelines for the Protection of Human Subjects of Research*. Washington, DC: U.S. Government Printing Office; 1979.

9. Council for International Organizations of Medical Sciences (CIOMS). *International Ethical Guidelines for Health-related Research Involving Human Subjects*. Geneva, Switzerland: World Health Organization; 2016. https://cioms.ch/wp-content/uploads/2017/01/WEB-CIOMS-EthicalGuidelines.pdf. Accessed July 11, 2017.

10. International Council for Harmonization of Technical Requirements for Pharmaceuticals for Human Use (ICH). *Guideline for Good Clinical Practice E6 (R2)*. International Conference on Harmonization; 2016. http://www.ich.org/fileadmin/Public_Web_Site/ICH_Products/Guidelines/Efficacy/E6/E6_R2_Step_4_2016_1109.pdf. Accessed August 11, 2017.

11. Code of Federal Regulations, Department of Health and Human Services. *Title 45: Public Welfare; Part 46: Protection of Human Subjects*. hhs.gov. http://www.hhs.gov/ohrp/policy/ohrpregulations.pdf. Accessed August 11, 2017.

12. Policy for the Protection of Human Subjects. Federal Register Vol. 82, No. 12. Rules and Regulations. https://www.federalregister.gov/documents/2017/01/19/2017-01058/federal-policy-for-the

-protection-of-human-subjects. Published January 19, 2017. Accessed August 11, 2017.

13. Crombie IK, McMurdo ME, Irvine L, Williams B. Overcoming barriers to recruitment in health research: concerns of potential participants need to be dealt with. *Br Med J*. 2006;333:398.

14. Hewison J, Haines A. Overcoming barriers to recruitment in health research. *Br Med J*. 2006; 333:300-302.

15. Gelsinger P. Forward: Jesse's intent. In: Bankert EA, Amdur RJ. (eds.). *Institutional Review Board: Management and Function*. 2nd ed. Sudbury, MA: Jones and Bartlett Publishers; 2006:xix.

16. Colletti AS, Heagerty P, Sheon AR, Gross M, Koblin BA, Metzger DS, et al. Randomized, controlled evaluation of a prototype informed consent process for HIV vaccine efficacy trials. *J Acquir Immune Defic Syndr*. 2003;32:161-169.

17. Grady C, Touloumi G, Walker AS, Smolskis M, Sharma S, Babiker AG, et al. A randomized trial comparing concise and standard consent forms in the START trial. *PloS One*. 2017;12(4). doi: 10.1371/journal.pone.0172607.

Chapter Questions

1. What key principle of ethical research was described in the 1947 Nuremberg Code? Was this principle followed in the Tuskegee Syphilis Study?

2. Which of the following ethical principles were included in the 1964 and 1975 Declarations of Helsinki?

    a. Informed consent should be given freely.
    b. Human subjects research should be reviewed by an independent committee.
    c. The risks of participating in a study should not exceed the benefits.
    d. All of the above

3. Describe the major principles of human subjects research identified in the 1979 Belmont Report.

4. What is meant by the term *informed consent*?

CHAPTER 18

Answers to Chapter Questions (Chapters 1–17)

▶ Chapter 1: The Approach and Evolution of Epidemiology

1. A. Public health is a multidisciplinary field whose goal is to promote the health of populations through organized community efforts.

    B. Epidemiology is the study of the distribution and determinants of disease frequency in human populations and the application of this study to control health problems. Disease refers to a broad array of health-related states and events, including diseases, injuries, disabilities, and death.

    C. A population is a group of people with a common characteristic.

    D. A measure of disease frequency quantifies how often a disease arises in a population. Its calculation involves establishing the disease definition, developing a mechanism for counting the diseased cases (the numerator), and determining the size of the underlying population (the denominator).

    E. Disease distribution refers to the pattern of disease according to the characteristics of person (Who is getting the disease?), place (Where is it occurring?) and time (How is it changing over time?).

    F. Disease determinants are factors that cause either a healthy person to become sick or a sick person to recover.

    G. Disease control is the ultimate aim of epidemiology and refers to the reduction or elimination of disease occurrence. It is accomplished through epidemiological research and surveillance.

H. A hypothesis is a tentative explanation for an observation, a phenomenon, or a scientific problem that can be tested by further investigation.

2. Public health focuses on preventing diseases in communities, and medicine focuses on treating diseases at the individual level.

3. Public health achievements that have improved life expectancy include the routine use of vaccinations for infectious diseases, improved sanitation and clean water, modification of risk factors for coronary heart disease and stroke, improved access to family planning and contraceptive services, and antismoking campaigns.

4. The main objectives of epidemiology are to study the natural course of disease, determine the extent of disease in a population, identify patterns and trends in disease occurrence, identify the causes of disease, and evaluate the effectiveness of measures that prevent and treat disease.

5. Epidemiologists quantify the frequency of disease by developing a definition of the disease, instituting a mechanism for counting cases of disease within a population, and determining the size of that population. It is only when the number of cases are related to the size of the population that we know the true frequency of disease.

6. A. John Graunt summarized the patterns of mortality in 17th-century London and discovered the regularity of deaths and births.

B. John Snow conducted one of the first observational studies in the neighborhoods of 19th-century London and discovered that contaminated drinking water was the cause of cholera.

C. Richard Doll and Austin Bradford Hill conducted groundbreaking studies on cigarette smoking and lung cancer in the 1950s.

D. James Lind conducted one of the earliest experimental studies on the treatment of scurvy among sailors. Using sound experimental principles, he found that the consumption of oranges and lemons was the most effective remedy for scurvy in this population.

E. William Farr was the compiler of Statistical Abstracts in Great Britain from 1839 through 1880. In this capacity, he pioneered many activities encompassed by modern epidemiology, including the calculation of mortality rates using census data for denominators.

7. Today's subspecialties are defined in terms of the exposure (e.g., environmental exposures), the disease (e.g., cancer), and the population being studied (e.g., the elderly).

8. Modern epidemiology examines risk factors at the molecular level (e.g., biological markers of exposure, genetic markers), the societal level (e.g., social factors such as racism), and across the life span (from birth through old age).

▶ Chapter 2: Measures of Disease Frequency

1. A. Cumulative incidence
    B. Prevalence
    C. Incidence rate
    D. Prevalence
    E. Cumulative incidence
2. A. Prevalence quantifies existing cases; incidence quantifies new cases.
    B. The main similarity is that they both quantify the number of new cases of disease that develop in a population at risk during a specified period of time. The main difference is that the incidence rate is a true rate that directly integrates person-time of observation into the denominator, and cumulative incidence is a proportion whose denominator is the population at risk at the start of the observation period. Time in cumulative incidence is expressed only by words that go along with the proportion.
    C. A dynamic population is defined by a changeable state or condition, and therefore its membership is transitory; a fixed population is defined by a life event, and therefore its membership is permanent.
3. A. 0% and 100%
    B. 0% and 100%
    C. Zero and infinity. Infinity is, in theory, the highest value of the incidence rate when person-time is essentially zero. This could happen, for instance, if everyone in a population died instantaneously following a highly noxious exposure (e.g., cyanide).
4. No. It is also necessary to know the size of the population and the amount of follow-up time in each city.
5. D. All of the above
6. A. 5/100
    B. 0/100
    C. $3/(100-5)=3/95$. Remember that only the population at risk at the beginning of October is eligible for the denominator.
7. When the population is in steady state, $P = IR \times D$, where P is prevalence, IR is incidence rate, and D is average duration. Thus, $P = 500/100,000$ person-years $\times 3$ years or $1,500/100,000$.

8. $(20 \times 5 \text{ years}) + (10 \times 1 \text{ year}) + (70 \times 10 \text{ years}) = 100 + 10 + 700 = 810 \text{ person-years}$.

9. A. City A = 25/25,000 over 1 year or 50/50,000 over 1 year. City B = 30/50,000 over 1 year.
    B. City A has the higher cumulative incidence.

10. The following calculation assumes that everyone is followed for the entire 2 years and that all cases occurred at the end of the second year: $60/(100,000 \text{ persons} \times 2 \text{ years}) = 60/200,000$ person-years or 30/100,000 person-years. Different assumptions can be made regarding the length of follow-up for cases and noncases and the time of case occurrence.

11. The incidence rate was 12/100,000 person-years, which is equivalent to $x/250,000$ person-years. Solving for x, we arrive at 30 new cases.

12. A. Dynamic. This is a changeable condition; people are continually entering and leaving the city.
    B. Fixed. This is a permanent characteristic; once a man has the surgery, he is forever part of this group.
    C. Fixed. This is also a permanent characteristic; same rationale as answer B.
    D. Dynamic. This is a changeable characteristic. New graduates are entering practice, others are leaving by retirement, and so on.

13. A. Increases prevalence
    B. Decreases prevalence
    C. Decreases prevalence

14. A. True
    B. False
    C. False
    D. True
    E. True

15. A. i. 4/1,000.
        ii. 6/996. Remember that the population size has decreased by 4 because of death.
        iii. 4/994. Again, the population is smaller.
    B. 6/996. Only those who do not have the disease of interest are at risk.
    C. 6/1,000. Everyone in the population is at risk of dying.

▶ Chapter 3: Comparing Disease Frequencies

1. A. They are both ways to compare measures of disease frequency to assess the effect of an exposure on a disease. The ratio measure gives information on the strength of

the relationship between an exposure and a disease; the difference measure describes the excess number of cases of disease that are associated with the exposure.

B. Both provide information on the absolute effect of the exposure or the excess risk of disease. However, the risk difference gives the number of cases of disease among the exposed that may be attributable to the exposure, and the population risk difference gives the number of cases of disease in the total population that may be attributable to the exposure.

2. A. $30/100,000$ person-years/$45/100,000$ person-years $= 0.67$.

B. Women who engage in regular physical activity have 0.67 times the risk of ovarian cancer (or a 33% reduced risk of ovarian cancer) compared with women who do not engage in regular physical activity.

C. $30/100,000$ person-years $- 45/100,000$ person-years $= -15/100,000$ person-years. Note that the incidence rate difference is negative.

D. The excess rate of ovarian cancer among women who do not engage in regular physical activity is $15/100,000$ person-years. Or, if regular physical activity prevents ovarian cancer, then 15 cases per 100,000 person-years of follow-up would be eliminated if the women engaged in regular physical activity.

E. Null value for the incidence rate ratio is 1.0, and the null value for the incidence rate difference is 0.0.

3. A crude rate describes the disease frequency in a population using only raw data. For example, a crude prevalence is calculated by dividing the total number of cases in the population at a point in time by the total number of individuals in the population at a point in time. An age-adjusted rate is a summary rate used to compare disease frequencies across populations with different age distributions. Often, direct standardization is used to calculate age-adjusted rates.

4. An age-specific rate is a rate that applies only to a particular age group. For example, the incidence rate of HIV infection among 15- to 24-year-olds is an age-specific rate. As described above, an age-adjusted rate is a summary rate that accounts for the age differences when comparing populations. The numeric value of the age-adjusted rate depends on the particular weights used for the adjustment.

5. A. Crude heart disease death rate in the low-income country equals $(0.30 \times 2/100,000$ person-years$) + (0.40 \times 20/100,000$ person-years$) + (0.30 \times 40/100,000$ person-years$) = 20.6/100,000$ person-years. Crude heart disease death rate in the high-income country equals $(0.20 \times 2/100,000$ person-years$) + (0.30 \times 20/100,000$

person-years) + (0.50 × 40/100,000 person-years) = 26.4/100,000 person-years.

B. The age-adjusted rate is better because the age structures of the two populations are different.

6. A. Cumulative incidence (CI) among the delegates equals $a/(a+b) = 125/1,849 = 0.068$ (in 41 days). CI among the nondelegates equals $c/(c+d) = 3/762 = 0.004$ (in 41 days).

B. Cumulative incidence ratio equals $CI_{delegates}/CI_{nondelegates} = 0.068/0.004 = 17.0$.

C. The risk of Legionnaires' disease was 17 times greater among delegates than among nondelegates. Or, a delegate had 17 times the risk of contracting Legionnaires' disease as did a nondelegate.

D. Cumulative incidence difference equals $CI_{delegates} - CI_{nondelegates} = 0.068 - 0.004 = 0.064$ (in 41 days)

E. If delegate status is a "cause" of Legionnaires' disease, then 64 cases per 1,000 delegates would be eliminated if the delegates had been nondelegates. Note that delegate status is not the actual cause of Legionnaires' disease but reflects which part of the hotel that the individual entered during the convention. Further investigation found that the organism that causes Legionnaires' disease was present in certain air conditioners.

F. Attributable proportion equals $[(CI_{delegates} - CI_{nondelegates})/CI_{delegates}] \times 100\% = [(0.068 - 0.004)/0.068] \times 100\% = 94\%$.

G. This means that 94% of the cases of Legionnaires' disease among the delegates could be attributed to their delegate status.

7. A. False
   B. False
   C. True
   D. False
   E. True
   F. False

8. A. Yes
   B. Yes
   C. Yes
   D. No (This measure requires information about the proportion of the population that is exposed.)

9. A. The mortality rate ratio and difference for lung cancer are 14 and 130/100,000 person-years, respectively. The mortality rate ratio and difference for coronary heart disease are 1.6 and 256/100,000 person-years, respectively.

   B. Smoking is a stronger risk factor for lung cancer than coronary heart disease deaths (mortality rate ratios: 14 for lung cancer vs. 1.6 for coronary heart disease).

    C. Smoking has a greater public health impact via deaths from coronary heart disease (mortality rate differences: 130/100,000 person-years for lung cancer vs. 256/100,000 person-years for coronary heart disease). This means that 130 deaths from lung cancer for every 100,000 person-years would have been averted vs. 256 deaths from coronary heart disease for every 100,000 person-years.

    D. The reason for these different findings is the much higher mortality rate from coronary heart disease in the study population.

▶ Chapter 4: Sources of Public Health Data

1. D
2. C
3. B
4. There may be differences in the reliability and completeness of data on infant deaths and differences in the reliability and completeness of data on livebirths. This includes undercounting deaths and births because they are not reported to civil registers and inaccuracies regarding the age of the death.

▶ Chapter 5: Descriptive Epidemiology

1. A. i. There was about a 60% increase in the prevalence of gastroschisis from 2000 through 2009. The increase during 2000–2005 is steeper than that during 2006–2009. In fact, the prevalence decreases slightly from 2006–2007 to 2008–2009.

        ii. The prevalence of gastroschisis decreased dramatically with maternal age. It decreased by about 25% from ages 19 and under to 20–24 years and by another 72% from ages 20–24 years to 25 years and older.

        iii. The prevalence of gastroschisis was 1.9 times higher among White mothers as compared with Black mothers.

        iv. The prevalence of gastroschisis was 1.5 times higher among male infants as compared with female infants.

B.   There are many possible hypotheses. For example, the prevalence of gastroschisis increased over time because risk factors for the defect also increased over time. Gastroschisis has been associated with maternal alcohol consumption, illicit drug use, and use of acetaminophen and vasoactive drugs.

C.   There are many possible answers. For example, these data could be used to support increased screening activities for gastroschisis among teenaged White women who come to prenatal care.

2.   A.   A disease cluster is an aggregation of relatively uncommon events or disease in space and/or time in amounts that are believed or perceived to be greater than could be expected by chance.

B.   An outbreak is the occurrence of cases of an illness, specific health-related behavior, or other health-related events clearly in excess of normal expectancy. *Outbreak* is a synonym for *epidemic* that often refers to a localized epidemic.

C.   An epidemic is the occurrence of cases of an illness, specific health-related behavior, or other health-related events clearly in excess of normal expectancy. A worldwide epidemic is known as a pandemic.

▶ Chapter 6: Overview of Epidemiological Study Designs

1.   A.   In an observational study, the investigator "watches" as subjects themselves choose which group they will be in (exposed or unexposed); in an experimental study, the investigator assigns participants to their exposure groups.

B.   Both the exposures and outcomes have already occurred at the start of a retrospective cohort study. The outcomes have not yet developed at the start of a prospective cohort study. Thus, a retrospective cohort study investigates prior outcomes, and a prospective cohort study investigates future outcomes.

C.   A cohort study defines subjects according to their exposure level and follows them for disease occurrence. A case–control study defines cases of disease and controls and compares their exposure histories.

2.   A cross-sectional study examines the relationship between diseases and other variables at one particular time. Subjects are commonly selected without regard to exposure or disease

status. Its main limitation is that one cannot infer the temporal sequence between the exposure and disease.

3. The temporal inference problem in cross-sectional studies is avoided if an unalterable characteristic, such as a genetic trait, is the focus of the investigation or if the exposure measure reflects past exposure.

4. An ecological study examines the rates of disease in relation to a population-level factor. Thus, the units of analysis are populations rather than individuals. The lack of information about individuals leads to a limitation known as the "ecological fallacy," which means that the association observed on an aggregate level does not necessarily represent the association that exists on the individual level.

5. An ecological study is preferred when there is an interest in studying the impact of contextual effects among communities and cultures. For example, an ecological study may be preferred for examining the effect of racial segregation on rates of hypertension in urban communities.

6. A. Case–control
   B. Retrospective cohort
   C. Case–control
   D. Case–control
   E. Prospective cohort
   F. Case–control

7. A. Ecological
   B. Cross-sectional
   C. Case–control
   D. Experimental
   E. Retrospective cohort

8. A. True
   B. True
   C. False
   D. False
   E. False
   F. False
   G. True

▶ Chapter 7: Experimental Studies

1. A. A process by which the investigator assigns subjects to the treatment and comparison groups. Subjects have an equal chance of being assigned to either the treatment or comparison group.
   B. The group of people to whom the study results may be applied or generalized.

    C.   The study subject does not know whether he or she is in the treatment or comparison group.

    D.   Both the study subject and the investigator administering the treatment do not know the subject's group assignment.

    E.   The run-in period occurs before enrollment and randomization to determine which participants are able to comply with the study regimen. Potential participants are placed on the test or control treatment for a certain period of time to assess their tolerance to and acceptance of the treatment and to obtain information on compliance.

    F.   A placebo is an inactive substance, such as a sugar-coated pill, that is given as a substitute for an active substance. A sham is a bogus procedure that is designed to resemble a legitimate one. Both placebos and sham procedures permit the study participants and caregivers to be masked.

    G.   Equipoise is a state of mind characterized by genuine uncertainty about the appropriate course of action, that is, to give or withhold a particular treatment. It is ethical to conduct an experimental study only when there is a state of equipoise in the expert community.

2.   A.   In individual trials, the treatment is allocated to particular people; in community trials, the treatment is allocated to entire communities.

    B.   Preventive trials investigate measures that stop or delay the onset of disease; therapeutic trials investigate measures that treat existing disease.

    C.   Simple designs test one treatment; factorial designs test two or more treatments.

3.   A.   There are several possible answers. For example, design a simple protocol, enroll motivated and knowledgeable participants, exclude subjects who might have difficulty complying, present a realistic picture of the required tasks at enrollment, maintain frequent contact with study subjects, and use items such as pill packs to make it easier to comply with the treatment regimen.

    B.   Randomize a large number of study subjects.

    C.   Mask investigators to group assignment.

4.   An intent-to-treat analysis includes all individuals who were randomly allocated to the treatment and comparison groups, regardless of whether they completed or even received their assigned regimen. This type of analysis preserves the baseline comparability and gives information on the effectiveness of the treatment under real-life conditions.

5.   Unique features include random assignment of subjects to the treatment and comparison groups to control for confounding

and reduce biased allocation and the use of placebo controls to permit masked assessment of the outcomes.

6.   They are expensive to conduct, physicians and patients may be reluctant to participate, and a state of equipoise must exist.

7.   A.   True
      B.   False
      C.   True
      D.   True
      E.   False
      F.   True

8.   A

9.   A.   No
      B.   No
      C.   No
      D.   No

10.   A.   White men aged 50–64 living in the United Kingdom. This is because their baseline risk of prostate cancer is most similar to the U.S. men in the study. Because race and age greatly influence a man's risk of prostate cancer, the results may not be as generalizable to U.S. Black men and older U.S. men who have higher rates of this cancer. In fact, older men are more likely to have latent disease, making prevention via vitamin supplementation less likely.

▶ Chapter 8: Cohort Studies

1.   A.   An open, or dynamic, cohort is conducted in a population defined by a changeable characteristic, such as residence in a specific place. Thus, its members come and go, depending on whether they have the characteristic.
      B.   A fixed cohort is defined by an irrevocable event, and therefore it does not gain any new members.
      C.   A retrospective cohort study looks back in time and examines exposures and outcomes that have already occurred by the time the investigator begins the study.
      D.   A prospective cohort study looks forward in time and examines future outcomes in relation to past or current exposures.
      E.   An ambidirectional cohort study has both prospective and retrospective components.
      F.   A standardized mortality ratio (SMR) study is a special type of cohort study in which the mortality experience

of an exposed group is compared with that of the general population. It is commonly conducted in occupational settings.

2. The main similarity is that both types of studies compare two or more exposure groups, which are followed to monitor outcome rates. The main difference is that the investigators allocate the exposure in experimental studies and the participants choose their exposures in cohort studies.

3. The ideal but unattainable comparison group would consist of exactly the same individuals in the exposed group had they not been exposed. This concept is known as the counterfactual ideal because it is impossible for the same person to be exposed and unexposed simultaneously.

4. Of the three types of comparison groups, the internal comparison group comes closest to the counterfactual ideal because it comes from the same source population as the exposed group and so is most comparable. However, internal comparison groups are often difficult to identify. The general population is the next best option mainly because it is stable and easy to obtain. Its limitations can include lack of comparability to the exposed group and lack of information on confounders. The comparison cohort is the least preferable option. Although it may be comparable to the exposed group, results from such a study are difficult to interpret because the comparison cohort often has other, possibly noxious, exposures.

5. B

6. A. Yes
    B. No
    C. No
    D. Yes

7. Losses to follow-up decrease the number of individuals who can be included in the analysis and therefore reduce the statistical power of the study. Also, if those who are lost have different rates of disease than those who remain, the study results may be biased.

8. Person-time is accrued for each individual in a cohort study. It begins when the follow-up period of the study begins. It ends when one of the following occurs: the individual develops the outcome under study, dies, or is lost or the follow-up period for the study ends.

9. A. True
    B. False
    C. False
    D. True

10. A. Yes
    B. No
    C. No
    D. No
    E. No

▶ Chapter 9: Case–Control Studies

1. A. TROHOC is the word *cohort* spelled backward. Some epidemiologists have used TROHOC as a disparaging term for case–control studies because they believe that case–control studies are inferior to cohort studies because they move from effect to cause rather than from cause to effect. The TROHOC fallacy means that it is incorrect to consider the logic of a case–control study to be backward because the key comparison is identical to that of a cohort study: between exposed and unexposed groups.

    B. The odds ratio can be defined in two ways: (1) the odds of being a case among the exposed compared with the odds of being a case among the nonexposed or (2) the odds of being exposed among the cases compared with the odds of being exposed among the controls.

    C. A case–crossover study is a new variant of the case–control study that is used to study the acute effects of transient exposures. Here, cases serve as their own controls, and the exposure frequency during a hazard period is compared with that during a control period.

2. It is desirable to conduct a case–control study when the exposure data are difficult or expensive to obtain, the disease is rare, the disease has long induction and latent periods, little is known about the disease, and the underlying population is dynamic.

3. A

Mother exposed to overt incidents of racism during pregnancy	Preterm delivery	
	Yes (cases)	No (controls)
Yes	90	50
No	410	950
Total	500	1,000

    B.   Odds ratio equals ad/bc = $(90 \times 950)/(50 \times 410) = 4.2$.

    C.   Black women exposed to overt incidents of racism during pregnancy had 4.2 times the odds of preterm delivery compared to Black women who did not have these experiences.

    D.   There are many possible answers. The basic principle is that the controls should be comparable with the cases. They should satisfy the "would criterion." That is, if they had a premature delivery, they would end up as a case in the study. For example, one could select women who delivered full-term infants at the same facilities as the cases.

    E.   The purpose of the control group is to provide information on the exposure distribution in the source population that produced the cases.

4.   Advantage: They usually come from the same source population as the cases, and therefore they are likely to be comparable. Disadvantages: They are time consuming and expensive to identify, they are usually not as cooperative as hospital controls, and their recall of prior exposures may not be as accurate as that of cases.

5.   In survivor sampling, the investigator selects controls from survivors who did not become cases during the observation period. In base sampling, the investigator selects controls from the population at risk at the start of the observation period. In risk-set sampling, the investigator selects controls from the population at risk as the cases are diagnosed.

6.   Advantages: Case–control studies take less time and money to conduct than cohort and experimental studies, they are well suited for studying rare diseases and diseases with long induction and latent periods, and they can provide information on a large number of possible risk factors. Disadvantages: The possibility of bias is increased, and it may be difficult to establish the correct temporal relationship between the exposure and disease because the data are retrospective.

7.   A.   False
       B.   False
       C.   False
       D.   False
       E.   False
       F.   False
       G.   True

8.   The odds ratio is used because the numbers of exposed and unexposed individuals needed for the risk and rate denominators are unavailable in most case–control studies.

▶ Chapter 10: Bias

1. A. Recall bias occurs when the level of accuracy differs between the compared groups. It occurs in a case–control study when cases remember or report their exposures differently (more or less accurately) from controls. It occurs in a retrospective cohort study when individuals who are exposed remember or report illnesses differently than those who are unexposed.

   B. The healthy worker effect occurs in occupational studies when disease and death rates in a working population are compared with those among the general population. The rates of disease and death among workers are typically lower than those in the general population because there is a higher proportion of ill people in the general population.

   C. Control selection bias is a type of selection bias that occurs in case–control studies when the controls do not accurately represent the exposure distribution in the source population that produced the cases. It occurs when different criteria are used to select cases and controls and these criteria are related to the exposure.

2. In nondifferential misclassification, inaccuracies that occur on one axis (exposure or disease) are independent of the other axis. For example, if there is an error in exposure misclassification, it occurs with equal likelihood among diseased and nondiseased individuals. In differential misclassification, inaccuracies that occur on one axis (exposure or disease) are dependent on the other axis. For example, if there is an error in exposure misclassification, it occurs more often in the case group than the control group. Nondifferential misclassification of dichotomous variables (i.e., variables with two categories) biases the results toward the null. Differential misclassification can bias the results either toward or away from the null.

3. A. Nondifferential misclassification of the exposure. Some women who filled the health maintenance organization's prescriptions for antihistamines may not have used them, and other women may have obtained antihistamines from outside sources. This type of misclassification is as likely to occur among cases as among controls; therefore, it is nondifferential and biases results toward the null.

   B. Recall and interviewer bias. Subjects were not asked to recall their exposures, and interviews were not used to obtain the exposure data.

4.   A.   Yes
     B.   Yes
     C.   No
     D.   Yes (because it is a prospective cohort study with nearly 100% follow-up)

5.   A.   Interviewer bias: Mask interviewers to the study hypothesis and to the disease or exposure status of the study subjects, and carefully design the interview instrument.
     B.   Recall bias: Mask study subjects to the study hypothesis, use diseased controls if conducting a case–control study, and carefully design an interview instrument.
     C.   Ensure that selection of cases and controls is independent of exposure (in a case–control study) and that selection of exposed and unexposed groups is independent of outcome (in a retrospective cohort study), and obtain high follow-up and participation rates (all types of studies).
     D.   Use the most accurate source of information, and use sensitive and specific criteria to define the exposure and disease.

6.   A.   True
     B.   False
     C.   True
     D.   False
     E.   False
     F.   False
     G.   False
     H.   False
     I.   True
     J.   True
     K.   True

7.   D

8.   A

▶ Chapter 11: Confounding

1.   A.   Confounding is a mixing of effects between an exposure, an outcome, and a third extraneous variable that is termed the confounder. Confounding distorts the crude relationship between an exposure and an outcome because of the relationships between the confounder and the exposure and the confounder and the disease.
     B.   Residual confounding means that an association remains confounded even after some confounders have been controlled. It arises from lack of information on all

confounding variables, classifying confounders in overly broad categories, or mismeasuring confounders.

C. Positive confounding means that the true crude association is exaggerated, and negative confounding means that the true crude association is underestimated.

D. A directed acyclic graph (DAG) is a visual representation of the relationship between the exposure, disease, and confounding and mediating variables.

2. A confounder is associated with the exposure in the source population that produced the cases and an independent cause or predictor of the outcome under study. The latter means that it is associated with the disease among both exposed and unexposed individuals. In addition, a confounder cannot be an intermediate step in the causal pathway between the exposure and disease. An intermediate variable is often called a mediator.

3. A. Yes
   B. Yes
   C. No
   D. No
   E. No
   F. Can't tell

4. Here is one possible DAG. You might come up with other DAGS depending on your thoughts about the relationship between theses variables.

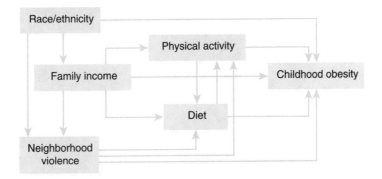

5. Randomization is the act of assigning or ordering using a random process. It means that everyone in the study has an equal chance of being assigned to one of the groups (such as treatment vs. comparison). The main advantage of randomization is that it controls for both known and unknown confounders if the sample size is sufficiently large. Its main disadvantage is that it can be used only in experimental studies. Matching is the process of making the distribution of confounders

identical in the compared groups while selecting the study subjects. It is good for controlling for confounding by complex nominal variables, such as neighborhood or sibship, and for controlling confounding in small studies. Its main disadvantages include the difficulty and expense of finding appropriate matches. Restriction means that the investigator limits admission into a study to individuals who fall within a specific category or categories of a confounder. Its main advantages are simplicity and relatively low expense, and its disadvantages include difficulty in identifying a sufficient number of subjects (this depends on the number and characteristics of the restrictions) and limiting the generalizability of the study.

6. Stratification is the process of evaluating the association within homogeneous categories of a confounder. Its main advantages are that it is straightforward and easy to carry out. It also allows epidemiologists to view the raw data. Its chief disadvantage is that it cannot control for numerous variables simultaneously because a large number of strata are generated relative to the number of study subjects. Multivariable analysis is a method for controlling confounding by constructing a mathematical model that describes the association between the exposure, the outcome, and the confounders. Its main advantage is that it can control for many confounders simultaneously. Its main disadvantage is that one can no longer view the raw data.

7. Epidemiologists usually compare the crude/confounded measure of association with the adjusted measure of association. If there is an appreciable difference between the two (i.e., at least a 10% difference), confounding is considered present.

8. A. Restriction
   B. Matching
   C. Stratified analysis

9. A. True
   B. False
   C. True
   D. False
   E. False
   F. True
   G. True

▶ Chapter 12: Random Error

1. A. Chance is an uncontrollable force that seems to have no assignable or predictable cause.
   B. Precision is the lack of random error. It is defined either as the state or quality of being exact or the ability of a measurement to be consistently reproduced.

C. Statistical inference is a method for generalizing results from a sample to a parent population.

2. The main assumption is that the null hypothesis is true.

3. Its chief limitation is the use of a purely arbitrary cutoff for deciding whether to reject the null hypothesis.

4. P values are affected by both the magnitude of the association and the study size. Thus, when results are summarized only by P values, it is impossible to determine whether a P value is small because the measure of association is strong or because the sample size is large. It is also impossible to determine whether a P value is large because the association is weak or the sample size is small.

5. According to a recent statement from the American Statistical Association, the use of P values for scientific conclusions and policy decisions can lead to mistaken beliefs and poor decisions.

6. A. Compared with olive oil users, there was a 1.8-fold increased odds (or an 80% increased odds) of coronary heart disease among margarine users.

   B. The strict statistical interpretation is as follows: If this study were repeated 100 times and 100 point estimates and confidence intervals were calculated, 95 of the 100 confidence intervals would contain the true point estimate. Or, assuming no bias or confounding, we could say that we have 95% confidence that the true measure of association lies within the interval 0.8 to 4.3, or that we have 95% confidence that the results are consistent with hypotheses that the strength of the association lies between 0.8 and 4.3.

   C. This confidence interval is rather wide because it extends from a small decrease in odds (0.8) to a moderate increase in odds (4.3).

   D. Assuming that the null hypothesis is true and that there is no bias or confounding, there is a 10% chance of seeing this result (an odds ratio of 1.8) or one more extreme (an odds ratio greater than 1.8).

7. Confidence intervals are not confounded statistics as are P values. They do a better job separating the influence of the sample size from the influence of the strength of the association. This is because the width of the interval is influenced mainly by the sample size, and the general position of the interval reflects the magnitude of the association.

8. The normal distribution is used for continuous variables, and the binomial and Poisson distributions are used for discrete variables with two mutually exclusive outcomes. In addition, the Poisson distribution is usually reserved for rare events.

9. A. True
    B. False
    C. True
    D. False
    E. True
    F. False
10. Study A
11. C
12. C

▶ Chapter 13: Effect Measure Modification

1. A. Effect measure modification occurs when the strength of an association varies according to the level of a third variable, which is called the effect modifier. The word *measure* is a key part of the term because effect measure modification depends on the particular measure of association that is used.

    B. Heterogeneity of effect is another term for effect measure modification. Homogeneity of effect means that effect measure modification is absent.

    C. Synergy is a type of effect measure modification in which the excess relative risk among individuals with two factors is greater than the sum of the excess relative risks among individuals with only one factor.

    D. Antagonism is a type of effect measure modification in which the excess relative risk among individuals with two factors is less than the sum of the excess relative risks among individuals with only one factor.

2. Confounding is a nuisance that epidemiologists try to eliminate from their studies. Effect measure modification is a natural phenomenon of scientific interest that epidemiologists try to describe and understand.

3. One can determine whether a factor is an effect measure modifier in a stratified analysis by comparing the stratum-specific measures of association to one another. If they are appreciably different, either by visual inspection or a statistical test result, then effect measure modification is present. One can also determine whether effect measure modification is present by examining the excess risk ratios. In contrast, one determines whether a factor is a confounder by comparing the crude and adjusted measures of association.

4.　A.　Yes
　　B.　The excess odds ratio of having both factors $(50 - 1 = 49)$ is much greater than the sum of the two excess odds ratios for each factor alone (excess odds ratio for smoking: $10 - 1 = 9$; excess odds ratio for asbestos: $5 - 1 = 4$; sum of excess odds ratios: $9 + 4 = 13$). Note that the odds ratio provides an estimate of the risk ratio in a case–control study.

5.　A.　2.8
　　B.　Male odds ratio: 2.0. Female odds ratio: 2.0.
　　C.　Yes
　　D.　No
　　E.　The stratum-specific (unconfounded) odds ratios are different from the crude (confounded) odds ratio. Therefore, confounding is present. However, the stratum-specific odds ratios are identical, and therefore there is no effect measure modification.

6.　A.　False
　　B.　True
　　C.　False

▸ Chapter 15: The Epidemiological Approach to Causation

1.　A.　A cause of disease is an event, condition, or characteristic that preceded the disease and without which the disease either would not have occurred or would have occurred later.
　　B.　A risk factor is another term for a determinant or cause of a disease.
　　C.　A component cause is a participating factor in a sufficient cause. It is depicted as a slice of a "causal pie."
　　D.　A sufficient cause is a set of conditions without any one of which the disease would not have occurred. It is depicted as a whole "causal pie."
　　E.　A necessary cause is a component cause that is a member of every sufficient cause.

2.　The overall induction period begins with the action of the first causal component and ends with the action of the last causal component and the simultaneous biological onset of disease. The latent period follows the induction period and so begins with the biological onset of disease and ends with the disease diagnosis.

3.   A.   True
      B.   True
      C.   False
      D.   True
      E.   True
      F.   False
      G.   False
      H.   False
4.   A.   Analogy
      B.   Biological plausibility and coherence
      C.   Coherence, consistency, and experiment
      D.   Consistency and coherence
      E.   Biological gradient, strength of association
5.   A.   False
      B.   True
      C.   True
      D.   False
      E.   False
      F.   True

▶ Chapter 16: Screening in Public Health Practice

1.   A.   Natural history of a disease is the course of a disease from its inception to its resolution.
      B.   The portion of the preclinical phase of a disease that can be identified by a screening test.
      C.   The criterion of positivity is the cutoff at which the screening test result is considered positive.
      D.   Sensitivity is a measure of a screening test's validity. It is the probability that a screening test classifies as positive those individuals who have preclinical disease.
      E.   Specificity is also a measure of a screening test's validity. The complement of sensitivity, it is the probability that a screening test classifies as negative those individuals who do not have preclinical disease.
      F.   Predictive value of a positive test is a way to measure a screening program's feasibility. It is the proportion of individuals with a positive test who have preclinical disease.
      G.   Lead time is the amount of time that the diagnosis of disease is advanced by screening.
2.   Primary prevention occurs before the pathological onset of disease, and its aim is to block the start of disease. Secondary prevention takes place from the pathological onset of disease to the occurrence of clinical symptoms. Its aim

is to delay the onset and duration of symptomatic disease and improve survival. Tertiary prevention takes place after clinical symptoms develop. Its aim is to slow or block the progression of disease and therefore reduce disease sequelae and improve survival.

3. Serious diseases with fairly long and prevalent detectable pre-clinical phases for which treatment is more effective at earlier stages.

4. A.

Screening test	Prostate cancer		
	Yes	No	Total
Positive	800	3,200	4,000
Negative	100	95,900	96,000
Total	900	99,100	100,000

B. Prevalence equals 900/100,000, or 0.9%.
C. Sensitivity equals 800/900, or 88.9%. It means that 88.9% of men who had prostate cancer tested positive on the screening test.
D. Specificity equals 95,900/99,100 = 96.8%. It means that 96.8% of the men who did not have prostate cancer tested negative on the screening test.
E. Predictive value positive equals 800/4,000, or 20%. It means that 20% of the men who tested positive truly did have prostate cancer.
F. A total of 3,200 men underwent unnecessary biopsies, and 100 men were falsely reassured that they did not have prostate cancer.

5. A. Age 30–60, or 30 years
B. Age 40–60, or 20 years
C. Age 45–60, or 15 years
D. Yes. She would have died at age 70 years if no screening had been done. Instead, she died at age 80 years.

6. The three types of bias are lead-time bias, length-bias sampling, and volunteer bias. Lead-time bias means that survival among screened individuals may appear longer than that for nonscreened individuals just because they were diagnosed earlier. Length-bias sampling means that survival among screened individuals may be longer than that for nonscreened individuals because screening tends to identify less aggressive forms of the disease. Volunteer bias is a form of confounding that occurs only in observational studies of screening

programs. It means that people who get screened tend to have different characteristics than those who do not get screened. These characteristics may be related to survival.

7.   A.   False
     B.   True
     C.   True
     D.   True
     E.   True
     F.   True
8.   A

▶ Chapter 17: Ethics in Research Involving Human Participants

1.   Voluntary consent of the human subject is absolutely essential. Informed consent was never obtained from participants in the 50-year Tuskegee Syphilis Study.

2.   D

3.   The three major principles identified in the Belmont Report include respect for persons, beneficence, and justice. Respect means that you allow participants to decide for themselves what will and will not happen to them. Beneficence means that you maximize the possible benefits and minimize the possible harms of research. Justice means that the burdens and benefits of the research are fairly distributed among all segments of the population.

4.   Informed consent is an educational and decision-making process in which potential volunteers must be effectively informed of the purpose, procedures, and possible risks and benefits associated with participation in a study.

Glossary

Note: The chapter(s) in which the key term appears in main discussion are included after the definition in parentheses.

Absolute measure of comparison Difference between two measures of disease frequency; describes the excess frequency of disease associated with the exposure among exposed individuals or the total population. (3)

Accuracy The lack of random and systematic error. (12)

Adjusted measure of association Measures of association that incorporate control of confounders. (11)

Agent-based modeling A method of analysis that uses computer simulations to study the complex interactions among individuals, their physical and social environments, and time. (6)

Age-specific mortality rates Total number of deaths from all causes among individuals in a specific age category per 100,000 population in the specific age category; usually expressed for a 1-year period. (2)

Alternation assignment Systematic method of group assignment in an experimental study that is based on the order of enrollment. (7)

Alternative hypothesis (H$_A$) In statistical hypothesis testing, states that there is an association between the exposure and disease. (12, 13)

Ambidirectional cohort study A cohort study that has both prospective and retrospective components. (6, 8)

Analogy One of Hill's guidelines for assessing causation, which involves making an analogy or a similarity between the observed association and any others. (15)

Antagonism A type of effect measure modification that occurs when the excess relative risk among individuals with both factors is less than the sum of the excess relative risks of each factor considered alone; thus, one factor reduces or even cancels out the effect of the other factor. (13)

Association There are two meanings for this term: (1) statistical dependence between two variables or (2) an essential attribute of a cause, meaning that the causal factor must occur together with the putative effect. (3, 15)

Attack rate Number of new cases of disease that develop (usually during a defined and short time period) per number in healthy population at risk at start of the observation period. Usually refers to infectious diseases. (2)

Attributable proportion among the exposed (AP$_e$) Excess proportion of disease among the exposed population. (3, 9)

Attributable proportion among the total population (AP$_t$) Excess proportion of disease among the total population. (3, 9)

Attributable risk (attributable rate) Another term for *risk difference* or *rate difference*; however, some epidemiologists think that this term should be discarded because it implies a definite causal relationship. (3)

Bernoulli trial In hypothesis testing that involves random variables with two possible outcomes, a Bernoulli trial is a random variable that takes on the value of 1 with a probability of "p" and a value of 0 with a probability of "$1 - p$." (12)

Bias An alternative explanation for an association; a systematic error in the design or conduct of a study that causes an erroneous association between the exposure and disease. (10, 11, 13, 15)

Biological gradient One of Hill's guidelines for assessing causation. It states that an association is more likely to be causal if its strength increases as the exposure level increases. (15)

Biomarkers Exposure data based on biological measurements in blood, urine, bone, toenails, etc. (8, 9)

Binomial distribution A theoretical probability distribution that describes a random variable with two possible discrete outcomes. (12)

Biostatistics Branch of statistics that applies statistical methods to medical and biological phenomena. (12)

Birth defect rate Number of children born with defects per 10,000 births. (2)

Blocking In an experimental study, randomization is conducted in groups or blocks of a certain size. (7)

Candidate population People who are at risk of getting a specified disease. (2)

Case Individual who has the disease in a case–control study; usually defined on the basis of a combination of signs and symptoms, physical and pathological examinations, and results of diagnostic tests. (6, 9)

Case–base sampling A method of sampling controls in a case–control study. Controls are sampled from the population at risk at the beginning of the case ascertainment period. (9)

Case–control study A type of epidemiological study in which cases of disease are identified and enrolled and a sample of the source population that gave rise to the cases is also identified and enrolled (i.e., the controls). Exposure histories of the two groups are compared. (9)

Case–crossover study A variant of the case–control study, which is used to study the effect of transient exposures on the risk of acute events. Cases serve as their own controls, and the exposure frequency during a hazard period is compared to that from a control period. (9)

Case fatality rate Number of deaths among cases per number of cases of disease. (2)

Catchment population Population served by a medical facility. (2)

Causal inference A judgment about causation using accumulated knowledge. (15)

Cause An event, condition, or characteristic that preceded the disease and without which the disease either would not have occurred at all or would not have occurred until some later time. (15)

Cause-specific mortality rate Number of deaths from a specific cause per 100,000 population. Usually expressed for a 1-year period. (2)

Census A complete count of a population. (4)

Chance An uncontrollable force with no apparent cause that arises from unforeseeable and unpredictable processes. (10, 11, 12, 15)

Chi-square test Used in statistical hypothesis testing involving discrete data. (12, 13)

Closed cohort A cohort that is defined by an irrevocable event; does not gain or lose members. (6, 8)

Coherence One of Hill's guidelines for assessing causation, which states that the cause-and-effect interpretation of data should not seriously conflict with generally known facts of the natural history and biology of the disease. (15)

Cohort A group of people with a common characteristic or experience. (6, 8)

Cohort study A type of epidemiological study in which subjects are defined according to their exposure level and followed for disease occurrence; also called follow-up, incidence, or longitudinal study. (6, 8)

Community trial A type of experimental study in which the treatment is allocated to an entire community. (7)

Comparison cohort A type of comparison group in a cohort study that consists of unexposed members of another cohort. (8)

Comparison group A group of individuals to whom the exposed group is compared; may also be called the reference group, referent group, or unexposed group. (3, 6, 7, 11)

Component cause Part of the sufficient-component causal model; a participating factor in a sufficient cause. (15)

Compliance Occurs when participants in an experimental study exactly follow the study protocol. (7)

Confidence interval Quantifies the variability around a measure of disease frequency or measure of association. Commonly defined as the range of possible values within which the true magnitude of effect lies with a stated level of certainty (e.g., 95%). Strict statistical definition of a 95% confidence interval is as follows: If a study were repeated 100 times and 100 point estimates and 100 confidence intervals were calculated, 95 out of 100 confidence intervals would include the true measure of association. (12)

Confounding Mixing of effects between an exposure, an outcome, and a third extraneous variable known as a confounder; a confounder is an independent risk factor for the disease that is also associated with the exposure and is not a step on the causal pathway between the exposure and disease. (10, 11, 13, 15)

Consistency One of Hill's guidelines for assessing causation, which states that an association is more likely to be causal if it has been observed repeatedly by different persons in different places and circumstances and at different times. (15)

Control An individual who serves as a comparison for a case–control study. (6, 9)

Control group A sample of the source population that produced the cases whose purpose is to estimate the exposure distribution in the source population; also called referent group. (9)

Control selection bias A type of selection bias that arises in case–control studies when controls do not accurately represent the exposure distribution in the source population that produced the cases. (10)

Counterfactual ideal The perfect comparison group for a group of exposed individuals consists of exactly the same individuals had they not been exposed. Because the same individuals cannot be simultaneously exposed and unexposed, the ideal is counter to fact. (8, 9, 11)

Criterion of positivity Point on a continuum (from clearly normal test results to clearly abnormal results) at which a screening test result is considered positive. (16)

Critical period Period of time when an individual is susceptible to the action of an exposure. (9)

Crossover trial A type of experimental study in which two or more study treatments are administered one after another to each group. (7)

Cross-sectional study A type of epidemiological study that examines the relationship between exposure prevalence and disease prevalence in a defined population at one particular time. (6)

Crude measure of association A measure of association that is based on raw data and does not incorporate any adjustment for confounding. (11)

Cumulative incidence Proportion of a candidate population that becomes diseased over a specified period of time. (2)

Descriptive epidemiology This branch of epidemiology assesses the frequency of disease in a population and determines the characteristics of diseased individuals and whether the occurrence of disease varies by place and time. (5)

Detectable preclinical phase (DPCP) The portion of the preclinical phase of a disease that can be identified by a screening test. (16)

Determinists Epidemiologists who think that every event, act, or decision is the inevitable consequence of prior events, acts, or decisions. (12, 15)

Differential misclassification A type of information bias in which classification errors on one axis (exposure or disease) are related to the other axis (exposure or disease). (10)

Direct standardization A method for controlling confounding. Involves calculating a weighted average of category-specific rates with the weights being equal to the proportion of the standard population in each category. (3)

Directed acyclic graph (DAG) A visual representation of the relationship between an exposure, a disease, and confounding and mediating variables. (11)

Direction An essential attribute of a cause, which means that there is an asymmetrical relationship between the cause and effect. (15)

Disease Absence of health; includes specific illnesses, disabilities, and injuries. (1, 2, 6)

Disease cluster An aggregation of relatively uncommon events or disease in space and/or time in amounts that are believed or perceived to be greater than could be expected by chance. (5)

Disease control Reduce or prevent disease. Epidemiologists accomplish disease control through epidemiological research and surveillance. (1)

Disease determinants Factors that bring about a change in health, that is, factors that either cause a healthy individual to become sick or a sick person to recover. (1)

Disease distribution Analysis of disease patterns according to person, place, and time. (1)

Disease frequency How often a disease arises in a population; measures of disease frequency include incidence and prevalence. (1)

Disease odds ratio The ratio of the odds of being a case among the exposed (a/b) to the odds of being a case among the nonexposed (c/d). (9)

Dose–response relationship The risk of disease increases as the intensity or duration of exposure increases. (8)

Dropouts Participants who withdraw from an experimental or observational study. (7, 8)

Dynamic population A population that is defined on the basis of a changeable state or condition and therefore membership is transient; also called open population. (2, 8)

Ecological fallacy An association observed between variables on an aggregate level does not necessarily represent the association that exists at the individual level. (6)

Ecological study An epidemiological study that examines the relationship between exposure and disease with population-level rather than individual-level data. (6)

Effect measure modification Strength of the association between an exposure and a disease differs according to the level of another variable (the effect modifier); also known as *heterogeneity of effect*. (13)

Efficacy analysis A type of analysis in experimental studies in which only individuals who comply with the treatment protocol are included; provides information on the effect of the treatment under ideal conditions. (7)

Epidemic Occurrence of cases of an illness, specific health-related behavior, or other health-related events clearly in excess of normal expectancy. (5)

Epidemiology Study of the distribution and determinants of disease frequency in human populations and the application of this study to control health problems. (1)

Equipoise State of mind characterized by genuine confidence that a treatment may be worthwhile to administer it to some individuals and genuine reservations about the treatment to withhold it from

others; needed for the ethical conduct of experimental studies. (6, 7, 16)

Experiment One of Hill's guidelines for assessing causation, which states that there is evidence of causation if an intervention initiated by the investigator that modifies the exposure through prevention, treatment, or removal results in less disease or no disease at all. (15)

Experimental study An epidemiological study in which the investigator actively manipulates which groups receive a preventive or a therapeutic treatment. (7)

Exposed group Individuals with a particular characteristic; may also be called the index group. (3, 6, 11)

Factorial trial A type of experimental study in which each group gets two or more treatments. (7)

Fixed cohort A cohort that is defined on the basis of an irrevocable event; does not gain members and losses may occur. (6, 8)

Fixed population A population whose membership is defined on the basis of an irrevocable event and whose membership is permanent. (2)

Follow-up Observation of subjects over time to assess their changes in health. (7, 8)

General cohort A cohort that is assembled to study a common exposure. (8)

Generalizability A judgment in which the investigator relates the conclusions of a study beyond the study setting and population to a broader setting and population. (7, 10)

Hawthorne effect Participants in an experimental study either consciously or unconsciously change their behavior just because they are being studied. (7)

Hazard period Term used in case–crossover studies, which is the period of increased risk following an exposure. (6, 9)

Health A state of complete physical, mental, and social well-being. (2)

Healthy worker effect A type of selection bias in cohort studies that results from comparing an exposed group of workers to the general population; occurs because death and disease rates among a working population are usually lower than those of the general population. (6, 8, 10)

Heterogeneity of effect Strength of the association between an exposure and a disease differs according to the level of another variable (the effect modifier); also known as *effect measure modification*. (13)

Hill's guidelines for assessing causation Nine guidelines to help determine whether associations are causal but not to provide indisputable evidence for or against causation: strength of the association, consistency, specificity, temporality, biological gradient, plausibility, coherence, experiment, and analogy. (15)

Homogeneity of effect Strength of the association between an exposure and a disease does not differ according to the level of another variable. Thus, effect measure modification is absent. (13)

Hypothesis A tentative explanation for an observation, phenomenon, or scientific problem that can be tested by further investigation. (5)

Hypothesis testing Used to assess the role of random error in epidemiological research; considered a "uniform decision-making criterion" that is superior to subjective impressions of the data. (12)

Incidence Measures the occurrence of new disease. The frequency of new cases of disease that develop in a candidate population over a specified time period. (2)

Incidence rate The occurrence of new cases of disease arising during at-risk person-time of observation. A true rate. (2)

Individual trial A type of experimental study in which the treatment is allocated to individual persons. (7)

Induction period The interval between the action of a cause and disease onset. (8)

Infant mortality rate Number of deaths of infants under one year of age per 1,000 livebirths. Usually expressed for a 1-year period. (2)

Information bias An error that arises from systematic differences in the way that information on exposure and disease is obtained from study groups. (10)

Informed consent The process of obtaining agreement from study participants. (7, 17)

Institutional review board Committee that reviews all studies to ensure that the research is ethical and legitimate. (7, 17)

Intent-to-treat analysis A type of analysis in experimental studies; includes all individuals who were randomly allocated to a treatment and provides information on the effectiveness of a treatment under everyday practice conditions. (7)

Internal comparison group A comparison group in a cohort study that comprises unexposed members of the same cohort. (8)

Interviewer bias A type of information bias in which there is a systematic difference in soliciting, recording, or interpreting interview information. (10)

Latent period Interval between disease onset and clinical diagnosis. (8)

Lead time Amount of time that the disease diagnosis is advanced by screening. (16)

Lead-time bias A bias that overestimates the benefit of screening whereby survival time appears to be longer among screened individuals because their diagnoses were made earlier, not because they lived longer. (16)

Length-bias sampling A bias that overestimates the benefit of screening; occurs because screening tends to identify cases with less aggressive forms of disease and who have a long clinical course and better survival. (16)

Life expectancy The average number of years of life remaining to a person at a given age. (5)

Livebirth rate Total number of livebirths per 1,000 population. Usually expressed for a 1-year period. (2)

Losses to follow-up Participants in an experimental or cohort study who can no longer be located or contacted by the investigator. (7, 8)

Masking (also called blinding) In experimental studies, a method for reducing information bias whereby the subject is unaware of his or her group assignment, called single masked, or both the subject and the investigator administering the treatment are unaware of the group assignment, called double masked. (7)

Matching A method for controlling for confounding whereby study subjects are selected so that potential confounders are distributed in an identical manner. (11)

Mean Measure of central tendency; the average. (12)

Measurement error Nonsystematic error in assessing the exposure and outcome that contributes to both nondifferential misclassification and random error. (12)

Measures of association General term to describe absolute and relative measures of comparison. Also called *measures of effect*. (10)

Median Measure of central tendency; the middle-most observation of the distribution. (12)

Mediator A variable that is a step in the causal pathway between an exposure and a disease. (11)

Migrant studies A study that compares the rates of disease among natives of a homeland to those among immigrants and those among natives of an adopted country. (5)

Misclassification An error in classifying the exposure or the disease; also called measurement error. (10, 11)

Mode Measure of central tendency; the most commonly occurring observation. (12)

Morbidity rate Number of existing or new cases of a disease per 1,000 population. Usually expressed for a 1-year period. Morbidity is a general word that can apply to a disease, condition, or event. (2)

Mortality rate Total number of deaths from all causes per 100,000 population. Usually expressed for a 1-year period. (2)

Multivariable analysis A method for controlling many confounders simultaneously; involves the construction of a mathematical model that describes the relationship between exposure, disease, and confounders. (11)

Natural history of a disease Course of a disease from its inception to its resolution. (16)

Negative confounding Confounding that pulls the crude measure of association toward the null. (11)

Noncompliance The failure of a study participant to observe the requirements of the protocol. (7)

Nondifferential misclassification A type of information bias whereby errors on one axis (exposure or disease) are unrelated to the other axis (exposure or disease). (10)

Normal distribution A theoretical probability distribution that describes continuous random variables; also known as the *Gaussian or bell-shaped distribution*. (12)

Null hypothesis (H_0) In statistical hypothesis testing, states that there is no association between the exposure and disease. (12, 13)

Observational study An epidemiological study in which the investigator passively observes as nature takes its course; includes cohort, case–control, cross-sectional, and ecological studies. (6)

Odds The probability that an event will occur divided by the probability that it will not occur. (6, 9)

Odds ratio The ratio of two odds; used to estimate the risk ratio in a case–control study. (6, 9, 10)

Open population A population that is defined on the basis of a changeable state or condition and therefore membership is transient; also called dynamic population. (6, 8)

Outbreak Occurrence of cases of an illness, specific health-related behavior, or other health-related events clearly in excess of normal expectancy. Synonym for epidemic that often refers to a localized epidemic. (5)

P value In hypothesis testing, the probability of obtaining the observed result and more extreme results by chance alone given that the null hypothesis is true; measures the consistency between the observed data and the null hypothesis. (12, 13)

Parallel trial An experimental study in which each group receives one treatment and the treatments are administered concurrently. (7)

Period prevalence Measures the frequency of existing disease. The proportion of the total population that is diseased during a specified duration of time (e.g., 1-year). (2)

Person-time The amount of time that an at-risk person is under observation in an epidemiological setting. (2)

Placebo A pharmacologically inactive substance given as a substitute for an active substance, especially when the person taking or receiving it is not informed whether it is an active or inactive substance. (7)

Placebo effect The beneficial effect produced by an inactive control treatment; thought to arise from the power of suggestion. (7)

Plausibility One of Hill's guidelines for assessing causation, which states that there should be an existing biological or social model to explain an association. (15)

Point prevalence Measures the frequency of existing disease. The proportion of the total population this is diseased at a single point in time. (2)

Poisson distribution A theoretical probability distribution that describes discrete, rare events. (12)

Population A group of people with a common characteristic such as place of residence, gender, age, or use of certain medical services. (1, 2)

Population at risk Members of the population at risk are capable of developing the outcome/disease of interest. This population typically excludes individuals who already have the disease of interest and individuals who are immune. Candidate population is a synonym. (2)

Population rate or risk difference The excess rate or risk of disease in the total population. (3)

Positive confounding Confounding that pulls the crude measure of association away from the null. (11)

Precision The lack of random error; the state of being precise or exact. (12)

Predictive value A measure of screening program feasibility. Predictive value positive is the proportion of individuals who test positive who have preclinical disease. Predictive value negative is the proportion of individuals who test negative without preclinical disease. (16)

Prevalence Measures existing cases in the total population. It is the proportion of the total population that is diseased. (2)

Preventive trial An experimental study in which a prophylactic agent is given to healthy or high-risk individuals to prevent disease occurrence. (7)

Primary outcome The main condition that a study has been designed to evaluate. It is an important factor in calculating sample size. (7)

Primary prevention Activities that maintain health and avoid disease through individual or community efforts. (16)

Probabilists Epidemiologists who believe that random error or chance is an important, even chief, explanation for events. (12, 15)

Proportion Division of two related numbers. Numerator is a subset of denominator. (2)

Proportional mortality ratio (PMR) The ratio of the observed proportion of deaths due to a particular cause to the expected proportion based on the general population. (8, 10)

Propositi Exposed subjects in an experimental or cohort study and cases in a case–control study. (14)

Prospective cohort study A cohort study in which participants are grouped on the basis of past or current exposure and followed into the future to observe the outcomes of interest. (6, 8)

Public health A multidisciplinary field whose goal is to promote the health of the population through organized community efforts. (1)

Random error An unsystematic error that arises from chance; an uncontrollable force that seems to have no assignable cause. (10, 11, 12, 13, 15)

Random sample A sample whose selection has a probabilistic element. (12)

Randomization A method used to control confounding in experimental studies; an act of assigning or ordering that is the result of a random process. (7, 11)

Range A measure of dispersion; the difference between the highest and lowest values in a data set. (12)

Rate Division of two numbers; time is always in the denominator. (2)

Rate or risk difference Absolute measure of comparison; measures excess rate or risk of disease in the exposed or total population. (3)

Rate or risk ratio Relative measure of comparison; measures strength of relationship between exposure and disease. (3)

Ratio Division of two unrelated numbers. (2, 10)

Recall bias A type of information bias whereby a differential level of accuracy in the information provided by compared groups occurs. (10)

Reference population The population to whom particular study results are generalizable. (7)

Referent group Another term for control group, so named because it "refers to" the exposure distribution in the source population. (9)

Reliability Ability of a test to give the same result on repeated testing. (16)

Relative measure of comparison Ratio of two measures of disease frequency; gives information about the strength of the relationship between an exposure and a disease. (3)

Residual confounding Confounding that remains even after some confounding variables have been controlled; refers to incomplete control of confounding. (11)

Restriction A method for controlling confounding whereby the admissibility criteria for study subjects are limited. (11)

Retrospective cohort study A cohort study in which both the exposure and outcome have already occurred when the study begins; studies past exposures and outcomes. (6, 8)

Risk factor An individual, environmental, or societal characteristic that influences a person's health. (15)

Risk set sampling A method for selecting controls in a case–control study. Controls are selected from the population at risk as the cases are diagnosed. (9)

Sampling variability Samples from a population differ in part by chance because the inclusion of particular individuals in a sample is partly determined by chance. (12)

Screening Presumptive identification of an unrecognized disease or defect by the application of tests, examinations, or other procedures that can be applied rapidly. (16)

Secondary outcome Additional events of interest in a study. (7)

Secondary prevention Activities that delay onset of the symptomatic or clinical phase of a disease. (16)

Seesaw effect A higher proportion of deaths from one cause must be counterbalanced by a lower proportion of deaths from another cause. This is a problem in PMR studies. (8)

Selection bias An error that arises mainly from systematic differences in selecting the study groups. (10)

Self-selection bias Bias arising in retrospective studies with low and moderate participation rates from refusal and nonresponse by participants that is related to both the exposure and disease or agreement to participate that is related to both the exposure and disease. (10)

Sensitivity A measure of the validity of a screening test whereby the probability that a test correctly classifies as positive individuals who have preclinical disease. (16)

Sham procedure A bogus procedure designed to resemble a legitimate one. (7)

Significance level In statistical hypothesis testing, an arbitrary cutoff for a P value used to decide whether the null hypothesis should be rejected; P values less that 0.05 are commonly called statistically significant. (12)

Simple trial A type of experimental study in which each group receives a treatment consisting of one component. (7)

Source population Population from which study subjects are drawn; also known as *study base*. (6, 7, 8, 9)

Special cohort A cohort that is assembled to study the health effects of rare exposures. (8)

Specificity One of Hill's guidelines for assessing causation, which states that a cause should lead to a single effect and vice versa. Also, a measure of the validity of a screening test whereby the probability that a test correctly classifies as negative individuals who do not have preclinical disease. (15, 16)

Standard deviation A measure of dispersion; expresses the variation of individual values around a sample mean. (12)

Standard error A measure of dispersion; expresses the variation of sample means around the parent population mean. (12)

Standardized mortality (or morbidity) ratio (SMR) The ratio of the observed number of cases of death or disease to the expected number based on general population rates. (8, 10)

Statistical inference Process of making generalizations from a sample to the source or parent population. (12)

Statistical power The ability of a statistical test to correctly reject the null hypothesis when the alternative hypothesis is true. (7, 12)

Steady state Describes a situation in which the number of people entering the population is equal to the number leaving. (2)

Stratification A method for controlling confounding whereby individuals are separated into homogeneous categories of a confounder. (7, 11)

Strength of association One of Hill's guidelines for assessing causality which states that strong or large associations are more likely to be causal than weak associations (15)

Student t test Used in statistical hypothesis testing for continuous variables. (12)

Study Includes both surveillance and epidemiological research on factors that cause or prevent disease. (6)

Study base Population from which study subjects are drawn; also known as *source population*. (9)

Sufficient cause Part of the sufficient-component causal model defined as a complete causal mechanism that inevitably produces disease and usually consists of several component causes. (15)

Surveillance Monitoring aspects of disease occurrence and spread that are pertinent to effective control. (6)

Survival rate Number of living cases per number of cases of disease. (2)

Survivor sampling A method for sampling controls in a case–control study. Controls are selected from the noncases or survivors at the end of the observation period. (9)

Synergy A type of effect measure modification that occurs when the excess relative risk among individuals with both factors is greater than the sum of the excess relative risks of each factor considered alone; thus, two factors work in concert to produce more disease than one would expect based on the action of either factor acting alone. (13)

Temporality One of Hill's guidelines for assessing causation, which means that true causes must precede their effects. (15)

Tertiary prevention Activities that slow or block the progression of a disease, thereby reducing impairments and disabilities and improving the quality of life and survival among diseased individuals. (16)

Therapeutic trial A type of experimental study in which treatment is given to diseased individuals to reduce the risk of recurrence and improve survival and quality of life. (7)

Time order An essential attribute of a cause that means that a cause must precede its effect. (15)

Treatment group The group that is allocated the agent under investigation in an experimental study. (6, 7)

Two-by-two table Used to organize epidemiological data to facilitate making comparisons. Usually cross-tabulates two exposure categories (yes or no) by two disease categories (yes or no). (3)

Unexposed group Individuals without a characteristic (also called reference, referent, or comparison group). (3, 6)

Validation The process investigators use to verify or corroborate the occurrence of the outcome using several sources. (7)

Validity Lack of random error, bias, and confounding. (6, 8, 10)

Variance A measure of dispersion of individual values around a mean. (12)

Volunteer bias A bias that affects the evaluation of screening programs that occurs when the decision to be screened is influenced by a person's "health awareness," which in turn may be related to his or her subsequent morbidity and mortality. (16)

Would criterion Guiding principle for the valid selection of controls in a case–control study. If the would criterion is met, then a member of the control group who gets the disease under study "would" end up as a case in the study. (9)

Years of potential life lost Number of years that an individual was expected to live beyond his or her death. (2)

Index

Note: Italicized page locators indicate figures; tables are noted with *t*.